MAYO CLINIC
Guide to a
Healthy
Pregnancy

SECOND EDITION

MAYO CLINIC

Medical Editor
Myra J. Wick, M.D., Ph.D.

Editorial Director
Paula M. Marlow Limbeck

Managing Editor
Anna L. Cavallo

Senior Product Manager
Christopher C. Frye

Illustration, Photography and Production
Jacqueline (Jackie) M. Carr, Michael A. King, Kent McDaniel, Matthew C. Meyer, Kevin J. Ness, Gunnar T. Soroos, Malgorzata (Gosha) B. Weivoda

Editorial Research Librarians
Abbie Y. Brown, Erika A. Riggin, Katherine (Katie) J. Warner

Proofreaders
Miranda M. Attlesey, Alison K. Baker, Julie M. Maas

Indexer
Steve Rath

Contributing Reviewers
Summer V. Allen, M.D.; Yvonne S. Butler Tobah, M.D.; Paula D. Chantigian, M.D.; Margaret L. Dow, M.D.; Laura L. Elliott, M.D.; Margaret C. Gill, M.D.; Thomas G. Howell Jr., M.D.; Melissa A. Kurke, R.N., I.B.C.L.C.; Julie A. Lamppa, APRN, CNM; Margaret E. Long, M.D.; Matthew R. Meunier, M.D.; Deborah Miller, APRN, C.N.P.; Rose J. Prissel, M.S., RDN; Rubin Raju, M.D., M.B.B.S.; Enid (Yvy) Y. Rivera-Chiauzzi, M.D.; Laura M. Rust, M.S., LCGC; Shana S. Salik, M.P.H., APRN; Susan M. Skinner, APRN, CNM; Hans P. Sviggum, M.D.; Daniel J. Swartz, M.D.; Cara N. Syth, M.D.; Mari Charisse (Charisse) Trinidad, M.D.

Published by Mayo Clinic

© 2018 Mayo Foundation for Medical Education and Research (MFMER)

For bulk sales to employers, member groups and health-related companies, write to Mayo Clinic, 200 First St. SW, Rochester, MN 55905, call 800-430-9699, or send an email to *SpecialSalesMayoBooks@mayo.edu.*

Library of Congress Control Number: 2018943136

ISBN 978-1-893005-60-0

Second Edition

Printed in the United States of America

2 3 4 5 6 7 8 9 10

Introduction

There are few events in anyone's life that rival the significance and the joy of childbirth. This new person you're bringing into the world will become so important to you that you'll do anything to nurture and protect him or her. Your interest in this book reflects your eagerness to form this unbreakable bond right from the start — to do all you can to help ensure a healthy pregnancy and a wonderful beginning to your child's life.

Mayo Clinic Guide to a Healthy Pregnancy is an authoritative reference manual that you can trust. And in this second edition, you'll find new and updated information to answer your questions about everything from the basics to newer trends, recommendations and technologies in prenatal care and childbirth.

This book is the work of a team of pregnancy experts who find nothing in medicine more exciting to experience than the development and birth of a child. It's our sincere wish that you find this book helpful and meaningful as you anticipate your new baby.

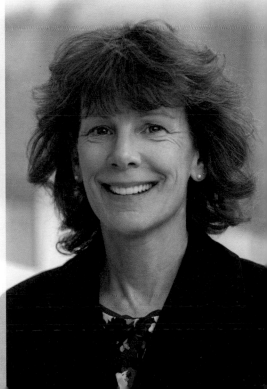

Myra J. Wick, M.D., Ph.D., is a specialist in the Department of Obstetrics and Gynecology and the Department of Clinical Genomics at Mayo Clinic in Rochester, Minn. She is also an associate professor at Mayo Clinic College of Medicine and Science. As a mother of four children, Dr. Wick can relate to pregnancy from both a doctor's and a mother's perspective.

How to use this book

Mayo Clinic Guide to a Healthy Pregnancy is a comprehensive how-to manual that provides answers and explanations to all of the questions and concerns of expectant parents. To help you easily find what you're looking for, the book is divided into six sections.

Part 1: Enjoying a healthy pregnancy
How to get pregnant, eating and exercise during your pregnancy, what you should know about medications — this section covers it all. Here you'll also find answers to many of the questions you've been wondering about.

Part 2: Pregnancy month by month
This section provides weekly and monthly insights into your baby's development and your own physical and emotional changes. It also includes detailed information on labor and childbirth.

Part 3: Baby is finally here
For first-time parents, caring for a newborn can be nerve-racking. The information and advice in Part 3 can help you get through those first couple of weeks.

Part 4: Important decisions of pregnancy
During pregnancy, you may be confronted with a number of decisions, big and small. Part 4 is designed to help you determine the best option for you in your particular situation.

Part 5: Symptoms guide
Here you'll find helpful self-care tips for backache, fatigue, heartburn, leg cramps, swelling and many more common concerns of pregnancy. The symptoms are listed alphabetically to help you easily find them.

Part 6: Complications of pregnancy and childbirth
Most pregnancies proceed smoothly, but sometimes problems can develop in mother or baby. The most common complications, and how they're treated, are discussed here.

Contents

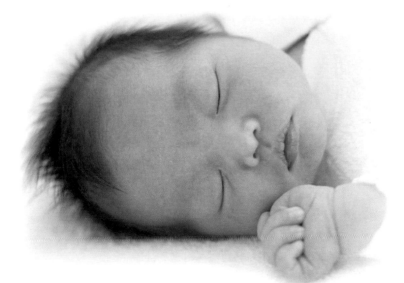

PART 1

Enjoying a healthy pregnancy

CHAPTER 1

Preparing to become pregnant

So you think you want to be a parent — at least sometime in the near future. How exciting! Having a child is a wonderful experience that will enrich your life forever. But the decision to have a child shouldn't be taken lightly. Parenthood is a lot of work, and the best way to approach it is by preparing yourself so that you're as ready as possible for this big change.

Thinking ahead can give you and your baby the best possible beginning. If you're reading this book and are still in the planning stages before becoming pregnant, you're giving yourself a head start on the exhilarating, sometimes bewildering path toward parenthood. Taking steps to be healthy and informed now can help set you up to enjoy a healthy pregnancy.

This introductory chapter includes some key concepts and actions to take that can help make your transition to pregnancy as smooth as possible. If you already know you're pregnant, congratulations! You may want to page through this chapter and begin with Chapter 2.

IS THE TIME RIGHT?

When your friends with children tell you to say goodbye to lazy weekends and impromptu nights out, and hello to nighttime feedings and loads of baby laundry, they're not kidding. Having a baby is life-changing. In most ways it's wonderful, but life will never be the same. Although there's probably never a perfect time to have a baby, some phases of your life may be more conducive to pregnancy and new parenthood than others.

Questions to ask Here are some questions you might ask yourself in determining whether the time is right:

- Why do I want to have a baby?
- Does my partner feel the same way I do? Do we share the same ideas about how to raise a child? If not, have we discussed our differences?
- How will having a baby affect my current and future lifestyles or career? Am I ready and willing to make those changes?

- Is there a lot of stress in my life right now that could interfere with my ability to care for myself and enjoy my pregnancy? What about for my partner? Is stress an issue?
- Emotionally, are we ready to take on parenthood?
- Financially, can we afford to raise a child? If I'm single, do I have the necessary resources to care for a child by myself?
- Does my health insurance plan cover maternity and newborn care?
- If I decide to return to work, do I have access to good child care?

If you haven't thought about any of these issues so far, it doesn't mean you'll have an unhealthy pregnancy or be unable to care for a child. But the sooner you set the stage for a successful outcome, the better your odds. That's true whether you're still in the planning stages, are trying to conceive or already have a baby on the way.

IS YOUR BODY READY?

You don't have to be exceptionally fit to have a child, but if you're healthy to begin with, you have a better chance of enjoying a healthy pregnancy.

So how do you know if your body is ready for pregnancy? Have your care provider give you the green light. Make a preconception appointment with your obstetrician-gynecologist, family physician, nurse-midwife or other care provider who will be guiding you through your pregnancy.

A preconception visit gives you and your care provider a chance to identify any potential risks to your pregnancy and establish ways to minimize those risks, as well as discuss general health issues.

If possible, have your partner attend the preconception visit with you. Your partner's health and lifestyle — including family medical history and risk factors for infections or birth defects — are important because they, too, can affect you and your baby.

At your appointment, your care provider will likely conduct a complete physical examination, including a blood pressure check and possibly updating your pap smear and pelvic exam. Some of the subjects you might talk about include:

Contraception If you've been using birth control pills, a vaginal ring, the patch, a contraceptive implant or an intrauterine device (IUD), you may be able to conceive shortly after discontinuing use. Some women become pregnant before their next period. (Not to worry — an expected due date can still be determined accurately without knowing the timing of ovulation.) If a waiting time is desired after stopping contraception, use condoms or another barrier method until you're ready to become pregnant. For most women, a normal menstrual cycle will return within three months of stopping birth control.

If you've been using contraceptive injections (Depo-Provera), you can try to conceive as soon as you stop receiving regular injections — but it could take up to 10 months or more for fertility to return.

Immunizations Infections such as chickenpox (varicella), German measles (rubella) and hepatitis B can be dangerous in pregnancy. If your immunizations aren't complete or you're not sure if you're immune to certain infections, your preconception care may include testing for immunity and receiving one or more vaccines, preferably at least a month before you try to conceive.

Chronic medical conditions If you have a chronic medical condition — such as diabetes, asthma or high blood pressure — you'll want to make sure the condition is under control before you conceive. In some cases, your care provider may recommend adjusting your medication or other treatments before pregnancy. He or she may also discuss any special care you may need during your pregnancy.

Medications and supplements Tell your care provider about any medications, herbs or supplements you're taking. He or she may recommend changing doses or stopping them altogether before you conceive.

This is also the time to start taking prenatal vitamins. Why so early? A baby's neural tube, which becomes the brain and spinal cord, develops during the first month of pregnancy, possibly before you

---

PRENATAL VITAMINS

One thing you'll be advised to do right away as you prepare for pregnancy is to start taking prenatal vitamins. If you're wondering whether this daily routine really matters, rest assured that it does!

It's best to start taking prenatal vitamins one to three months before conception. Prenatal vitamins help ensure you're getting enough folic acid, calcium and iron — essential nutrients during pregnancy.

▶ *Folic acid helps prevent neural tube defects.* These defects are serious abnormalities of the brain and spinal cord. The critical development of the baby's neural tube, which becomes the brain and spinal cord, occurs during the first month of pregnancy, when you may not even know you're pregnant.

▶ *Calcium promotes strong bones and teeth for both mother and baby.* Calcium also helps your circulatory, muscular and nervous systems operate normally.

▶ *Iron supports the development of blood and muscle cells for both mother and baby.* Iron helps prevent anemia, a condition in which blood lacks adequate healthy red blood cells. Many chewable gummy prenatal vitamins don't contain iron, so check labels.

▶ *Some research suggests that prenatal vitamins may reduce the risk of low birth weight.*

Prenatal vitamins are available over-the-counter in most pharmacies. Typically, a prescription for prenatal vitamins isn't necessary.

Taking prenatal vitamins prior to conception may help reduce nausea and vomiting in pregnancy. However, if your prenatal vitamins make you feel queasy, try taking them at night or with a snack. Chewing gum or sucking on hard candy right after may help, too. If they seem to make you constipated, drink plenty of water, and include more fiber in your diet and physical activity in your daily routine. Also, ask your care provider about using a stool softener.

If these tips don't help you tolerate prenatal vitamins, ask about other options. Another type of prenatal vitamin, or taking separate folic acid, calcium and iron supplements, may cause fewer side effects.

even know that you're pregnant. Taking prenatal vitamins before conception is the best way to help prevent neural tube defects, which can result in spina bifida and other spinal or brain disorders.

Sexually transmitted infections Sexually transmitted infections can increase the risk of infertility, ectopic pregnancy — when the fertilized egg implants itself outside the uterus, such as in a fallopian tube — and other pregnancy complications. If you're at risk of a sexually transmitted infection, your care provider may recommend preconception screening, followed by treatment if needed.

Family history Certain medical conditions or birth defects run in families and ethnic populations. If you or your partner has a family history of a genetic disorder or may be at risk, your care provider may refer you to a medical geneticist or a genetic counselor for a preconception assessment (see Chapter 20).

Previous pregnancies If this isn't your first pregnancy, your care provider may ask about previous pregnancies. Be sure to mention any complications you may have had, such as high blood pressure, gestational diabetes, preterm labor or birth defects. If you had a previous pregnancy that involved a neural tube defect, your care provider may recommend a higher daily dose of folic acid than what's found in most prenatal vitamins.

If you have any concerns or fears about another pregnancy, share them with your care provider. He or she will help you identify the best ways to boost your chances of a healthy pregnancy.

Lifestyle Healthy lifestyle choices during pregnancy are essential. Your care provider will likely discuss the importance of eating a healthy diet, getting regular exercise and getting adequate sleep. Good nutrition and exercise create the ideal environment for creating a

ADDITIONAL NUTRIENTS

While prenatal vitamins can help you meet most of your nutrient needs, there are a couple of nutrients you may want more of. Talk with your care provider about these:

▶ *Vitamin D.* This vitamin is especially important during the third trimester, when calcium demands increase. Most prenatal vitamins don't contain optimal amounts of vitamin D. In addition to your prenatal vitamin, drink vitamin D-fortified milk or look for other calcium-rich foods containing vitamin D. If you don't drink milk daily or eat calcium-rich foods such as yogurt, salmon or kale, it may be wise to take calcium and vitamin D supplements.

▶ *Omega-3 fatty acids.* Standard prenatal vitamins don't include omega-3 fatty acids. The benefits of omega-3 fatty acids on fetal development are uncertain, but there's some evidence they may promote fetal brain development. If you're unable to or choose not to eat fish or other foods high in omega-3 fatty acids, talk to your care provider to see if supplementation with omega-3 fatty acids might be appropriate.

healthy baby. If you're a snack-food junkie, you might give up some of the junk food before you become pregnant and replace it with healthy fruits, vegetables and hearty whole grains. If your idea of exercise is a short jaunt from your car to work, make it a point to go for a walk or bike ride each day, or sign up for an exercise or yoga class. This will help prepare your body for pregnancy.

If you're underweight or overweight, your care provider may recommend addressing your weight before you conceive. As you prepare for pregnancy, it's also important that you avoid alcohol, illegal drugs and exposure to toxic substances. If you smoke, ask your care provider about resources to help you quit.

HOW TO GET PREGNANT

Sure, some couples seem to get pregnant simply by talking about it. For others, it takes plenty of patience and a bit of good fortune. If you're wondering how to give yourself the best chance of becoming pregnant, here's what you need to know.

Conception is based on an intricate series of events. Every month, hormones from your pituitary gland stimulate your ovaries to release an egg (ovulate). For most women, ovulation occurs within four days of the midpoint of a menstrual cycle. Once the egg is released, it travels to the fallopian tube to encounter any sperm that may be present.

Your fertile period is the period of time when egg and sperm are most likely to meet. This window of opportunity is governed by two factors:

▶ The life span of sperm inside the woman's reproductive tract (no more than five days)
▶ The life span of the egg (24 hours)

Your best chance of becoming pregnant is to have intercourse one or two days preceding ovulation. But how can you tell when you're ovulating?

The simplest and most effective solution is to have frequent intercourse. If you consistently have sex every two to three days, you're likely to hit a fertile period at some point. But if you'd like to know more precisely when your fertile period is, there are ways to do this.

When you're most fertile Following are some simple measures you can take that may help you predict your fertile period, including the five days leading up to ovulation and the 24 hours following it. You can use these methods separately or together. For example, some women find that combining the first three methods — tracking cycle days, changes in cervical mucus and basal body temperature — gives them a better prediction of their fertile period.

Calendar tracking Use an app, your day planner or another simple calendar to track your cycle each month. Mark the first day of menstrual bleeding (not spotting) as Day 1, and also note the number of days each period lasts. The last day of your cycle is the day before your next period.

After tracking your menstrual cycles for several months, once you know your average cycle length, you can get a general idea of when you're most likely to ovulate. The phase of your cycle that follows ovulation (the luteal phase) is generally fixed at 14 days. So if your cycle is 30 days long, you'll likely ovulate on day 16 (30 days - 14 days = day 16).

Using this example, your fertile window would fall between days 12 and 17. If you have sex every two days during this period, you're likely to have sperm ready

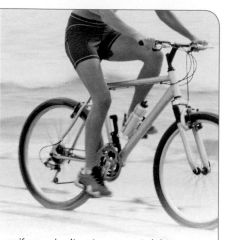

MAXIMIZING YOUR FERTILITY

To increase your chances of being successful when you're trying to conceive, here are some simple do's and don'ts.

Do:

▶ *Make healthy lifestyle choices.* Maintain a healthy weight, include physical activity in your daily routine, eat a healthy diet, limit caffeine and keep stress under control. These same good habits will serve you and your baby well during pregnancy.

▶ *Have sex regularly.* For healthy couples who want to conceive, frequent intercourse may be all it takes to become pregnant.

▶ *Have sex once a day or every other day near the time of ovulation.* Daily intercourse during the days leading up to ovulation may increase your odds of becoming pregnant. Although a man's sperm concentration will drop slightly with daily sex, the reduction isn't usually an issue for healthy men.

▶ *Consider preconception planning.* Your care provider can assess your overall health and help identify lifestyle changes that may improve your chances for a healthy pregnancy. Preconception planning is especially helpful if you or your partner have any health issues that could affect your ability to become pregnant.

Don't:

▶ *Stress.* Sometimes, trying to conceive can seem more like work than fun. Try not to become stressed if you don't get pregnant right away or even after the first two or three tries. Even with optimum timing, your chances of getting pregnant in a given cycle are about 50 percent at the most, and often closer to 25 to 30 percent. With frequent sex, most healthy couples conceive within one year.

▶ *Smoke.* Using tobacco may affect hormone levels, which could cause changes in the cervical mucus and make it difficult for sperm to reach the egg. Smoking may also increase the risk of miscarriage, decrease birth weight and deprive your developing baby of oxygen and nutrients. If you smoke, ask your care provider to help you quit before conception. E-cigarettes aren't a safe alternative, as the nicotine they contain still poses serious health risks.

▶ *Drink alcohol.* Alcohol may reduce fertility and, if you do conceive, may be harmful to the fetus.

▶ *Take medication without your care provider's OK.* Certain medications may not be safe when you're trying to conceive. Others may not be safe once you're pregnant.

and waiting when ovulation occurs, giving you the best chance of conception.

If your cycles are routinely shorter than 23 days or longer than 34 days, this may be an indication that you're not ovulating. Let your care provider know, as you may benefit from evaluation.

▶ *Pros.* Calendar calculations can be handled by an app or done simply on any calendar.

▶ *Cons.* Many factors may affect the exact timing of ovulation, including illness and exercise. Counting days is often inaccurate, especially for women who have irregular cycles.

Cervical mucus changes Just before ovulation, you might notice an increase in clear, slippery vaginal secretions, if you look for it. These secretions typically resemble raw egg whites. After ovulation, when the odds of becoming pregnant are slim, the discharge will become cloudy and thicker or will disappear entirely.

▶ *Pros.* Vaginal secretions resembling egg whites are often an accurate sign of impending fertility. Simple observation is all that's needed.

▶ *Cons.* Judging the texture or appearance of vaginal secretions can be fairly subjective.

Body temperature Your basal body temperature is your body's temperature when you're fully at rest. Ovulation causes a slight increase in basal temperature — typically less than one degree. You should be most fertile during the two to three days before your temperature rises. Your basal body temperature then remains higher after ovulation until just before your next period.

HEALTHY SPERM

Male fertility depends on sperm quality and quantity, which can be affected by a variety of factors. Men may not be able to control everything that could improve their fertility, but there are steps that can be taken to maximize fertility and help ensure their sperm are top performers.

▶ *Limit alcohol and don't smoke.* Drinking alcohol, smoking cigarettes and chewing tobacco may decrease sperm count as well as sperm movement.

▶ *Eat a healthy diet, including lots of fruits and vegetables.* These foods are rich in antioxidants, which may help improve sperm health. A balanced diet helps to avoid vitamin deficiencies.

▶ *Reduce stress.* Stress might interfere with certain hormones needed to produce sperm. Stress can also decrease sexual function.

▶ *Get regular exercise.* Physical activity is good for reproductive health as well as overall health. However, men who exercise to exhaustion show a temporary change in hormone levels and a drop in sperm quality.

▶ *Be weight conscious.* Too much or too little body fat may disrupt production of reproductive hormones, which can reduce sperm count and increase the percentage of abnormal sperm. Men at a healthy weight are most likely to produce lots of high-quality sperm.

Use a digital thermometer to monitor your basal body temperature. Some are specifically designed for this. Take your temperature every morning before you get out of bed. Record the readings and look for a pattern to emerge. Go high-tech or low — recording in an app or on paper both work.

Remember, by the time you see a change in temperature, ovulation will likely have already occurred. But by tracking your temperature each day for a few months, you may be better able to predict the days before you ovulate, when odds for conception are best.

- *Pros.* It's simple, and the only cost is the thermometer. It can be helpful in determining when you've ovulated and identifying if the timing is consistent from month to month.
- *Cons.* The temperature change can be subtle, and the increase comes after ovulation has already happened —

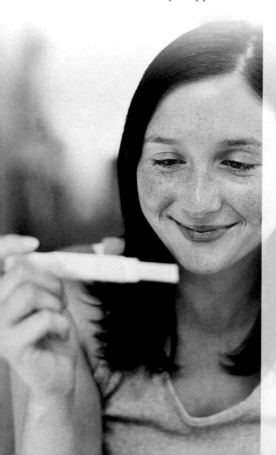

too late for conception. Your temperature may also be affected by a fever, alcohol use or too little sleep. It can be inconvenient to take your temperature every morning, especially if you have irregular sleeping hours.

An ovulation predictor kit Over-the-counter ovulation kits test your urine for the surge in hormones that takes place before ovulation. For the most accurate results, follow the label instructions on how to perform the test.

- *Pros.* Ovulation kits can identify the most likely time of ovulation. These kits are available without a prescription in most pharmacies.
- *Cons.* Timing sex too precisely around predicted ovulation can invite being too late. For some women, the cost of ovulation kits is prohibitive.

If you're having trouble If you're in your early 30s or younger, you have regular periods every 23 to 34 days, and you and your partner are in good health, try to conceive on your own for a year before consulting a doctor.

If you're age 35 to 39, it's recommended that you seek help if after six months of trying you haven't been successful, in order to avoid further delays.

If you're age 40 or older, or you or your partner know or suspect that fertility issues may be a problem in your efforts to conceive a child, your doctor may want to begin testing or treatment right away.

Infertility affects men and women equally — and treatment is available. Depending on the source of the problem, your gynecologist, your partner's urologist or your family doctor may be able to help identify the problem and suggest treatment. In some cases, a fertility specialist may offer the best hope.

ARE YOU PREGNANT?

Maybe your period is a day or two late, or maybe it's just a gut feeling you have, but you think you might be pregnant. How will you know? A big clue, obviously, is if you miss your period. But you may experience certain signs and symptoms even before then. A home pregnancy test can give you a more reliable answer, when used according to directions.

Early symptoms For some women, early signs and symptoms of pregnancy begin in the first few weeks after conception. Don't get too hung up on early symptoms, though. Some can indicate that you're getting sick or that your period is about to start. Likewise, you can be pregnant without experiencing any of these symptoms.

Tender, swollen breasts Your breasts may provide one of the first symptoms of pregnancy. As early as two weeks after conception, hormonal changes can make your breasts tender, tingly or sore. They may also feel fuller and heavier.

Fatigue Fatigue also ranks high among early symptoms of pregnancy. During early pregnancy, soaring levels of the hormone progesterone can cause you to feel unusually tired.

Slight bleeding or cramping Sometimes a small amount of spotting or vaginal bleeding is one of the first symptoms of pregnancy. Known as implantation bleeding, it happens when the fertilized egg attaches to the lining of the uterus, usually about 10 to 14 days after fertilization. This type of bleeding is usually a bit earlier, spottier and lighter in color than a normal period and doesn't last as long. Some women also experience abdominal cramping early in pregnancy that's similar to menstrual cramping.

Nausea with or without vomiting Morning sickness, which can strike at any time of the day or night, is one of the classic symptoms of pregnancy. For some women, the queasiness begins very early — two to three weeks after conception. Pregnant women also have a heightened sense of smell, so various odors — such as foods cooking, perfume or cigarette smoke — may cause waves of nausea in early pregnancy.

Increased urination You may find yourself urinating more often. Early in pregnancy, this is due to an increase in blood volume, meaning more fluid going through your kidneys to your bladder.

Food aversions or cravings You might find yourself turning up your nose at certain foods, such as coffee or fried foods. Food cravings are common, too. Like many other symptoms, they most likely can be chalked up to hormonal changes.

Headaches and dizziness Hormonal changes may trigger mild headaches. Dehydration and not getting enough sleep can also contribute to the frequency of headaches. In addition, as your blood vessels dilate and your blood pressure drops, you may feel lightheaded or dizzy.

Mood swings The flood of hormones in early pregnancy can make you unusually emotional and weepy. If you're not feeling well or not getting enough sleep, those may be part of the issue. Let your care provider know if you or your family have concerns about your mood.

Home pregnancy tests If this seems like a lot of work, relax. An easier way to find out if you're pregnant is to take a home pregnancy test. These user-friendly tests are widely available at drugstores and pharmacies. They work by detecting the level of human chorionic gonadotropin (HCG), a hormone associated with pregnancy, in your urine.

Taking the test is pretty simple. It usually involves holding a test stick in your urine stream or dipping the stick into a cup of collected urine. The results window on the stick will show a control line (to indicate the test is working) and the test result, typically a line or plus sign for positive results. On a digital test, the window will read "pregnant" or "not pregnant." Check the test's packaging to see what each result should look like.

Home pregnancy tests are generally considered very accurate, but there are a few things to keep in mind to make sure you're getting the best results:

- Because the amount of HCG increases day by day in early pregnancy, wait until the first day of a missed period to take the test. It will give you a more credible result.
- Test first thing in the morning, when your urine is the least diluted.
- Positive results are more likely to be correct than are negative ones.
- Follow the directions supplied with the test exactly. Waiting too long or not long enough to read the test often produces unreliable results.

If you have a positive result on your home pregnancy test, contact your care provider. In some cases, he or she may want to confirm the results with a laboratory test (of either urine or blood) that's more sensitive to HCG. Or your care provider may schedule you for your first prenatal appointment without another test. In either case, let the excitement begin!

CHOOSING A CARE PROVIDER

Whether pregnancy is a new adventure for you or you're an old hand at it, finding the right care provider to help you prepare for childbirth can make a big difference in your experience.

Plenty of options are available for obstetrical care, birth locations and birth preferences. The challenge sometimes lies in deciding which options to choose. The nature of your pregnancy and your own personal preferences can serve as your guides. Take the time to think carefully about your options. Once you've made the decision, you'll know that you chose your care provider for a reason. Trust his or her abilities to safely guide you and your baby through the birthing process, and allow your provider to give you the best possible care.

There are many people who provide maternity care. Here's a brief look at each specialty.

Obstetrician-gynecologists Doctors of obstetrics and gynecology are commonly referred to as ob-gyns. They specialize in the care of women during pregnancy and also provide general reproductive care, including care of a woman's reproductive organs, breasts and sexual function. Ob-gyns generally have advanced surgical training to deal with problems in women that may require surgery. Because of their emphasis on women's health, ob-gyns are the doctors women most frequently see.

Practice Ob-gyns often work in a group practice consisting of various medical professionals, including nurses, certified nurse-midwives, nurse practitioners, physician assistants, dietitians and social workers. Ob-gyns may work in a clinic or hospital setting.

GIVING BIRTH IN A HOSPITAL

When deciding on a care provider, you might also think about where you want to have your baby. This decision is often closely tied to your choice of a care provider and where he or she practices. Most women in the United States have their babies in a hospital. In many places, the hospital birth experience is evolving, with updated facilities and services to accommodate a variety of birth preferences. Talk with your care provider about choosing your birth location.

Most of today's hospitals treat childbirth less like a medical procedure and more like a natural process. Some hospitals now refer to their maternity unit as a birth center and offer a relaxed setting in which to have your baby, with options such as:

▶ *Birthing rooms.* These are homelike suites where you can labor and deliver. The father or labor partner can be an active part of the birthing team. In some cases, you may be able to recover in the same room after giving birth.

▶ *Rooming-in.* In this arrangement, the baby stays with you almost all of the time instead of being taken to the nursery. Rooming-in is increasingly common for healthy newborns. Experienced staff are available to help you with feeding and caring for the baby.

Advantages If you already see an ob-gyn for your general health care, he or she may be a natural choice for continuing to provide care during your pregnancy and childbirth. Many women choose an ob-gyn for obstetrical care because if a problem or complication arises during pregnancy, they won't have to switch care providers.

Issues to consider An ob-gyn can meet all the needs of most pregnant women, except perhaps those with extremely high-risk pregnancies. In such a case, your ob-gyn may refer you to a maternal-fetal medicine specialist.

You might choose an ob-gyn if:

▶ You have a higher-risk pregnancy. You may be high-risk if you're over age 40 or you develop gestational diabetes or high blood pressure (preeclampsia) during pregnancy.

▶ You're carrying twins.

▶ You have a pre-existing medical condition, such as diabetes, high blood pressure or an autoimmune disorder.

▶ You want the reassurance that if a problem arises, you won't need to be transferred to a different provider.

Midwives Midwives provide preconception, maternity and postpartum care for women at low risk of complications. Throughout much of the world, midwives are the traditional care providers for women during pregnancy. In the United States, the use of midwives is steadily increasing.

In general, midwives follow a philosophy that builds on the view that women have been having babies for millennia, and they don't always need all of the technological intervention that's available with today's health care.

Certified nurse-midwives have received formal training in midwifery and well-woman care beyond their nursing degree. Most nurse-midwives at health-care facilities and birth centers in the United States are certified by the American Midwifery Certification Board (AMCB). Independent midwives may not have any medical credentials.

Practice Midwives may work in a hospital setting, in a birthing center or in your home. They may practice solo, but they're often part of a group practice, such as a team of obstetric care providers. Most midwives are associated with an ob-gyn in case problems occur.

Advantages Midwifery care may offer a more natural, less regimented approach to pregnancy and childbirth than does traditional care. A midwife may also be able to provide greater individual attention during pregnancy and may be more likely to be present during labor and delivery than is a doctor.

If your child's birth is attended by a midwife in a hospital, you'll have access to the pain relief options available at the hospital.

Issues to consider When considering a midwife, ask about the person's training, certification and licensure in your state. Most midwives associated with a hospital are certified nurse-midwives. If a midwife works independently, also make sure she or he has a backup arrangement with a hospital so that you can have access to obstetrical skills and equipment in case problems develop.

If you're interested in giving birth outside of a hospital, make sure you've discussed risks and suitability with your care provider. (See "Considering an out-of-hospital birth" on page 29.) It's important to be aware of the risks associated with delivery outside of a hospital. You'll also want to create an emergency plan with your midwife. Include details such as the name and phone number of your midwife's backup doctor, the hospital you'll be taken to, how you'll get there in a safe and timely way, and the name and phone numbers of the people who need to be alerted. This can reduce stress later if you need to be transferred during labor.

You might choose a midwife if:

▶ You're free of health problems and you expect a low-risk pregnancy.
▶ You prefer a more personalized approach to the birthing process.
▶ You desire a less regimented birthing process.
▶ You desire fewer interventions.

Family physicians Family physicians provide care for the whole family through all stages of life, including pregnancy and birth. Some family physicians, however, choose not to handle pregnancies.

Practice Family physicians may work solo, or they may be part of a larger group practice that includes other family physicians, nurses and other medical professionals. Family physicians are usually associated with a hospital where they can perform deliveries.

Advantages If you've had the same family doctor for a while, he or she will probably know you well and be familiar with your family and medical history. Thus, a family doctor may view your pregnancy as part of the larger picture of your life. Another advantage of a family doctor is that he or she can continue to treat you and your baby after birth.

Issues to consider Family physicians can cover most obstetrical care, but if you've had problems with a pregnancy before, your family physician may refer you to a

CONSIDERING AN OUT-OF-HOSPITAL BIRTH

While most women in the United States give birth in a hospital, some women choose to give birth at a standalone birthing center or in their own homes.

Talk with your care provider in choosing a birthing location. Being pregnant for the first time, being pregnant with multiples, having a previous cesarean delivery and other risk factors are considered in weighing the safety and recommendations for each woman. For all women, a certified midwife or physician attending the birth and ready access to a nearby hospital are critical for a safe outcome.

Birthing center Birthing centers can be independent facilities, or they may be affiliated with a hospital. Most birthing centers are run by certified nurse-midwives or teams of obstetrical care providers, and they strive to provide a more natural birthing experience for low-risk, routine pregnancies, without overuse of medical intervention. Because of the reduced need for personnel and equipment, birthing centers may be more cost efficient. You might consider a birthing center if your pregnancy is low-risk, you're looking for a homelike experience and there's an affiliated medical center nearby. Be sure to check on the licensing and credentials of the providers, as well as your insurance coverage. If you're worried that complications could arise, a birthing center may not be the best choice. If you do experience complications, you'll likely need to be transferred to a hospital, and that takes time.

Home In the United States, each year about 1 percent of women have their babies at home. The trend for home births has been growing in recent years and remains somewhat controversial, as the risks even for women with healthy pregnancies are greater than in a hospital. Midwives are almost always the care providers for home deliveries. Women who choose to deliver at home often wish to avoid medical interventions and the hospital environment. The disadvantage is that if problems arise, they may not be recognized early on. In certain situations, delay of care could compromise the health or life of mom and baby.

Research suggests there may be certain benefits to women in these settings compared with hospital births, including fewer interventions, such as labor induction or episiotomy, and fewer perineal tears. However, the possible benefits of a home birth must be weighed against a higher risk for both mom and baby.

Keep in mind: Current research findings reflect that women who plan to give birth out of hospitals generally have fewer risk factors than those planning hospital births, leading to differences in outcomes. In addition, out-of-hospital birth statistics may not include cases in which a woman is transferred from home or a birthing center to a hospital due to complications.

Further research is needed to better determine the benefits and risks of out-of-hospital births in the United States. Meanwhile, care providers can help review risks for those considering birth outside a hospital setting.

specialist in obstetrics or use a specialist as a backup provider. The same may be true if you have diabetes, high blood pressure or another medical problem that may complicate your pregnancy.

You might choose a family physician for your prenatal care if:

- You and your doctor don't foresee any problems with your pregnancy.
- You want your doctor to be involved with all members of your family.
- You enjoy the continuity in care from prenatal appointments throughout childhood and beyond.

Maternal-fetal medicine specialists Also called perinatologists, these specialists are trained in the care of high-risk pregnancies. They deal with the most severe pregnancy complications.

Practice Maternal-fetal medicine specialists often work as part of a group practice, and they're generally associated with a hospital, university or clinic.

Advantages This highly specialized doctor is familiar with the complications of pregnancy and adept at recognizing problems. When women with major medical concerns become pregnant, their physicians often consult with maternal-fetal medicine specialists to optimize care for both the mother and her baby.

Issues to consider Maternal-fetal medicine specialists concentrate solely on the problems that occur with pregnancy.

A maternal-fetal medicine specialist rarely serves as the primary health care provider for a pregnant woman. This specialist is brought in at the request of another care provider. You may be referred to a maternal-fetal specialist if:

- You have a severe medical condition complicating your pregnancy, such as

an infectious disease, heart disease, kidney disease or cancer.

- You've previously had severe pregnancy complications.
- You plan on having prenatal diagnostic or therapeutic procedures, such as chorionic villus sampling, amniocentesis, or fetal surgery or treatment.
- You're a known carrier of a severe genetic condition that may be passed on to your baby.
- Your baby has been diagnosed before birth with a medical condition, such as spina bifida.

How to decide Navigating the health care system to find the right care provider can be a daunting process. Here are some suggestions that may be helpful.

Ask for help Try these approaches:

- Check with your insurance company to find out which hospitals and services are covered. The "find a doctor" feature on your health plan's website may be helpful.
- Consult with your regular doctor and other medical professionals.
- Ask family and friends whom they would recommend.
- Check the website of the clinic or hospital you prefer to find out who provides maternity care.
- Contact the labor and delivery unit at the hospital you prefer and ask for a recommendation.

Issues to consider Ask yourself these questions:

- Is the care provider certified by a medical board or the board of nurse-midwifery?
- Is the provider's office a convenient distance from home or work?
- Is the care provider going to be able to deliver my baby in the place I want to

give birth — at a particular hospital or birthing center, or my home?

▶ Does the care provider work in a solo or group practice? If it's a group practice, how often will I see him or her? How often will I see others from the practice?

▶ Who will replace my care provider if he or she isn't available in an emergency or when labor begins?

▶ Is the care provider available to answer questions in between my scheduled appointments?

▶ Do I want my care provider to be able to treat my entire family?

▶ Did the individual listen to my concerns and answer my questions?

▶ Did the individual seem open and caring?

▶ Is the care provider covered by my insurance company?

DELAYED PREGNANCY AND FERTILITY

Just because you're a little older doesn't mean you've missed the boat. Many women today put off pregnancy to go to school, start a career, travel or simply enjoy time to themselves in their younger years. If you're in your 30s or even 40s, you can still have a healthy pregnancy and a healthy child.

In fact, if you're in your mid- to late 30s and hoping to become pregnant, you're in good company. Over the past several decades, the average age of first-time moms in the United States has increased. In 1970, the average first-time mom was 21.4 years old. Today, the average first-time mom is 26 years old. Though the numbers vary quite widely from state to state and for different ethnic groups, this upward trend is widespread,

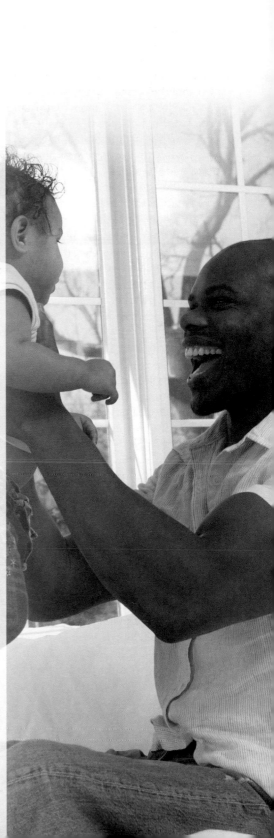

occurring in all ethnic groups and all 50 states. In countries such as Switzerland, Ireland, Italy, Japan and South Korea, the average age is even higher, around 30.

During this same time period, the proportion of first-time moms who are 35 and older has increased dramatically, from about 1 percent of all first births to about 9 percent. Some women are becoming moms even in their late 40s or 50s with the help of assisted reproductive technologies such as in vitro fertilization of donor eggs, preserved eggs or frozen embryos. In 2015, more than 2,600 American women had their first child between the ages of 45 and 54. Most women at this age will need the assistance of reproductive technologies to become pregnant.

Issues to consider The age of 35 is often viewed as the critical age when it comes to getting pregnant. While the biological clock is a fact of life, there's nothing magical about the age of 35. It's simply an age at which certain factors become worthy of discussion. For example:

Becoming pregnant may take longer You're born with a limited number of eggs. As you reach your early 30s, your eggs may decline in quality and quantity — you may ovulate less frequently, even if you're still having regular periods. An older woman's eggs also aren't fertilized as easily as a younger woman's eggs. Does this mean you can't get pregnant? Of course not. But pregnancy is less certain, and it may simply take longer. If you're 35 to 40 and haven't been able to conceive for six months, or you are not getting your period regularly, ask your care provider for advice. He or she may suggest fertility testing at that point. Over age 40, it's worth discussing and testing without any wait.

A multiple pregnancy is more likely The chance of having twins increases with age. The use of assisted reproductive technologies, such as in vitro fertilization, also plays a role. Since these procedures typically enhance ovulation, they're more likely to result in twins or other multiples.

Risk of gestational diabetes increases This type of diabetes occurs only during pregnancy, and it's more common as women get older. Tight control of blood sugar through diet, exercise and other lifestyle measures is essential. Sometimes, medication is needed as well. Left untreated, gestational diabetes can cause a baby to grow too large, which increases the risk of problems during delivery. A baby may also have difficulty maintaining a high enough blood sugar level after birth.

Chances of a cesarean delivery increase Older mothers have a higher risk of pregnancy-related complications that may lead to a C-section delivery.

Risk of chromosomal abnormalities increases Babies born to older mothers have a higher risk of certain chromosome conditions, such as Down syndrome. Babies of older fathers are also at higher risk of certain disorders.

Risk of miscarriage is higher Miscarriage risk increases as you get older, in part due to the higher likelihood of chromosomal abnormalities. Rates of miscarriage continue to increase with age, reaching 20 percent at age 35, 40 percent at age 40 and 80 percent by age 45.

Making healthy choices Steps toward a healthy pregnancy are the same for women age 35 and older as for younger women. To reduce your risk of complications and help ensure a healthy pregnancy at an older age:

▶ *Seek regular care.* See your care provider before you conceive, as well as during your pregnancy.

▶ *Choose a healthy lifestyle.* Eat a balanced diet, stay physically active and strive for the right amount of weight gain for your pregnancy.

▶ *Avoid risky substances.* This includes alcohol, tobacco, illegal drugs and even some prescription medications.

▶ *Read up on prenatal testing.* Ask your care provider's advice about the benefits and risks of each test. Although most prenatal tests simply confirm that a baby is healthy, their results can alert you to other possibilities.

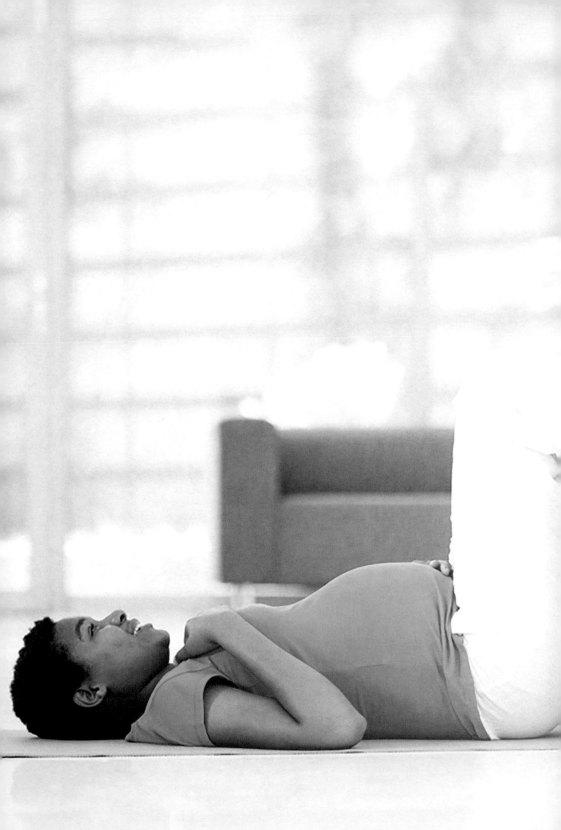

CHAPTER 2

Healthy choices during pregnancy

A new baby on the way is a great reason to take stock of your current lifestyle. Pregnancy provides many women with the motivation to eat well, exercise more and minimize risky habits. And if you make healthy habits a priority now, it'll be that much easier to maintain them after the baby arrives, meaning you'll lose the pregnancy weight faster, have more energy to devote to your new baby and get back to your old (or new and improved!) self in record time.

If you already practice a healthy lifestyle, you're one step ahead of the game. And even if all of your choices haven't been spot on in the past, pregnancy is a good time to start fresh.

This chapter will show you how to make the best choices for you and your growing baby during pregnancy. As an added bonus, your healthy choices may have a positive effect on other family members, as well. If you start eating better and exercising more, others around you may, too.

PREGNANCY DIET

During your pregnancy, you'll be eating for two (you and your baby). But don't think of this as eating twice as much. You don't actually need additional calories each day until the second trimester. Instead, think of it as eating twice as well.

If your diet isn't as healthy as you would like it to be, or if you tend to skip meals or you eat a limited variety of foods, start making changes now. In fact, it's a good idea to make healthy eating a part of your pregnancy planning from the start. Eating well helps create ideal conditions for early fetal development. Over the course of your pregnancy, there are certain nutrients you'll need more of, too, such as iron, calcium, folic acid, and other essential vitamins and nutrients.

Don't worry! Eating right doesn't mean taking the fun out of eating or that you have to follow a rigid diet. To get proper nourishment, you want to enjoy a variety of foods.

Making every bite count Truth be told, there's no magic formula for a healthy pregnancy diet. In fact, the basic principles of healthy eating recommended for everyone apply to pregnant women as well. What are those principles? Eat plenty of vegetables, fruits and whole grains. Choose lean protein and low-fat dairy products. And select a variety of foods. If you can remember these key principles, you and baby will be well on your way to a balanced diet.

Eating a variety of foods over three meals — and snacking on healthy foods if you're hungry between meals — is a good way to get the nutrients you need. The chart on pages 38 and 39 breaks down the different food groups and how much of each to strive for daily when you're pregnant. Not sure how well your eating habits measure up? Writing down what you eat every day for a week or so can help you become more aware of your food choices and where you might make improvements.

Also pay close attention to ingredient lists and nutrition information on food labels. This information can help you keep track of sugars and fats, which add calories but little nutrition to your diet. It's also wise not to eat too many salty foods.

If you're pregnant with twins or other multiples, you'll likely need more nutrients and calories. Talk to your care provider or a dietitian about how many calories you'll need.

Foods to avoid During pregnancy, typical food safety guidelines still apply. However, there are certain foods you should limit or avoid because of health risks to your baby. The chance of a serious complication is small, but it's best to play it safe.

- *Seafood high in mercury.* Seafood is a good source of protein and iron, and the omega-3 fatty acids in many fish may possibly help promote fetal brain development. However, some seafood contains potentially dangerous levels of mercury, which can damage a baby's developing nervous system. These fish include swordfish, shark, king mackerel and tilefish.

  According to the Food and Drug Administration (FDA) and Environmental Protection Agency (EPA), pregnant women can safely eat up to 12 ounces of seafood a week. That equates to two average-sized portions or three smaller portions of shrimp, salmon, pollock, cod or canned light tuna. Limit albacore tuna and tuna steak to 6 ounces a week. For guidance on many other types of fish, check recommendations from the FDA.

- *Undercooked meat, poultry and eggs.* Pregnant or not, if you eat undercooked foods you may experience food poisoning. But because pregnancy causes changes in your immune system, you may get sicker than an individual who isn't pregnant. Although rare, it's possible your baby may get sick, too.

  To prevent foodborne illness, fully cook all meat and poultry before eating them. Use a meat thermometer to make sure the meat is done. If you're having steak, for example, the internal temperature should be at least 145 F.

  Cook eggs until the egg yolks and whites are firm, and avoid foods made with raw or partially cooked eggs. Raw eggs can be contaminated with salmonella bacteria.

- *Raw, undercooked or contaminated seafood.* It's also best to avoid raw fish and shellfish, such as oysters and clams, and refrigerated smoked seafood, such as lox. If you eat fish from local waters, pay attention to local fish advisories — especially if water pollution is a concern. If advice isn't available, limit the amount of fish from local waters you eat to 6 ounces a week, and don't eat other fish that week. Most seafood should be cooked to an internal temperature of 145 F.

▶ *Processed meats.* Meats can become contaminated during production, especially if a lot of processing is involved. Sliced deli meat, bologna, salami and hot dogs can be sources of a rare but potentially serious foodborne illness called listeriosis. Listeria, a type of bacteria, can grow in cold environments such as refrigerators but cannot tolerate heat. Make sure hot dogs and processed meats have been cooked to an internal temperature of 165 F or steaming just before serving. There's less risk if the meat is sliced from fully cooked roasts or turkeys, but heating the meat adds a level of safety.

▶ *Unpasteurized foods.* Low-fat dairy products can be a healthy part of your diet, but avoid anything containing unpasteurized milk because the products may lead to foodborne illness including listeriosis. Stay away from soft cheeses — Brie, feta, Camembert, chevre, blue cheese and Mexican-style soft cheeses, such as queso fresco and queso blanco — unless they're clearly labeled as being made with pasteurized milk. Also, don't drink unpasteurized juice.

▶ *Unwashed produce.* Raw fruits and vegetables are great to eat during pregnancy. Just make sure to wash them, especially if they come from a garden, farmers market or orchard, where they may not have been thoroughly cleaned.

▶ *Homemade fermented foods.* If you eat yogurt or kimchi for a healthy gut, there's no need to stop. The same goes for sauerkraut, tempeh and miso, but skip homemade options. During fermentation, microorganisms break down a food's carbohydrates into other compounds. While those "good bugs" are generally beneficial for people, there is a risk of other bacteria causing infection. Pasteurized versions of fermented foods are the safest option during pregnancy, because pasteurizing kills any bacteria. It's also best to avoid kombucha (a kind of fermented tea), as it may contain alcohol.

▶ *Large quantities of liver.* Liver is high in vitamin A. Small amounts of liver are OK to eat while pregnant; however, eating large amounts could lead to vitamin A toxicity and cause birth defects. Look at the vitamin A content in any supplements you're taking, too. Vitamin A in the form of beta carotene is not associated with toxicity, but preformed vitamin A (retinol) is. It can build up in your system from food, supplements and topical treatments, so pay attention to your total intake.

Vegetarian tips Wondering if your vegetarian diet will cause any problems for your baby? Relax. If you're in good health, there's no reason you shouldn't be able to follow your diet during pregnancy and have a healthy baby. The rules are the same for you as for nonvegetarians: Eat a wide variety of foods, and make sure to balance your daily nutrients.

If you normally include fish, milk and eggs in your diet, you'll have an easier time getting the iron, calcium and protein you need. If you're a vegan — you don't eat any animal products at all — you may need to plan what you eat more carefully. Vegans sometimes have difficulty getting enough zinc, vitamin B-12, iron and calcium in their daily diets. To help avoid this problem, try the following:

THE GOOD STUFF

Here's a guide to foods that are good to eat during pregnancy, and how much of each you should aim to get each day if you're staying active.

Food category	Daily amount during pregnancy	Good choices
Grains *Your body's main source of energy*	6 to 8 ounces 1 ounce = • ½ cup hot cereal or 1 cup cold cereal • ½ cup cooked pasta or rice • 1 slice whole-wheat bread	Whole-grain cereals, brown rice and bread, whole-wheat pasta, wild rice, quinoa, barley *Tip:* Trade sugary cereals and white bread for products that list whole grains first in the ingredients list.
Vegetables *Provide key vitamins and minerals, and fiber*	2½ or more cups 1 cup = • 1 cup cooked or raw vegetables • 2 cups raw, leafy vegetables count as 1 cup	Lettuce, spinach, peppers, sweet potatoes, squash, peas, green beans, broccoli, carrots, corn *Tips:* Make a veggie pizza. Add extra vegetables to your casserole.
Fruits *Naturally sweet and rich in nutrients and fiber*	2 or more cups 1 cup = • 1 medium-sized piece of fruit • 1 cup fresh, frozen or canned fruit • 1 cup 100 percent fruit juice • ½ cup dried fruit	Apples, bananas, grapes, pineapple, strawberries, blueberries, oranges, grapefruit, melon, peaches, raisins *Tip:* Top your cereal or yogurt with fresh fruit.

Source: USDA SuperTracker MyPlan, part of ChooseMyPlate.gov

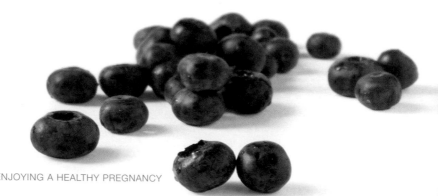

Food category	Daily amount during pregnancy	Good choices
Dairy products *Provide calcium, which helps build your baby's bones and teeth*	3 cups Each cup = • 1 cup milk • 1 cup yogurt • 1½ ounces cheese (or 2 ounces processed cheese, such as American)	Skim milk, low-fat cheese, low-fat yogurt, low-fat cottage cheese *Tip:* If you have trouble digesting dairy products, try soy milk fortified with calcium and vitamin D, lactose-free products, and foods naturally low in lactose.
Meat, poultry and fish *Provide plenty of protein, which is crucial for your baby's growth*	5½ ounces 1 ounce = • 1 ounce of cooked lean meat, poultry or fish • 1 egg • ¼ cup cooked beans • ¼ cup (2 ounces) tofu • 1 tablespoon peanut butter	Chicken, dried peas and beans, fish, lean beef, lean pork, peanut butter, eggs, tofu *Tips:* Eat whole-wheat toast with peanut butter for breakfast. Have salmon for dinner. Add chickpeas to your salad. Snack on a handful of soy nuts.
Oils *Dense sources of energy*	6 teaspoons Include oils in foods: • ½ avocado = 3 teaspoons oil • 1 ounce nuts = 3-4 teaspoons oil • 1 tablespoon peanut butter = 2 teaspoons oil	Olive oil, nuts, seeds, avocado, salad dressing, soft margarine (trans fat free), mayonnaise *Tip:* Opt for oils and fats from plant sources, which are typically low in saturated fat.
Added sugars *Extra calories that are low in nutrients*	Use sparingly	*Tip:* Any sugars not occurring naturally in a food (as in milk or fruit) count as added sugar, including honey and added fruit juice.

Tip: It's usually easier to eat well if you prepare more of your own food. Need recipe ideas? Check out the Healthy Recipes page at MayoClinic.org.

- *Eat at least 4 daily servings of calcium-rich foods.* Nondairy sources of calcium include broccoli, kale, beans, fortified juices, cereals and soy products. Vitamin D intake is also important to help you absorb calcium.
- *Add more energy-rich foods to your diet.* This is important if you're having trouble gaining enough weight. Good sources of calories include nuts, nut butters, seeds and dried fruit.
- *Seek advice on supplements.* Many vegans need a vitamin B-12 supplement. Supplementation with other nutrients commonly found in animal products also may be necessary, depending on your circumstances. To be sure of what's right for you, talk with your care provider and, if recommended, see a registered dietitian.

Taking supplements The best way to get the vitamins and minerals you need is from food. Yet during pregnancy, some women find it difficult to eat enough foods to supply them with adequate folic acid, iron and calcium, especially if they're coping with morning sickness. That's why prenatal vitamins are recommended.

Here's the scoop on those nutrients that are the most critical for healthy moms and babies. You'll get some of these nutrients by taking your prenatal vitamins, but it's still important that you eat well. Daily supplements can't take the place of a nutritious diet.

Folate and folic acid Folate is a B vitamin that helps prevent serious abnormalities of the brain and spinal cord (neural tube defects). The synthetic form of folate found in supplements and fortified foods is known as folic acid.

How much you need You want 600 to 800 micrograms (mcg) of folate or folic acid daily, from supplements and a variety of foods, during pregnancy. For at least one month before conception, 400 to 800 mcg is recommended.

Good sources Fortified cereals are great sources of folic acid. Leafy green vegetables, citrus fruits, and dried beans and peas are good sources of naturally occurring folate.

Calcium You and your baby need calcium for strong bones and teeth. Calcium also helps your circulatory, muscular and nervous systems run normally. If there's not enough calcium in your diet, the calcium your baby needs will be taken from your bones.

How much you need Aim for 1,000 to 2,500 milligrams (mg) a day of calcium. Pregnant teenagers need 1,300 to 3,000 mg daily.

Good sources Dairy products provide the richest sources of calcium. Simply drinking 3 cups of milk every day — a cup at each meal — will nearly meet your calcium needs. You can also get your calcium from other dairy products. Many nondairy milks, fruit juices and breakfast cereals are fortified with calcium, too.

Protein Protein is crucial for your baby's growth, especially during the second and third trimesters.

How much you need The recommended amount is 1.1 grams per kilogram of body weight. If you weigh 150 pounds, this is about 75 grams of protein daily.

Good sources Lean meat, poultry, fish and eggs are great sources of protein. Other options include beans and peas, tofu, dairy products, and peanut butter.

FOODS HIGH IN FOLATE (FOLIC ACID)

Food	Serving size	Folate/folic acid content
Cereal	¾ to 1 cup 100 percent-fortified ready-to-eat cereal	400 micrograms
Spinach	½ cup cooked spinach	130 micrograms
Beans	½ cup canned Great Northern beans	106 micrograms
Asparagus	4 boiled spears (about ⅓ cup, chopped)	90 micrograms
Peanuts	1 ounce dry roasted	40 micrograms
Oranges	1 medium orange (¾ cup)	39 micrograms

FOODS HIGH IN CALCIUM

Food	Serving size	Calcium content
Cereal	1 to ⅓ cups 100 percent-fortified ready-to-eat cereal	1,000 milligrams
Yogurt	8 ounces plain, low-fat yogurt	415 milligrams
Milk	1 cup fortified 1 percent milk	305 milligrams
Juice	6 ounces orange juice fortified with calcium and vitamin D	262 milligrams
Cheese	1 ounce part-skim mozzarella cheese	200 milligrams
Salmon	3 ounces canned pink salmon with bones	180 milligrams
Spinach	½ cup cooked spinach	120 milligrams

Source: USDA National Nutrient Database for Standard Reference, Release 28

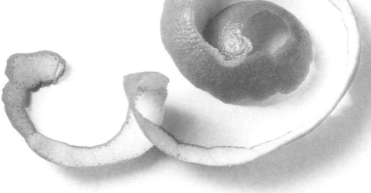

FOODS HIGH IN PROTEIN

Food	Serving size	Protein content
Poultry	½ boneless, skinless cooked chicken breast	29 grams
Cottage cheese	1 cup 1% cottage cheese	28 grams
Fish	3 ounces wild Atlantic salmon	22 grams
Milk	1 cup 1% milk	8 grams
Peanut butter	2 tablespoons creamy peanut butter	7 grams
Eggs	1 large hard-boiled egg	6 grams

FOODS HIGH IN IRON

Food	Serving size	Iron content
Cereal	1 to 1⅓ cups 100 percent-fortified ready-to-eat cereal	18 milligrams
Beans	1 cup boiled soybeans	9 milligrams
Spinach	1 cup boiled spinach	6½ milligrams
Trail mix	1 cup trail mix with chocolate chips, nuts and seeds	5 milligrams
Meat	3 ounces lean beef tenderloin	3 milligrams
Poultry	3 ounces turkey, dark meat	1 milligram

Source: USDA National Nutrient Database for Standard Reference, Release 28

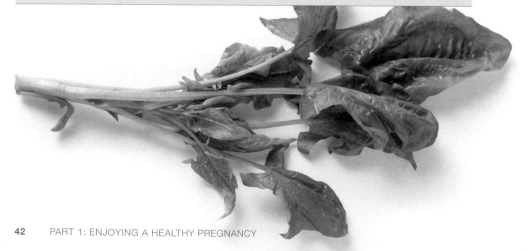

GETTING YOUR D

Vitamin D is important because it helps your body absorb calcium, which in turn keeps your bones strong and protects you from diseases such as osteoporosis. Sunlight is a great source of vitamin D, as are dairy products and fish.

Getting adequate vitamin D is important during pregnancy. Some studies suggest that vitamin D deficiency in pregnancy may be associated with problems such as gestational diabetes, preeclampsia and low birth weight. Further research is still needed to confirm whether taking extra vitamin D reduces the risk of these complications during pregnancy.

Nutrition experts recommend that pregnant women get 600 international units (IUs) of vitamin D daily. The upper limit for pregnant women is 4,000 IUs. Talk to your care provider about your need for vitamin D, especially if you have limited exposure to sunlight. Spending just 15 minutes or so in the sun or drinking an extra glass of fortified milk or orange juice each day may be just what the doctor ordered.

Iron During pregnancy, your blood volume increases to accommodate changes in your body and to form your baby's blood supply. As a result, your need for iron nearly doubles. Your body uses iron to produce hemoglobin, a substance in red blood cells that carries oxygen. If you don't get enough iron, you'll likely notice. A common symptom of too little iron is fatigue.

How much you need The recommended amount is 27 milligrams of iron a day.

Good sources Lean red meat, poultry and fish are good sources of iron. Other options include iron-fortified breakfast cereals, nuts and dried fruit.

GAINING WEIGHT

Pregnancy is the one time in your life when you can gain as much weight as you want and not worry about it. Right?

Not quite. Most women should gain weight during pregnancy, but you want to aim within a healthy range. Healthy weight gain — not too much or too little — is good for both you and baby. Gaining within the right range for your body also makes it easier to shed the extra pounds after your baby is born.

What's healthy? There's no one-size-fits-all approach to how many pounds you should gain when you're pregnant. Healthy weight gain depends on a variety of factors, including your pre-pregnancy weight and body mass index (BMI). Your health and your baby's health also play a role.

You'll want to work with your care provider to determine what's right for you, but here are some general guidelines. Keep in mind that if you're carrying twins or other multiples, you'll need to gain more weight.

If you're overweight Although excess weight carries risks — such as gestational

YOUR WEIGHT GOAL

Pre-pregnancy weight	Recommended weight gain (pounds)
Underweight (BMI less than 18.5)	28 to 40
Healthy weight (BMI 18.5 to 24.9)	25 to 35
Overweight (BMI 25 to 29.9)	15 to 25
Obese (BMI 30 or greater)	11 to 20

DETERMINING YOUR BMI

Body mass index (BMI) is one measurement care providers use to assess your weight and health. Use this chart to determine your BMI.

	Healthy		Overweight		Obese			
BMI	19	24	25	29	30	35	40	45
Height	Weight in pounds							
4'10"	91	115	119	138	143	167	191	215
4'11"	94	119	124	143	148	173	198	222
5'0"	97	123	128	148	153	179	204	230
5'1"	100	127	132	153	158	185	211	238
5'2"	104	131	136	158	164	191	218	246
5'3"	107	135	141	163	169	197	225	254
5'4"	110	140	145	169	174	204	232	262
5'5"	114	144	150	174	180	210	240	270
5'6"	118	148	155	179	186	216	247	278
5'7"	121	153	159	185	191	223	255	287
5'8"	125	158	164	190	197	230	262	295
5'9"	128	162	169	196	203	236	270	304
5'10"	132	167	174	202	209	243	278	313
5'11"	136	172	179	208	215	250	286	322
6'0"	140	177	184	213	221	258	294	331
6'1"	144	182	189	219	227	265	302	340
6'2"	148	186	194	225	233	272	311	350
6'3"	152	192	200	232	240	279	319	359
6'4"	156	197	205	238	246	287	328	369

Asians with a BMI of 23 of higher may have an increased risk of health problems.

Based on Circulation, 2014;129(suppl 2):S102; NHLBI Obesity Expert Panel, 2013.

WHERE THE WEIGHT GOES

Let's say your baby weighs 7 or 8 pounds at birth. That accounts for some of your pregnancy weight gain. But where does the rest of the weight go? Here's a sample breakdown:

- Baby: 7 to 8 pounds
- Fat stores: 6 to 8 pounds
- Increased blood volume: 3 to 4 pounds
- Larger breasts: 1 to 3 pounds
- Increased fluid volume: 2 to 3 pounds
- Larger uterus: 2 pounds
- Placenta: 1½ pounds
- Amniotic fluid: 2 pounds

diabetes and high blood pressure — pregnancy isn't the time to try to lose weight. Talk with your health care provider to find out how much weight gain is appropriate for you.

If you're underweight For women who are underweight, it's essential that they gain a reasonable amount of weight during their pregnancies — especially during the second and third trimesters. Without the extra weight, your baby may be born earlier or smaller than expected. This increases the risk of complications.

If you've had an eating disorder Many pregnant women experience body image issues as their bodies change shape. For some, new or returning symptoms of an eating disorder may appear in pregnancy. Eating disorders such as anorexia nervosa or bulimia nervosa can deprive you and your baby of vital nutrients.

If you've previously been treated for an eating disorder, or if you're struggling with your body image while pregnant, let your care provider know. He or she can help you determine an appropriate weight-gain goal and discuss healthy lifestyle habits and proper nutrition during pregnancy. It might also be helpful to see

a registered dietitian or a mental health provider for additional support.

Slow and steady In the first trimester of your pregnancy, don't worry too much about gaining weight. If you start out at a healthy weight, you need to gain only a few pounds in the first few months.

Steady weight gain is more important in the second and third trimesters. This often means gaining 3 to 4 pounds a month until delivery. An extra 300 calories a day — half of a peanut butter and jelly sandwich and a glass of skim milk — is often enough to maintain healthy weight gain. If you began your pregnancy underweight, your care provider may suggest additional calories.

STAYING ACTIVE

Pregnancy seems like a perfect excuse to sit back and relax, doesn't it? The fatigue, back pain and swelling sometimes associated with pregnancy all seem to be pointing you emphatically toward the couch.

But the truth is sitting around won't help matters. In fact, it's quite the opposite. Exercise can help reduce common pregnancy complaints, such as back pain. It can boost your energy level and reduce your risk of gestational diabetes and pregnancy-related high blood pressure. It can also set you up to lose the baby weight more easily after your baby arrives, and it may help lower your risk of postpartum depression.

Perhaps best of all, regular exercise can help you prepare for labor and childbirth by increasing your stamina and muscle strength. If you're in good physical condition before giving birth, you're less likely to need medical intervention, and you may even shorten your labor and recovery times.

To be safe, talk with your care provider early in pregnancy about which type of exercise may be best for you.

Baby, let's move! Try to spend at least 30 minutes each day exercising. But you don't have to do all 30 minutes at once. Even shorter or less frequent workouts can help you stay in shape and prepare for labor.

Walking is a great exercise. It provides moderate aerobic conditioning with minimal stress on your joints. Other good choices include swimming, rowing, cy-cling on a stationary bike, cross-country skiing, Pilates and yoga. Just avoid heated yoga classes, due to a risk of overheating, and skip or modify movements as needed.

Strength training also is beneficial, as long as your care provider has OK'd it. Make sure you discuss safe weight limits for lifting to avoid injury.

If you haven't exercised for a while, begin with as little as five minutes of physical activity a day and increase to 10 minutes the next week, then 15 minutes, and so on. If you exercised before getting pregnant, you can probably continue similar workouts through most of your pregnancy — as long as you're feeling comfortable and your care provider says it's OK. In general, you should be able to carry on a conversation while you're exercising. If you can't, you're likely pushing yourself too hard.

Remember to stretch gently before and after each workout. Drink plenty of fluids to stay hydrated, and be careful to avoid overheating. No matter how dedicated you are to being in shape, don't exercise to the point of exhaustion.

Working in workouts You're pregnant and tired. When do you have time to

---

WHEN EXTRA CAUTION IS NEEDED

Although exercise during pregnancy is generally good for both mothers and babies, you'll want to talk with your care provider first about what's appropriate for you. Your care provider may limit your physical activity if you're at risk of preterm labor in the current pregnancy, or if you have any of the following conditions:

- Severe anemia
- Pregnancy with multiples
- Certain types of heart or lung disease
- Preeclampsia
- Placenta previa (see page 447)

- Vaginal bleeding
- Premature rupture of membranes
- Cervical problems
- Poorly controlled diabetes
- High blood pressure

exercise? The truth is, you're more likely to stick with an exercise plan if it involves activities you enjoy and fits into your daily schedule. Consider these tips:

- *Start small.* You don't need to join a gym or buy expensive workout clothes. Just get moving. Try a daily walk through your neighborhood. Vary your route to keep it interesting.
- *Find a partner.* Exercise is often more fun if you team up with a friend or involve the whole family. A partner can also hold you accountable.
- *Schedule it.* When do you have time and energy during the day? Block out that time and set a reminder.
- *Use a headset.* Listen to music or a book while you exercise. Use lively songs to energize your workout.
- *Try a class.* Many fitness centers and hospitals offer classes designed for pregnant women.
- *Get creative.* Don't limit yourself to just one thing. Consider hiking, rowing or dancing.
- *Give yourself permission to rest.* Your tolerance for strenuous exercise will probably decrease as your pregnancy progresses.

Athletes and pregnancy If you're a regular jogger, runner or swimmer, it's likely you'll be able to continue these activities throughout most of your pregnancy, with your care provider's approval. Worries such as overheating have proved largely unfounded in studies of women

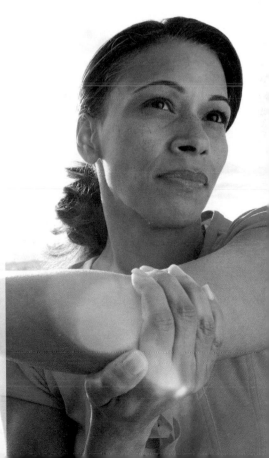

who exercise at a low to moderate intensity. Concerns of preterm labor due to strenuous exercise and reduced blood flow to the baby haven't been proved either. Recent research has shown that for many women with low-risk pregnancies who were already regular exercisers, even high-intensity activity is generally safe. So keep it up! Just stay on alert for any signs of overexertion.

In addition, it is especially important to stay hydrated and replace fluids you lose during exercise. Dehydration may cause mild contractions in some women.

Most active women, even competitive athletes, tend to decrease the intensity of exercise, especially toward the end of their pregnancies. As your weight increases, your center of gravity shifts and your ligaments become looser, so modify your routine as needed to avoid injury.

Activities to approach with care
After the first trimester, it's best to avoid floor exercises that require you to be on your back for a long period of time. The weight of the baby can cause problems with blood circulation.

While you're pregnant, avoid activities that carry a high risk of falling or abdominal injury. Gymnastics, horseback riding, downhill or water skiing, and vigorous racket sports have greater risk of injury. It's also wise to avoid high contact sports such as basketball or soccer. In addition to carrying a risk of falling or colliding with another person, these sports often require you to jump or change directions quickly. You may run a greater risk of straining the cartilage and ligaments that support your joints, which soften during pregnancy.

Underwater and high-altitude activities also can be a problem. Snorkeling is generally OK, but avoid scuba diving during pregnancy because the air de-

compression poses a potential risk to the baby. Activities such as hiking at altitudes higher than 6,000 feet above sea level can put you at risk of altitude sickness — especially if you're not yet acclimated to the elevation — which could endanger your health and your baby's.

Pregnancy exercises Childbirth is a wonderful experience, but the hours leading up to delivery can be a real workout. Your muscles and joints are moving and changing in all sorts of ways to make it possible for your baby to enter the world.

You can make childbirth more manageable by preparing your body for what's to come. Certain exercises help limber up the joints and muscles you'll rely on during labor and delivery. Some exercises can also help relieve the aches and pains that often accompany pregnancy, such as back pain or leg cramps.

In Part 2 of this book, each month a pregnancy exercise is introduced — a helpful stretching or flexibility maneuver. The idea is to start out with one exercise and add another to your routine each month, but you can also do them all at once or in whatever order you prefer. When the time comes and those contractions begin, your body will be ready!

PLAYING IT SMART

If you're accustomed to certain habits — maybe three cups of coffee a day, or a glass of wine with dinner — you'll now have to make some changes. While it's no fun to have restrictions placed on things you enjoy or even crave, like that midafternoon double latte, during pregnancy you need to play it safe. You likely know the key suspects to avoid — caffeine,

CAFFEINE COUNTER

Coffee and espresso	Caffeine (milligrams)
Brewed coffee, 8 ounces	95-190
Brewed coffee, decaffeinated, 8 ounces	2-5
Espresso, 1 ounce	47-75
Instant coffee, 8 ounces	27-135
Starbucks Caffè Mocha, grande, 16 ounces	175

Tea	Caffeine (milligrams)
Brewed tea	
Black tea, 8 ounces	30-80
Black tea, decaffeinated, 8 ounces	2-5
Iced Tea	
AriZona Green Tea, 16 ounces	15
Generic instant mix, unsweetened, 1 teaspoon	27
Honest Tea Organic Lemon Tea, 17 ounces	90

Soft drink, 12 ounces	Caffeine (milligrams)
Barq's Root Beer, regular	22
Coca-Cola Classic	34
Diet Coke	46
Dr. Pepper, regular or diet	41
Mountain Dew, regular or diet	54
Pepsi, regular or diet	34-38

Energy drink	Caffeine (milligrams)
5-hour Energy, 2 ounces	200
Monster Energy, 16 ounces	160
Red Bull, 8 ounces	75

Other	Caffeine (milligrams)
Candy	
Dark chocolate, 60-69 percent cacao solids, 1 ounce	24
Hershey's Milk Chocolate bar, 1.55 ounces	9
Ice cream	
Dreyer's or Edy's Slow Churned Coffee ice cream, 4 ounces	15
Haagen-Dazs Coffee ice cream, 4 ounces	29
Medication	
Anacin, 2 tablets	64
Excedrin Migraine, 2 tablets	130
NoDoz, Maximum Strength, 1 tablet	200

Based on USDA National Nutrition Database for Standard Reference, Release 2018; Center for Science in the Public Interest, 2016, 2017; Food and Chemical Toxicology, 2015.

alcohol, tobacco and illicit drugs. The good news is that becoming pregnant is a powerful motivator for many women to give up risky behaviors.

Caffeine It's best to avoid caffeine whenever possible during pregnancy. At the very least, limit how much you consume. Research on the subject has produced mixed results, but overall, studies show that a moderate intake — 200 milligrams (mg) or less a day, about the amount found in one to two cups of coffee — generally has no harmful effects on moms or babies.

However, the risk appears to increase with the amount of caffeine consumed daily. Recent studies suggest the higher the intake of caffeine, the greater the risk of low birth weight. Low birth weight can make it difficult for the baby to maintain a healthy body temperature and appro-

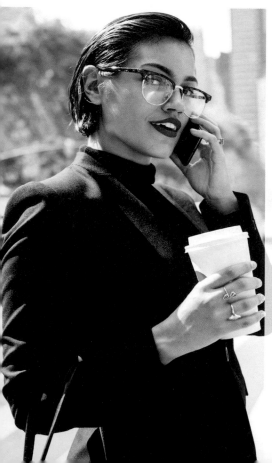

priate blood sugar levels, which can lead to other problems.

And remember, caffeine isn't limited to coffee. Tea, carbonated beverages, cocoa and chocolate also contain caffeine. To reduce the amount of caffeine you consume in a day, consider switching to decaffeinated beverages. Or with hot, brewed beverages, shorten the time you brew them. For instance, brewing a tea bag for just one minute instead of three minutes can reduce caffeine content by as much as half.

Alcohol If you drink alcohol, so does your baby. It doesn't matter if you drink beer, wine or other forms of liquor. Once in your bloodstream, alcohol passes through the placenta to your baby. Drinking during pregnancy increases your risk of miscarriage and fetal death. It can also cause permanent damage to your baby.

Fetal alcohol spectrum disorders (FASDs), including fetal alcohol syndrome, are a range of conditions caused by alcohol consumption. FASDs include serious birth defects such as facial deformities, heart problems, low birth weight and intellectual disability. Babies born with FASDs may also have permanent growth problems, experience short attention spans and learning disabilities, and have behavioral problems.

As soon as you know you're pregnant, don't drink alcohol. If you're planning to get pregnant, it's a good idea to stop drinking beforehand. Alcohol exposure can cause birth defects in the early weeks of your pregnancy, before you may know you're carrying a child.

Once your child is born, small amounts of alcohol can wind up in breast milk and be passed on to your baby through your milk. Therefore, it's best to limit alcohol use until you're finished breast-feeding.

Tobacco Smoking also is dangerous for you and your baby. Smoking during pregnancy increases the risk of stillbirth, premature birth, low birth weight and sudden infant death syndrome (SIDS).

Cigarette smoke contains literally thousands of harmful chemicals. Two toxins especially — carbon monoxide and nicotine — can reduce the flow of oxygen to the developing baby. In addition, nicotine, which causes your heartbeat and blood pressure to increase and your blood vessels to constrict, can decrease your baby's supply of nutrients.

It's best to stop smoking before you become pregnant. This may help you give up the habit permanently. However, it's never too late to quit. Even if you stop smoking late in pregnancy, you can reduce your baby's exposure to dangerous chemicals and protect him or her against some problems.

It's also wise to avoid being around the smoke of other smokers. Regular exposure to secondhand smoke appears to be capable of causing health problems for your child before and after birth.

E-cigarettes aren't a safe alternative to smoking during pregnancy. The nicotine they contain can still harm your baby's brain and lungs, and the flavorings used may not be safe for developing babies. If you need help to quit smoking or stop using nicotine products, talk to your care provider.

Illicit drugs Any and all illicit drug use can harm your baby. This includes everything from marijuana to cocaine, heroin, LSD, PCP, methamphetamine and any other kind of recreational or street drug. Keep in mind that even if marijuana use is legal where you live, it still poses risks for your baby.

Abuse of prescription drugs also is dangerous for both you and your baby.

See upcoming pages for additional information on medication use.

While you're pregnant, the drugs you take can pass from you to your baby. This can affect the development of the fetus and your child's future as he or she grows up. It can also cause fetal death or withdrawal symptoms in newborns that can lead to death if untreated.

MAKING SENSE OF MEDICATIONS

Hopefully, you will enjoy a smooth and uneventful pregnancy. However, you may still get colds and headaches and have to deal with allergies and aching joints. There are times when a pain reliever or an antihistamine could come in handy, but you'll want to be careful not to take anything that might hurt your baby.

So, are there some medications that are safe to use during pregnancy? And what if you're already taking a medication to treat an ongoing health condition? Should you stop taking it?

What's safe? As a general rule, it's best to use caution and avoid use of medications during pregnancy when possible. Some drugs can cause an early miscarriage or impair your baby's development. Very few drugs have been proved to be completely safe in pregnancy, but at the same time, many have been found to be safe enough that their benefits outweigh any tiny, unknown risk. It's best to check with your care provider before taking any medicine, be it prescription or over-the-counter. He or she can help you make the right decision based on your health history and the medication in question. A pharmacist also can provide general guidelines on medication safety.

A MEDICATION GUIDE FOR COMMON CONDITIONS

Condition	Generally safe	Use with caution	Avoid
Allergies Colds Flu	• Nasal sprays • Chlorpheniramine (Chlor-Trimeton) • Acetaminophen (Tylenol, others) • Cetirizine (Zyrtec) • Fexofenadine (Allegra) • Loratadine (Claritin)	• Medications containing pseudoephedrine (Sudafed, Claritin-D, others), especially during the first trimester • Medications containing dextromethorphan (Robitussin, Vicks NyQuil, Vicks DayQuil, others)	• Medications containing phenylephrine (Tylenol Allergy Multi-Symptom, others)
Constipation	• Psyllium (Metamucil) • Glycerin suppositories (Fleet)	• Docusate (Colace, Surfak) • Bisacodyl (Dulcolax) • Senna (Senokot)	• Mineral oil
Diarrhea		• Loperamide (Imodium A-D) for only short-term use in second and third trimesters; avoid in first trimester	• Bismuth subsalicylate (Pepto-Bismol)
Heartburn	• Antacids (Maalox, Tums) • Famotidine (Pepcid) • Ranitidine (Zantac) • Cimetidine (Tagamet HB)		• Medications containing aluminum or aspirin (Pepto-Bismol, Alka-Seltzer)
Hemorrhoids	• Psyllium (Metamucil)		
Pain and fever	• Acetaminophen (Tylenol, others)	• Ibuprofen (Advil, Motrin IB, others) only in first and second trimesters and no more than 48 hours of continuous use • Naproxen sodium (Aleve) only in first and second trimesters and no more than 48 hours of continuous use	• Aspirin (unless directed by your care provider)
Yeast infection	• Clotrimazole (Lotrimin AF, Mycelex)	• Miconazole (Monistat 3, Monistat 7) • Fluconazole (Diflucan)	

Although some medicines should be avoided, others may be recommended because of your needs. If you have a health condition that requires regular medication — such as asthma, hypothyroidism, high blood pressure or depression — don't stop or modify the medication until you talk with your care provider. He or she can help you evaluate what's safe to take before, during and after pregnancy. In many cases, continuing your medication may be the best choice. Or you may be advised to discontinue use or switch to a medication that poses less risk to you or your baby.

On the facing page is a list of common over-the-counter medications that are generally considered safe to use during pregnancy, as well as those that you should use with caution or under the supervision of your care provider, and some you should avoid. Be sure to ask your care provider if you have any questions about a drug. Also make sure that any care provider who's prescribing medication for you knows that you're pregnant.

What's not safe? Some medications have been shown to be extremely harmful to a developing fetus, even in the early weeks of pregnancy. Some of the most dangerous include:

▶ The acne medication isotretinoin (Claravis, Myorisan, others), formerly sold as Accutane
▶ The multiuse medication thalidomide (Thalomid)
▶ Some blood pressure medications (ACE inhibitors, ARBs and renin inhibitors)

If you're taking one of these medications, avoid becoming pregnant until you discontinue its use. Your care provider will advise you on the best way to stop taking a medication and how long you may need to wait before it's safe to conceive. Don't restart a drug without talking to your care provider.

QUESTION & ANSWER

I was taking birth control pills when I found out that I was pregnant. Did I hurt my baby?

Generally, taking birth control pills during early pregnancy isn't cause for great concern. While doing so isn't recommended, it happens fairly often among women who weren't expecting to become pregnant.

According to the American College of Obstetricians and Gynecologists, taking birth control pills during pregnancy doesn't increase the risk of birth defects. Some studies suggest a possible association between use of birth control pills near or after conception and an increased risk of low birth weight or premature delivery. However, these concerns generally haven't been observed in clinical experience.

Keep in mind that most babies are born healthy with no problems. However, if you're concerned about having taken birth control pills during early pregnancy, and you need more reassurance, talk to your care provider.

Opioid use during pregnancy Prescription opioid medications pose special concerns for women who are pregnant. These medications are an important option for managing pain, but using them repeatedly can lead to dependence. Addiction and overdose are serious risks.

Like any drugs, opioids taken during pregnancy might cross the placenta. Occasional use during pregnancy doesn't typically pose concerns for the baby, although using opioids close to delivery might cause the baby to experience slow and ineffective breathing (respiratory depression) after birth.

In contrast, many complications have been associated with opioid dependency during pregnancy. These include placental problems, preterm labor and premature birth, preeclampsia, and miscarriage or fetal death. And after you give birth, your baby could experience withdrawal symptoms.

If you have chronic pain while pregnant, your doctor will aim to avoid or minimize the use of opioids.

Pregnant women who are addicted to opioids should talk with their health care provider. Substitution therapy (treatment with a different drug) may be available as a safer option for the developing baby.

What about herbal products? It may be tempting to turn to herbal products to help alleviate your aches or other symptoms during this time when many traditional medications are off-limits. Perhaps some melatonin could help you sleep? But don't be misled by the idea that just because herbal products are "natural," they must be safe.

The fact is, herbal products need to be treated in the same manner as most medications — avoid them. Use a certain herb only if your care provider says it's OK to do so. Herbal products can be just as dangerous during pregnancy as traditional medications. They could even be more harmful because so little is known about many herbal supplements.

Unlike prescription and nonprescription drugs, herbal supplements sold in health food stores and pharmacies aren't tested and approved by the Food and Drug Administration. And they're not required to undergo clinical trials, in which the safety, purity and effectiveness of the product is determined.

Some herbal teas, supplements and alternative therapies have been specifically tied to negative pregnancy outcomes such as uterine contractions or preterm birth. For example, topical use of almond oil as a treatment for stretch marks has been associated with an increased risk of preterm birth. Overall, research and information on the safety of unconventional therapies in pregnancy have been very limited.

Pregnancy is generally a time to play it safe. If you're pregnant — or even if you're trying to become pregnant — it's important that you discuss all alternative and complementary therapies, including the use of herbs, with your care provider. Some, such as drinking ginger tea in moderation to treat nausea, may be safe. Your care provider may recommend that you forgo others until after baby is born.

WORKING WHILE PREGNANT

When you become pregnant, going to work can seem like agony if you're dealing with morning sickness and fatigue. Consider adjustments you may be able to make at your job, depending on your work situation. During the first three or four months of pregnancy, you may need more-frequent bathroom breaks, water

PROPER WAY TO LIFT

1. Kneel down next to the object, resting one knee on the floor.
2. Lift the object between your legs, keeping your back as straight as possible. Rest the object on your knee.
3. Keeping the object close to your body, use your leg muscles — not your back — to stand and lift.

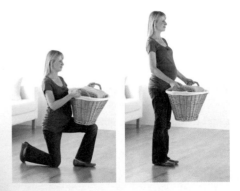

and snacks. Frequent changes in the timing of work shifts may be harder on you, too. Avoid hot environments to lessen issues with nausea and dizziness, and make sure your work schedule doesn't keep you from getting enough rest.

Once you move into your second trimester, things are likely to feel much better — queasiness usually subsides, your energy returns and you've got that pregnancy glow! During the second and third trimesters, try to make any changes needed to avoid heavy lifting and minimize the risk of falling at work. And remember to cut yourself some slack. You're growing a whole new person!

For some women, work can be a good way to occupy their minds while waiting for baby to arrive. Here are some tips to make pregnancy at work a little easier and a little more comfortable. These same tips also apply to chores you do at home.

Handling fatigue You may feel tired as your body works overtime to support your pregnancy, and resting during the workday can be tough. It may help to:

- *Eat foods rich in iron and protein.* Fatigue can be a symptom of iron deficiency anemia, but adjusting your diet can help. Choose foods such as red meat, poultry, seafood, leafy green vegetables, whole-grain cereal and pasta, beans, nuts, and seeds.
- *Take short, frequent breaks.* Getting up and moving around for a few minutes can reinvigorate you. Spending a few minutes with the lights off, your eyes closed and your feet up also can help you recharge.
- *Cut back on activities.* Scaling back can help you get more rest when your workday ends. Look for activities or chores you can cut back on or hand off to someone else.

- *Keep up your fitness routine.* Although exercise may be the last thing on your mind at the end of a long day, physical activity may help boost your energy level, especially if you sit at a desk all day. Take a walk after work or join a prenatal fitness class, as long as your care provider says it's OK.
- *Go to bed early.* Aim for eight to 10 hours of sleep every night. Later in your pregnancy, resting on your left side will improve blood flow to your baby and help prevent swelling. Place pillows between your legs and under your belly for increased comfort.

Sitting, standing, bending and lifting
Carrying around a growing baby can make everyday activities such as sitting, standing, bending and lifting uncomfortable. It can also cause constant pressure on your bladder, strain on your back, and swelling in your legs and feet.

Emptying your bladder frequently can help relieve pressure. Moving around every few hours can ease muscle tension and help prevent fluid buildup. But you may need to try other strategies to make yourself comfortable throughout your workday and prevent potential health hazards. Here's how to handle common on-the-job activities:

Sitting If you have an office job, the chair you sit in is important — and not just during pregnancy! While the weight of your body is increasing and shifting, you want a seat that you can adjust for height and tilt. Adjustable armrests, a firm seat and back cushions, and good back support can make long hours of sitting much easier and help you exit from the chair.

If a chair with these options isn't available, take steps to improve what you do have. For instance, if you need more cushioning or back support, use a small pillow or invest in a cushion designed to support the lower back. This type of cushion can also serve as a car seat support, which might make driving easier if you have a long commute.

While sitting, it's best to elevate your feet on a footrest or box to help take some of the strain off your back. This may also reduce your chance of developing varicose veins or clots in the veins of your legs. Using a footrest can also help reduce swelling in your feet and legs.

Standing During pregnancy, your blood vessels dilate to allow for greater blood circulation. This can cause blood to pool in your legs with too much standing, which can lead to leg pain and even dizziness. Standing for long periods of time can also put pressure on your back.

If standing is part of your job, put one foot on a box or low stool to take pressure off your back and decrease blood pooling. Switch feet every so often. It may help to wear support hose and take frequent breaks throughout the day. Wear shoes with low, wide heels rather than high heels or flats.

Bending and lifting Pregnant women typically cannot lift as much weight as they did prior to becoming pregnant. Talk with your care provider about how much weight you can safely lift. To prevent or ease back pain, follow proper form when bending and lifting (see page 55). In addition, avoid standing on ladders or stools to lift or reach things, as changes to your balance can increase the risk of falls.

If you have older children that weigh more than 30 to 40 pounds, you may need to limit or avoid lifting and carrying them during the second half of pregnancy. Start this transition early in your pregnancy to make it easier on your children. Offer other ways to be physically close,

such as sitting together and cuddling. Instead of lifting your children into a car seat, spot them as they climb in.

Avoiding harmful substances As long as you and the company you work for follow standard Occupational Safety and Health Administration (OSHA) practices regarding harmful substances, it's unlikely that your job will pose a risk to your baby.

To be safe, be aware of any substances you're exposed to at work — especially if you're in health care or manufacturing. Industries in the United States are required by federal law to have material safety data sheets on file that report hazardous substances in the workplace and to make this information available to employees.

Substances known to be harmful to a developing fetus include lead, mercury, ionizing radiation (X-rays) and drugs used to treat cancer. Organic solvents such as benzene are suspected of being harmful, although results of studies are inconclusive.

Tell your care provider about any part of your job that exposes you to chemicals, drugs or radiation. Also tell your care provider about any equipment you use to minimize your exposure. This may include gowns, gloves, masks and ventilation systems.

Your care provider can use this information to determine whether a risk exists and, if so, what might be done to eliminate or reduce it. Fortunately, it appears that environmental agents cause few birth defects. Of the small percentage of birth defects that can be traced to an environmental cause, most involve alcohol, tobacco or drugs used during pregnancy — not substances in the workplace. Nevertheless, avoid exposure to known or suspected harmful substances.

TRAVELING WISELY

You may worry your pregnancy will interfere with your travel plans or your summer vacation, but it doesn't have to. It's usually safe to travel while you're pregnant, as long as you're in good health and observe basic safety precautions. Generally speaking, the best time to travel is during the second trimester, when you're likely to have less morning sickness and your body is adjusted to carrying a baby. By the third trimester, you may find it more difficult to move around.

However, if you have a medical problem, such as heart disease, or a history of problems with pregnancy, your care provider may advise you to stay close to home in case an emergency arises.

Always talk to your care provider before setting out on an extended trip, as your mode of travel and destination may have implications for your pregnancy. If you travel often, such as for business, discuss your schedule with your care provider. Together you may find ways to make your trips more comfortable.

In planning or preparing for travel, find out what medical care will be available at your destination. Rural or island destinations may be hours away from obstetric care if an emergency arises. Flights across the ocean can also mean a long delay in care. While most women don't have pregnancy complications that lead to hospitalization or early delivery, it's best to consider what insurance coverage and social support would be available just in case.

Also consider the risk of diseases at your destination. And pay attention to the safety of food choices, which may be more difficult when you're away from home.

When choosing your mode of travel, consider how long it will take you to get to your destination. Generally, the fastest way is the best, but understandably, cost and other factors need to be considered.

Airplane travel Air travel during pregnancy is generally considered safe for women who have healthy pregnancies. Still, it's best to check with your care provider before you book that trip. And note

DESTINATIONS TO AVOID

When planning trips during pregnancy, consider your destination. A hot, humid climate may not be the best if you find it difficult to keep yourself cool these days. Travel to high altitudes may make breathing difficult because of the decreased oxygen level. This isn't good for you or baby. If the trip is going to require a lot of walking and standing, you may want to think twice. In planning activities, remember that scuba diving, snow or water skiing, rock climbing, and horseback riding are not recommended during much of pregnancy.

You also want to consider the risks of visiting regions with a high risk of exposure to infectious diseases, such as the Zika virus or Ebola virus. Travel to these regions often requires that you receive a number of vaccinations, and the risk of food- or waterborne illness may be greater. If you go to a high-risk region, make sure to get medical advice before you leave. Your provider will likely have updates on travel precautions from Centers for Disease Control and Prevention (CDC).

PROPER SEAT BELT USE

When buckling up, place the lap belt below your abdomen and over your upper thighs. Wear the diagonal shoulder strap between your breasts. Make sure the belt fits snugly.

that many airlines have restrictions on flying after 36 weeks.

Air travel may increase the risk of complications associated with certain conditions in pregnancy, such as sickle cell disease and clotting disorders. In addition, your care provider may restrict travel of any type after 36 weeks of pregnancy or if you're at risk of preterm delivery.

If you have flexibility in your travel plans, the best time to fly is usually during your second trimester — approximately weeks 14 to 28. This is when you're likely to feel your best, and the risks of miscarriage and premature labor are the lowest.

When you fly:
- *Check the airline's policy about air travel during pregnancy.* Guidelines for pregnant women may vary by carrier and destination.

Sea travel Ships and cruise liners are just as safe for pregnant women as are other forms of travel, and many vessels have medical facilities onboard. Make sure that your ship has a doctor or a nurse onboard at all times. Also check to see if the locations you visit are cities with medical facilities that can care for complications in pregnancy, in case you need emergency care. Most cruise liners accept women up to 24 weeks of pregnancy.

Keep in mind that the movement of the ship may increase problems with nausea and vomiting. In addition, be careful when walking on the ship's deck, where floors may be slippery. You don't want to slip or lose your balance and fall.

If you're worried about getting seasick, pack some seasickness bands. These are bands you wear on your wrist that use acupressure to help prevent an upset stomach. While the bands may be a good alternative to medication for some women, others may find they're not helpful.

Car travel When traveling by car, the main thing to remember — pregnant or not — is to always wear your seat belt. Trauma during a car accident is a leading cause of fetal death.

Wear the lap belt below your abdomen and over your upper thighs, and wear the diagonal shoulder strap between your breasts.

If you are traveling by car for a long distance, stop regularly to stretch. If possible, avoid staying in a seated position for more than two hours at a time, and limit total car time to six hours a day. Walking around for a few minutes every couple of hours will keep blood from pooling in your legs. This reduces the risk of blood clots forming. Chances are, you also may need to take frequent bathroom breaks.

Be sure to drink plenty of water to keep well-hydrated. This is true with any type of travel.

COMMON QUESTIONS

When you're pregnant, all sorts of questions seem to pop up — things that, until now, probably never crossed your mind. Is it OK to dye your hair? What about sitting in a hot tub? Here are some answers to commonly asked questions. You can find even more information online at MayoClinic.org.

? I tripped and fell. Do I need to see a doctor? It's easy to panic if you fall during pregnancy, but your body is designed to protect your developing baby. An injury would have to be severe enough to seriously hurt you before it would directly harm your baby.

The walls of your uterus are thick, strong muscles that help keep your baby safe. The amniotic fluid also serves as a cushion. In addition, during the early weeks of pregnancy, the uterus is tucked behind the pelvic bone, so there's even more protection. If you do fall, you can take comfort in knowing that your baby most likely won't be hurt. After approximately 23 weeks' gestation, a direct blow to the abdomen can possibly cause complications and should be evaluated.

If you're worried about the welfare of your baby after a fall, see your care provider for reassurance. Seek medical attention immediately if:

▶ Your fall results in pain, bleeding or a direct blow to the abdomen.
▶ You're experiencing vaginal bleeding or leaking of amniotic fluid.
▶ You feel severe pain or tenderness in your abdomen, uterus or pelvis.
▶ You have uterine contractions.
▶ You notice the baby isn't moving as much as normal.

In most cases, your baby will be fine. But your care provider may want to run some tests to make sure everything is OK.

? Should I get an annual flu shot? Yes, it's safe to get an influenza (flu) shot during pregnancy. In fact, the Centers for Disease Control and Prevention (CDC) recommends seasonal flu shots for anyone who will be pregnant during peak flu season — typically November through March — unless you have a severe allergy to eggs, or you've had a severe reaction to a previous flu vaccination.

Pregnancy puts extra stress on your heart and lungs. Pregnancy can also affect your immune system. These factors increase the risk not only of getting the flu but of developing complications of the flu, such as pneumonia and respiratory distress. A seasonal flu shot can help prevent these potential problems.

The flu vaccine is updated each year to protect against several strains of flu viruses that experts predict will be most common. There is still a chance you'll catch the flu after getting your shot, but being vaccinated can offer some protection against severe symptoms and complications — even for flu viruses not covered by the shot. In addition, mothers who are vaccinated during pregnancy can potentially provide protection to infants who cannot be vaccinated.

If offered a choice, be sure to request the shot and not the nasal spray vaccine. The flu shot is made from an inactivated virus, so it's safe for mothers and babies during any stage of pregnancy. The nasal spray vaccine is made from a live virus, which makes it less appropriate during pregnancy. In recent years, the CDC hasn't recommended the nasal spray vaccine because it was relatively ineffective in previous flu seasons.

If you're unsure about a flu vaccine, find out as much as you can about it. Go to websites you can trust, such as the CDC, and talk with your care provider.

? Are other vaccinations safe? Some are and some aren't. In addition to the seasonal flu vaccine, the CDC recommends you get a tetanus, diphtheria and acellular pertussis (Tdap) booster shot during each pregnancy, between 27 and 36 weeks, even if your vaccination was up to date before becoming pregnant.

If you're traveling abroad or you're at increased risk of certain infections, your care provider may recommend other vaccines during pregnancy, such as hepatitis A, hepatitis B, meningococcal or pneumococcal vaccines.

Vaccines to avoid during pregnancy include the live attenuated flu vaccine,

human papillomavirus (HPV), measles, mumps, German measles (rubella) and chickenpox (varicella).

? What's the best way to treat a cold? A cold can make you feel miserable. On top of that, pregnant women are advised against certain cold medications, such as decongestants, cough syrups and antihistamines (see page 52). So get set to make yourself as comfortable as possible while your body fights off the virus that's causing your discomfort. These tips may help:

▌ *Drink lots of fluid.* Water, juice and warm soup are all good choices. They help replace fluids lost during mucus production or fever.

▌ *Get plenty of rest.* Being run down puts a strain on your body.

▌ *Adjust your room's temperature and humidity.* Keep your room warm, but not overheated. If the air is dry, a cool-mist humidifier or vaporizer can moisten the air and help ease congestion and coughing. Be sure to keep the humidifier clean to prevent the growth of bacteria and molds.

▌ *Soothe your throat.* Gargling with warm salt water several times a day or drinking warm lemon water with honey may help soothe a sore throat and relieve a cough.

▌ *Use saline nasal spray.* To help relieve nasal congestion, try saline nasal spray. You can buy it over-the-counter, and it's safe and nonirritating.

▌ *Use acetaminophen for fever and body aches.* Acetaminophen (Tylenol, others) is a pain reliever and fever reducer that's generally considered safe to use during pregnancy.

? How do I treat allergies? As a first step, try to determine what you're allergic to and, if possible, avoid exposing yourself to those things. Some of the usual remedies for allergies — including certain antihistamines and decongestants — generally aren't recommended in pregnancy (see page 52). The best way to treat a runny or stuffy nose and other allergy symptoms is with these self-care measures.

▶ *Try cromolyn.* Cromolyn (NasalCrom) is a nonprescription nasal spray that reduces inflammation. It's effective for treating mild allergies and is often a good option for pregnant women.

▶ *Rinse your nasal passages.* Dissolve ¼ teaspoon salt in 1 cup of warm water. Place the solution in a special squeeze bottle you can purchase at a pharmacy, or use a large rubber-bulb syringe to administer the solution. Lean over the sink with your head down and to the side. Place the bottle or syringe into your upper nostril while holding the other nostril closed with your finger. Squeeze the bottle or syringe. The solution will move through your nasal passages and into your mouth. Spit the solution out and blow your nose. Tilt your head to the other side and repeat in the other nostril. Use of a neti pot is another option for rinsing nasal passages. Follow the package directions.

▶ *Breathe in steam from a hot shower or cool-mist humidifier.* Be sure to keep the humidifier clear of bacteria.

▶ *Use your fingers to massage your sinuses.* This can sometimes help relieve sinus congestion.

If your symptoms are more severe and these measures don't work, talk to your care provider.

? Can I use over-the-counter creams for acne? Pregnancy acne isn't a special form of acne. Many women simply have trouble with acne when they're pregnant. The likely culprit for most women is increased production of oil (sebum), which happens when your hormones go into overdrive. The best way to treat acne that occurs during pregnancy is to:

▶ *Wash your face twice a day.* Use a mild cleanser with lukewarm water.

▶ *Shampoo daily.* Be sure to keep your hair off your face.

▶ *Use oil-free cosmetics.* Look for descriptions such as water-based, noncomedogenic or nonacnegenic.

▶ *Avoid resting your hands on your face.* This can trap skin oils and sweat, which irritate acne.

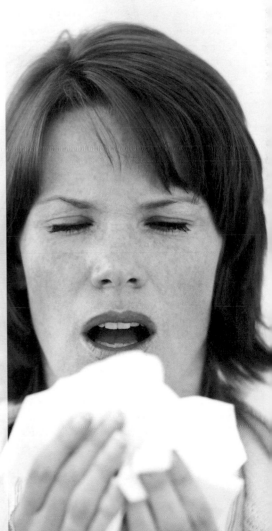

Any medication that's applied to your skin or swallowed can enter your bloodstream, so it's important to use caution during pregnancy — even with over-the-counter products.

The first drug of choice for pregnancy acne is often erythromycin (Erygel), a topical treatment available by prescription.

Azelaic acid is another option, available either by prescription (Azelex, Finacea) or over-the-counter. Other over-the-counter treatments considered safe include topical benzoyl peroxide, topical salicylic acid and topical glycolic acid. Still, it's best to talk with your care provider before using any acne treatments.

Certain acne medications should be avoided at all costs because they can cause birth defects. These include the medications adapalene (Differin), tazarotene (Avage, Tazorac) and isotretinoin (Claravis, Myorisan, others), formerly sold as Accutane.

? I'm lactose intolerant. How do I get enough calcium? For many women, the ability to digest lactose improves during pregnancy, especially as the pregnancy progresses. So even if you're normally lactose intolerant, you may find that while you're pregnant you can consume milk and other dairy products without bothersome symptoms.

The Institute of Medicine recommends a daily calcium intake of 1,000 milligrams (mg) for women age 19 and older, including pregnant women, and 1,300 mg for pregnant teens under age 19. It can be hard to meet this requirement if you don't consume milk and other dairy products, which are the best sources of calcium.

If you are lactose intolerant or dislike milk or other dairy products, consider the following suggestions:

▶ Most people who are lactose intolerant can drink up to a cup of milk with

meals without causing symptoms. If that amount bothers you, try reducing the portion to half a cup, twice a day.

▶ Try using lactose-free or lactose-reduced products, including milk, cheese and yogurt.

▶ Yogurt and fermented products such as cheeses are often better tolerated than is regular milk. The lactose in yogurt is already partially digested by the active bacteria cultures in yogurt.

▶ Try using lactase enzyme tablets such as Lactaid, which help with lactose digestion.

▶ Take calcium supplements.

▶ Choose a variety of other calcium-rich foods, such as sardines or salmon with bones, tofu, broccoli, spinach and calcium-fortified juices and foods.

? Can I color or highlight my hair? When you use hair dye, a small amount of the dye may penetrate your skin. Generally, however, the dye isn't thought to pose harm to a developing baby.

Few studies have examined women's use of hair dye before and during pregnancy. In studies on animals, even high doses of the chemicals in hair dye have not caused serious birth defects. Most researchers agree that use of hair products before or during pregnancy is safe.

If you decide to dye your hair during pregnancy, it doesn't hurt to play it safe. Have someone else apply the dye and make sure to rinse your scalp thoroughly after its application. If you're concerned about using hair dye during your pregnancy, avoid it or talk to your care provider to get more information.

? Is it safe to use hot tubs and saunas during pregnancy? A bath can help you relax and relieve sore muscles without posing any health hazards. But saunas should be avoided, and pregnancy and hot tubs can be a dangerous combination. Spending 10 or more minutes in a hot tub can raise your body temperature to 102 F, causing a condition known as hyperthermia. Some studies have shown an increased risk of miscarriage and neural tube defects in the babies of pregnant women exposed to high temperatures in the first four to six weeks of pregnancy. Exposure to high heat at any time during pregnancy also can cause you to overheat and lower your blood pressure, which could decrease your baby's oxygen supply and make you lightheaded, possibly causing you to fall.

If you choose to be in a hot tub during pregnancy, follow these steps:

- Limit time in the tub to less than 10 minutes.
- Avoid sitting near the inlet that provides newly heated water.
- Get out of the hot tub if you start to sweat or feel any discomfort.
- Stay out of the tub if you already have an elevated temperature due to a fever, exercise or previous sauna use.

? Is it safe to have an X-ray during pregnancy? It may surprise you, but having an X-ray during pregnancy is generally considered safe. In most cases, the benefits of the X-ray outweigh the potential risks.

When you have an abdominal X-ray during pregnancy, your developing baby is exposed to radiation. If the radiation causes changes in your baby's rapidly growing cells, it's possible that your baby could be at a slightly higher risk of birth defects or illnesses, such as leukemia, later in life.

Generally, however, having an X-ray during pregnancy is thought to pose only the most remote risk to a developing baby. Most X-ray exams — including those of your arms, legs, head, teeth or chest — won't expose your reproductive organs or your baby to radiation. A leaded apron and collar also can be worn to block any scattered radiation.

If you need an X-ray, let your care provider know that you are or might be pregnant. He or she might be able to do an ultrasound instead of an X-ray. Also, if you have a child who needs an X-ray exam, don't hold your child during the exam if you are or might be pregnant. Ask another person to take your place.

If you had an X-ray exam before you knew you were pregnant, don't panic. Remember, the risk is very small. It's highly unlikely that you received enough radiation to cause problems. If, however, you received a radiation treatment for a medical condition — such as radiation to treat cancer — the risks may be more significant. Share any concerns about radiation exposure with your care provider.

? Do I need to worry about using devices such as cellphones, computers or microwaves? These and many wireless devices give off electromagnetic energy as radiofrequency waves. The radiation from these devices is different from and much less than the radiation that comes from X-rays.

Still, researchers and environmental watchdogs have speculated that increasing exposure to these devices, such as holding a cellphone close to your head or body for extended periods, may expose you to harmful levels of electromagnetic energy over time and carry health risks.

There have been suggested links between heavy maternal cellphone use during pregnancy and miscarriage or other issues of fetal development. However, studies are limited and contradictory. Other studies have examined links between pregnancy problems and radiofrequency exposure such as living close to a cell tower. There's no scientific evidence to support such an association.

For now, evidence indicates no cause for alarm. But if you're concerned about exposure to radiofrequency energy, limit your cellphone use and store your cellphone away from your body while you're not using it, including overnight.

? What about the full-body scanners at airports? Are they safe for pregnant women? These modern scanners work in two ways. One type uses nonionizing electromagnetic radiation (millimeter waves), a form of energy similar to that used in radar images and radio signals. This type of radiation, which has been used for a century, has no known health effects.

The other type of scanner uses "back scatter" ionizing radiation, which exposes

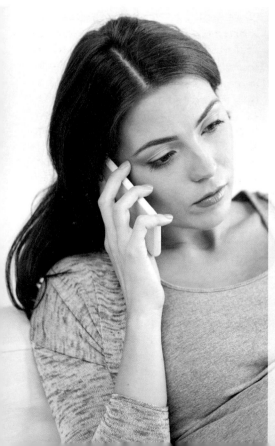

an individual to a very weak, very low-dose X-ray signal. The radiation emitted from the scanner is weak enough that the X-ray doesn't penetrate the body.

With either type of machine, there's no evidence of risk to the developing fetus.

? Is it OK to use DEET to prevent mosquito bites? DEET, the active ingredient in many common insect repellents, is safe as long as you follow the manufacturer's instructions. DEET provides effective protection against mosquitos and ticks that transmit diseases such as Zika virus, West Nile virus and Lyme disease. The benefits of avoiding these illnesses generally exceed the risks of the small amount of DEET that might enter your bloodstream through your skin. To stay on the safe side, minimize your time outdoors, especially during the first trimester, and consider what concentration of DEET you'll need for the amount of time you'll spend outside.

? Are basic household cleaners safe to use? Regular use of normal household cleaners hasn't been shown to harm a developing baby. Still, it's a good idea to stay away from oven cleaners that emit strong fumes in a contained space. And — pregnant or not — don't mix chemicals such as ammonia and bleach because the combination can produce toxic fumes.

When cleaning, avoid inhaling strong, caustic fumes. Wear protective gloves to avoid absorbing any chemicals through your skin. You might also consider switching to cleaners that don't contain any harsh, toxic chemicals.

? Are paint fumes harmful? In general, avoid exposure to oil-based paints, lead and mercury, all of which may be found in old paints that you may be stripping from surfaces. Also avoid other substances that have solvents, such as paint removers. Use water-based paint, which is generally considered safe in pregnancy. And even if you're just painting a small room or piece of baby furniture, work in a well-ventilated area to minimize breathing fumes. Don't eat or drink in the area where you're painting. In addition, be extra careful if you use a ladder. Your changing body shape may throw off your sense of balance.

? What's the concern about kitty litter boxes? Toxoplasmosis is an infection that can threaten the health of an unborn child. It's caused by a parasite called *Toxoplasma gondii.* The parasite multiplies in a cat's intestine after the cat eats an infected rodent or other small animal. The parasite is shed in cat feces for several weeks after infection, mainly into litter boxes and garden soil. You can get the parasite by touching your mouth after handling cat litter or soil where there are cat feces. You can also get the parasite from eating undercooked meat from infected animals.

If you have indoor-only cats, the risk of toxoplasmosis is lower. But to be safe during pregnancy, have another member of the family change the litter box. If you must handle the chore, wear rubber gloves and wash your hands thoroughly afterward. Also wear gloves when you garden.

? Is it true that pregnancy causes cavities? Dental health during pregnancy isn't a glamorous topic, but it's an important one. And often, these issues aren't discussed at prenatal appointments. Common dental health problems during pregnancy include:

▶ *Tooth decay.* During pregnancy, increased acidity in the mouth increases the risk of tooth decay. Vomiting dur-

ing pregnancy can aggravate the problem by exposing the teeth to more gastric acid.

▶ *Loose teeth.* Increased levels of progesterone and estrogen can affect the ligaments and bones that support the teeth, causing teeth to loosen.

▶ *Gum disease.* The hormonal changes of pregnancy can lead to gingivitis, an inflammation of the gums. Some studies suggest that severe gum disease in pregnancy may be associated with preterm birth and low birth weight.

So how do you keep your teeth and gums healthy during pregnancy? Stick to the basics. Brush and floss your teeth regularly. Rinse regularly with a fluoride mouthwash. If you have morning sickness, rinse your mouth with a solution of 1 teaspoon baking soda in 1 cup of water after vomiting.

? I enjoy water parks and amusement rides. Do I need to avoid them during pregnancy? While there's no consensus on avoiding water parks and amusement rides while you're pregnant, you may want to check with your care provider before riding a roller coaster or going down a rapid water ride. Research indicates that trauma during pregnancy that produces a forceful shearing effect — such as the sudden stop experienced in a car crash — can cause the placenta to separate from the uterus (placental abruption). This type of force may be experienced to a lesser extent in an amusement ride or water park slide.

Many theme park rides have restrictions for pregnant women. If you decide to go on a ride, be sure to check the restriction policy first.

Bottom line: You may want to stick with lounging in the pool rather than flying down a wild ride while you're pregnant.

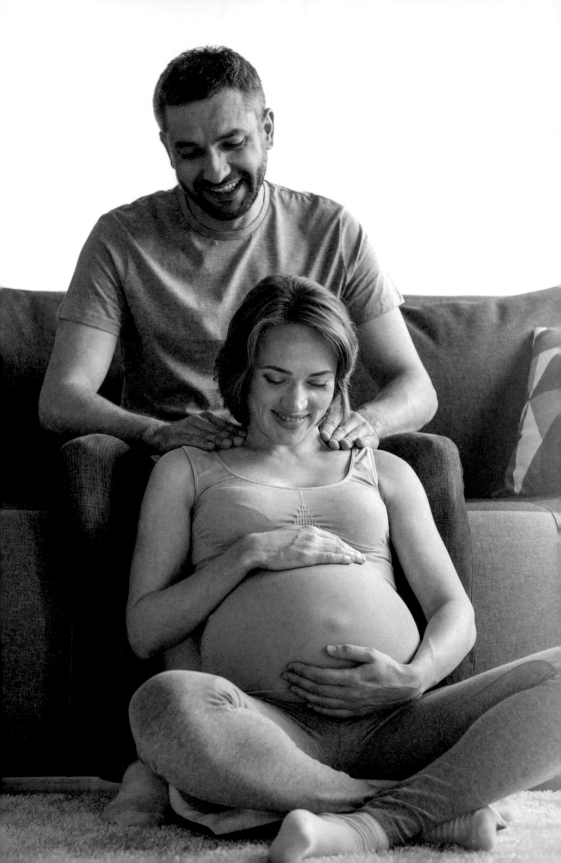

CHAPTER 3

For dads and partners

If you're an expectant parent — but not the pregnant one — you may be wondering how you fit into this adventure. At one point in time, the extent of most dads' involvement in expecting a baby was to help conceive and then pace the waiting room 10 months later in anticipation of news about the delivery. But most dads today are much more involved in their partner's pregnancy, from going along to the first prenatal visit to attending childbirth classes and being a labor coach in the delivery room.

Even though you're not the one growing a baby bump and getting all the attention, there's plenty you can do to feel less like a bystander and more like an active participant in your expanding family. The 10 months of pregnancy also offer a key preparation period for parenting, giving you valuable time to transition toward parenthood.

And although this chapter is aimed mainly at dads-to-be, much of this information can be applied to nonbiological parents or same-sex partners, as well.

HOW TO TAKE PART

Here are some ways to be involved in your partner's pregnancy right from the start:

Offer to run out and purchase the pregnancy testing kit It's never too early to get involved. If you and your partner have been trying to conceive, or even if you haven't, and your partner thinks she may be pregnant, offer to get the pregnancy testing kit so that you both can find out together. Seeing that positive test result appear is exciting confirmation that yes, you are pregnant!

Attend prenatal visits Even if you can't make it to all of the prenatal appointments, try to go to the first visit and the appointment that includes an ultrasound. There are many serious decisions to be made after the first visit, and it definitely helps to have both of you listening to the issues involved in certain optional tests. If you're the biological father, sharing your personal and family medical history with your partner's care provider can help him or her determine the best prenatal care for the baby. An ultrasound usually happens between weeks 18 and 20 of pregnancy. The procedure gives you a glimpse of the baby in utero and helps to confirm the baby's health.

Talk to your partner Nonpregnant partners often get most of their information directly from their pregnant partners. It's important that the two of you talk about your emotions and her physical sensations as you proceed through the pregnancy. It can give you a better sense of what she's going through and make you feel more knowledgeable about the pregnancy. Learning more about pregnancy on your own or with your partner can help you to be more aware of what she may be experiencing so you can help her feel supported.

Get to know your baby Talk and sing to your baby while massaging your partner's belly. There's evidence that babies recognize voices and sounds they've heard often in utero. Around 16 to 20 weeks, you may begin to feel the baby's movements through your partner's belly. This is often an exciting time for both parents.

Take a class Prenatal classes can help you and your partner find out what to expect during labor and delivery, as well as learn how to take care of a newborn.

Support your partner in a healthy lifestyle During pregnancy, team up with your partner to eat a balanced diet, exercise regularly and get plenty of rest. It's good for mother and baby, and it's good for you, too. If you smoke, don't smoke around your partner, as the chemicals in secondhand smoke can be harmful to the baby. Better yet, make a commitment to quit before the baby is born. If you both are used to drinking alcohol, support your partner's abstinence from alcohol during pregnancy by minimizing your own intake.

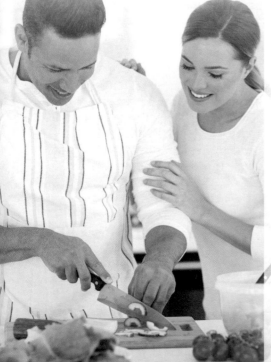

GETTING THROUGH THE FIRST TRIMESTER TOGETHER

Especially if this is a first pregnancy, those early weeks during the first trimester can be a challenge.

First, although your partner looks exactly the same as before — the belly doesn't start showing until week 12 or so — it might seem that she's not quite herself. She may:

▶ Constantly feel nauseated
▶ Vomit at the sight of food
▶ Ask why you would ever dream of making eggs and ham for her in the morning when the smell makes her feel sick

- Be ravenous two hours later
- Cry for no apparent reason
- Want you near her, but please, for heaven's sake, don't touch her
- Need a caramel decaf latte, with soy milk, right now!

This is partly in jest, of course, but undoubtedly your friends and family who've had babies could come up with many other examples of their partners' behaviors during that first trimester.

But consider this: An invisible, yet amazing transformation is taking place in your partner's body. Within two weeks of conception, hormones trigger your partner's body to begin preparing for the baby. Increased hormone production can lead to all sorts of symptoms, including nausea, tiredness, mood swings, food cravings and more.

To help ease the way for your partner (and yourself), consider these tips:

Minimize nausea triggers The common term for pregnancy-related nausea, *morning sickness*, can be a misnomer since some women feel queasy 24/7 during the first trimester. Nausea and queasiness usually tend to ease up by week 14, but in the meantime, it can be rough on your partner. Things that might help your partner feel a little better include making sure she has plenty of fluids (ginger ale may be a good choice) and fixing her smaller, frequent meals to keep her from getting too hungry, which can make nausea worse. Avoid foods and smells that tend to make her feel worse. These tactics can also help minimize heartburn and constipation.

YOUR SYMPTOMS (YOU GET 'EM TOO)

Researchers have shown that males of certain species, including human males, experience hormonal changes that enhance and accelerate their paternal instincts when they're in close contact with a pregnant partner. For example, in men:
- Levels of prolactin, a hormone that helps new mothers make milk but which is also present in men, increase just before the birth of the baby.
- Levels of cortisol, a hormone that your body produces in response to stress, also increase before childbirth and even more so during labor. This heightened stress response may help fathers focus on and bond with their newborns.
- Levels of testosterone, a male hormone, decrease right after the baby's birth, suggesting that the focus is on nurturing rather than competitive behavior.

Pregnancy-related hormonal patterns in men tend to mirror those of women in general. But while female hormonal patterns are closely tied to the number of days until birth, male hormonal changes are more closely linked to the female partner's hormonal changes. This suggests that closeness between partners affects the physiological changes men experience.

Some men also experience sympathy pains (couvade) during their partner's pregnancy, including weight gain, nausea, fatigue and emotional changes. So don't be surprised if you find your feelings and physical sensations mirroring those of your partner.

You might place plain crackers and whatever fluid your partner prefers on her night stand, in case she feels sick during the night or early in the morning. And if she suddenly changes her mind about what she can and can't eat or drink, try to go with the flow.

Help combat fatigue As your partner's body gears up for pregnancy, her heart will pump faster and harder, and her pulse will quicken. All the internal activity is likely to wear her out. Help her get as much rest as she can. Getting enough protein and iron in her diet and physical activity in her day also can help fight off fatigue. Good sources of protein and iron include lean meat, chicken, beans, nuts and eggs.

Ride out the mood swings Changing levels of hormones can put your partner on an emotional seesaw. This is normal. She may feel ecstatic one moment and weepy the next. Half the time, she may not know herself why she's feeling the way she is (and be just as frustrated as you). The key here is to ride out the storm. By the time the two of you reach the second trimester, your partner's hormone levels will have stabilized and the world will seem much calmer. In the meantime, offer plenty of support.

Remember it will pass Most women start to feel less queasy and more energetic once the second trimester begins. In fact, the second trimester is an enjoyable time for many couples, as the discomforts of early pregnancy are usually past and the belly is still a manageable size. This might be the time to do fun things together, such as go on a minivacation or get the nursery ready. Your pregnant partner can safely help paint if you're using latex paint in a well-ventilated area, al-though the smell might still be bothersome. She'll just need to avoid risky movements such as climbing on ladders or lifting heavy objects.

SEX DURING PREGNANCY

It's not unusual to have concerns about how sexual activity with your partner might change during pregnancy or how sex might affect the baby. Here are some answers to common questions about sex during pregnancy.

Is it OK to have sex during pregnancy? As long as the pregnancy is proceeding normally, and your partner wants to, you can have sex as often as you like. At first, hormonal fluctuations, fatigue and nausea may sap your partner's sexual desire, though not always. During the second trimester, increased blood flow to her sexual organs and breasts may rekindle her desire for sex. However, by the third trimester, weight gain, back pain and other symptoms may once again dampen her enthusiasm. Every couple is different, though. Consider what's best for the two of you.

Does sex during pregnancy harm the baby? Your baby is protected by the amniotic fluid in your partner's uterus, as well as the mucous plug that blocks the cervix throughout most of the pregnancy. Sexual activity won't affect the baby.

What are the best sexual positions during pregnancy? As long as you and your partner are comfortable, most sexual positions are OK during pregnancy. As the pregnancy progresses, experiment to find what works best. Rather than lying on top of your partner, you might want to lie next to her sideways or position yourself under or behind her. Let your creativity take over, as long as you keep mutual pleasure and comfort in mind.

What about oral sex? Oral sex is safe during pregnancy. There's a caveat, however. Make sure you don't blow air into her vagina. Rarely, a burst of air may block a blood vessel (air embolism) — which could be a life-threatening condition for mother and baby.

Are condoms necessary? Exposure to sexually transmitted infections during pregnancy increases the risk of complications and harm to the baby. Use a condom if you have a sexually transmitted infection or if you're having sex with more than one partner. You should also use a condom if you've traveled anywhere in the past six months where there's risk of the Zika virus — even if you're symptom-free — to protect your partner from exposure.

What if she doesn't want to have sex? This can be distressing, but try to remember that it won't be this way forever. There's more to a sexual relationship than intercourse. If sex is difficult, unappealing to her or off-limits, try cuddling, kissing or giving each other a massage.

Also, try to look at it from her perspective. Is she eyeing the mountain of laundry while you're doing your utmost to seduce her? Consider relieving some of the mundane stressors so that she has more energy to respond to your advances. Is she always tired at night? Consider having sex in the morning or on a lazy afternoon, or whatever time of day she feels best.

Be understanding of the discomfort she may be dealing with and all of the body changes she's facing. Remind her of how beautiful she is to you. Remember, thoughtfulness begets thoughtfulness, and if you respect her feelings, she may decide that she's not so averse to yours, after all.

After the baby is born, how soon can we have sex? Whether your partner gives birth vaginally or by cesarean delivery, her body will need time to heal. Many care providers recommend waiting four to six weeks before resuming intercourse. This allows time for the cervix to close and any tears or a repaired episiotomy to heal. Initially, the vagina may be tender and sex might be painful. A non-irritating lubricant will help until this resolves.

Staying intimate You can maintain intimacy in many ways. Stay connected during the day with short phone calls, email messages or text messages. Reserve a few quiet minutes for each other before the day begins or while you're winding down before bed. When you're ready to have sex after the baby is born, take it slow — and use a reliable method of contraception to prevent a subsequent pregnancy.

LABOR AND DELIVERY WORRIES

As your partner's due date approaches, excitement and nervousness build. Soon your baby will be here, but first you need to get through labor and delivery. As supporter, labor coach and general logistics coordinator, you have an important role to play. To get ready:

Educate yourself about childbirth Knowing the signs and symptoms of labor, and what to expect when your partner starts having contractions, can help you know when to go to the hospital. And don't be surprised or overly disappointed if there are one or two false labor episodes. This is very common, especially with first babies. Also, knowing what to expect in the delivery room can prevent surprises and help you adjust to rapid changes, if necessary.

For example, many men report feeling bewildered and excluded when the need for an emergency cesarean delivery arises and the room is suddenly filled with hospital staff. Knowing what to expect with an emergency cesarean section can help prevent some of those feelings. Read Chapter 14 to learn more about labor and childbirth and Chapter 15 to learn about cesarean birth.

Map your route Find the shortest and safest way to the hospital from your house or your partner's workplace. Create a backup plan in case of a traffic delay or bad weather. While you're at it, scout out the parking situation at the hospital (some hospitals have valet parking for pregnant patients) and know which way to go once you get inside. Last but not least, make sure your vehicle always has plenty of gas in the tank when the delivery date is near.

Install an infant car seat To bring your baby home, you'll need to put him or her in an infant car seat. For the most protection, the car seat should be rear facing and installed in the middle of the back seat.

Give yourself plenty of time to install the seat. Car seats can be deceivingly tricky, so make sure you follow the car seat manufacturer's instructions and that the car seat is installed correctly. If you have questions about proper installation or need a hand, check the National Highway Traffic Safety Administration's website to find a car seat inspection station near you. Be sure to follow the child passenger safety laws in your state.

Keep a copy of the birth plan If you and your partner have created an outline of your combined preferences during childbirth, such as options for handling pain — often called a birth plan — keep a copy with you, just in case. But be prepared to adapt if need be. For instance, your partner may decide she wants pain medication after all, once labor begins, even though she may have indicated otherwise in her birth preferences.

Pack your bags Have a bag with your partner's preferred toiletries, and maybe a new set of pajamas or some of her favorite music, ready to go. If you're staying with her and the baby, have your overnight bag ready, too.

Manage communications During and after the birth, you might find yourself serving as the issuer of the latest news and sender of pictures for friends and family! Still, consider limiting use of social media and cellphones during labor so that you can be present to what you and your partner are experiencing.

HELPING DURING LABOR

These days, most fathers and partners are present during labor and delivery. In general, hospitals don't restrict who can be present for the delivery, but they may restrict the number of people in the room. Decide ahead of time who your partner wants in the room in addition to you. It's OK if she prefers just the two of you. Too many bystanders can result in overcrowding, which can be a burden for both of you.

During labor and delivery, there's plenty that you can do to help your partner. Here are some suggestions from The

American College of Obstetricians and Gynecologists:

- Help distract your partner during the first stage of labor. Talk about your day, or watch a movie together.
- Unless she's been told to stay in bed, take short walks with your partner.
- Time her contractions.
- Offer to massage her back and shoulders between contractions.
- Help her with relaxation techniques.
- Support her during the pushing stage.

The important thing is to be there for her if she needs you, regardless of whether she's squeezing your hand off or using language that's not entirely polite.

After the delivery Often, this is the best part: the moment when you can finally engage with your child. At this stage you can be actively involved in bathing, changing and cuddling your newborn. If your partner is breast-feeding, you can offer her valuable moral support — it's not always easy the first time around — or if you're using formula, you can take turns giving the baby a bottle.

You can also help monitor visits from family and friends. Consider delaying visits until both of you have had some initial time with your newborn. If your partner gets tired and needs a rest, offer to take visitors for a walk through the halls of the maternity department. Help visitors sanitize or wash their hands before touching the baby.

Once your partner can eat and drink normally, bring her something from her favorite bakery or shop as a fun treat.

COMMON ANXIETIES

No one said this would be easy. Along with the excitement, having some anxiety is normal. As a new parent, you may worry about:

Limited paternity or family leave If you aren't able to take time off when the baby is born, it may be difficult to keep up your regular work schedule and find time to spend with your newborn.

New responsibilities Newborns require constant care and attention. On top of feedings, diaper changes and crying spells — tasks for which some new parents aren't prepared — parents must find time to do household chores and other daily activities. If you're used to a care-free, independent lifestyle, you may wonder if you'll be able to adjust.

Disrupted sleep Newborns challenge their parents' ability to get a good night's sleep. Sleep deprivation can quickly take a toll on new parents.

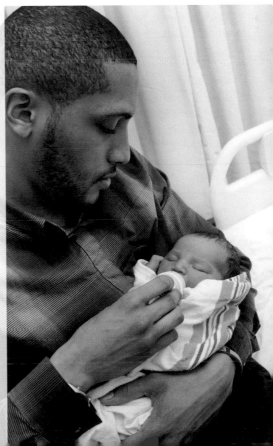

Less time with your partner Having a baby means sharing your partner's attention with a third party. This is something new, and feeling left out is not uncommon, especially if your partner breast-feeds the baby.

Less sexual activity A lull in your sex life with your partner can sometimes lead to resentment and strain your relationship.

Financial strain Children come with expenses that sometimes can seem daunting — delivery, health care, diapers, clothing, furniture and more.

Depression Research shows that some fathers, like some mothers, may experience depression shortly after a child's birth. If you're feeling depressed, don't hesitate to see a professional. Depression is treatable.

Take action You can help ease your anxieties by actively preparing for parenthood. For example:

Keep talking to your partner Discuss how the baby's arrival will likely affect your daily lives, your relationship with each other and even your careers. Feel free to share your dreams about the future, too.

Build a network of social support During pregnancy, the mother carrying the baby often gets support from care providers, family and friends. It's important that you to have a support network during this time, too — especially if the pregnancy was unplanned or you've heard negative stories about parenting. Seek out friends and family who can give you advice and encouragement as you prepare to become a parent.

Be proactive about financial issues Try to plan for the new costs you'll have through saving, budgeting and forgoing unnecessary expenses.

Consider what kind of parent you want to be Take time to think about the parenting you received. Consider what aspects of your relationship with your parents you might want to have with your own child and what you might do differently.

Stay involved Once your baby is born, look for ways to connect with your newly expanded family. For example:

Room with your family at the hospital If the hospital and your work schedule allow, consider staying with your partner and newborn until it's time to take the baby home. This will help you feel more like a key participant in the first few days of your baby's life. If you have other children, arrange for a fun night or nights with grandparents or other family members or friends so that you can devote full attention to mom and baby.

Take turns caring for the baby Take turns feeding and changing the baby. If your partner is breast-feeding, offer to change diapers in the middle of the night or bring the baby to your partner in bed. If she needs to use the bathroom when she wakes up, you can change the baby while she does that and then bring her the baby and a glass of water. This way you may shorten the time that you're both awake, instead of listening to the commotion as she does all of those things herself.

You could also bottle-feed pumped breast milk. Or you could burp the baby and put him or her to sleep after the breast-feeding sessions.

Play with the baby Once back home and settling into life with baby, women tend to provide low-key, soothing stimulation for their babies, while men often engage their little ones in noisier, more-vigorous activities. Both styles of play are important. Seeing your baby smile is its own reward.

Be affectionate with your partner Just because sex is off-limits temporarily doesn't mean you and your partner can't cuddle or kiss. Keep in mind that eventually your family will develop a routine, and you and your partner will have some time to yourselves again.

Keep the lines of communication open Continue talking to your partner about the changes you're experiencing, whether reality is matching your expectations and what you can do to support each other as your baby gets older. If one parent is away at work, share pictures and funny stories about the day via email. Try to find some time for just the two of you, too. It may not always be easy for your partner to ask for help, so encourage her to talk about any difficulties she may be feeling as a new mother.

Seek help If you're having trouble dealing with changes in your relationship or you think you may be depressed, talk to a counselor or other mental health professional.

Relax Parenting can be a challenge, but the more prepared you are for what lies ahead, the more confident and supported you'll feel once the baby arrives. Chapter 19 covers many aspects of preparing for parenthood, including how to handle the first few weeks, what to expect when it comes to your relationship with your partner and some tips on the financial aspects of raising a child. When you get a chance, have a look at that chapter. You may also want to look for recommendations of books, apps and other resources that can help you prepare.

YOU MADE IT

Congratulations! You're a parent, and a whole new path has opened up to you. Take it one step at a time. No one ever learned to raise a child all at once. It takes practice and patience. Most of all, be sure to enjoy yourself and your family along the way.

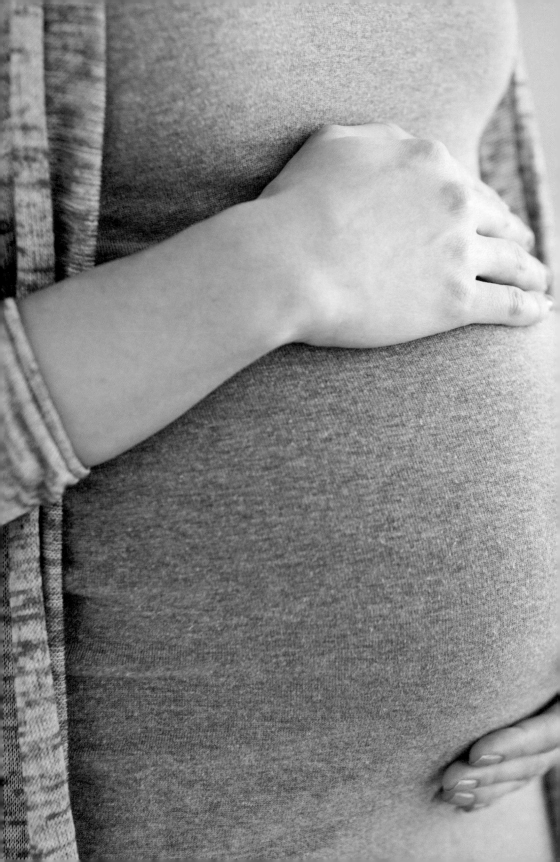

PART 2

Pregnancy month by month

You've always known pregnancy to last nine months, so why do we list 10 months? Nine months is the common measurement for pregnancy, but pregnancy doesn't divide itself evenly into months. In determining your due date and monitoring your progress, your care provider works from a 40-week calendar (explained further in Chapter 4). If you think of a pregnancy month as four weeks, take 40 divided by 4, and that equals 10 months. In actuality, though, most calendar months are a little more than four weeks, and those extra days add up. So, if you track your pregnancy by calendar months, it often comes out closer to nine months.

Your care provider is more interested in tracking your pregnancy in weeks, because months are too imprecise. If you say you're in your "third month," that could mean you're at week 9, 10, 11 or 12 of your pregnancy. To determine if your baby's growth is on track, your provider needs to know the exact week, or close to it. Also, some testing has a narrow window during which the test should be administered.

PREGNANCY CALENDAR

	BEFORE CONCEPTION	WEEK 1	2	3	4	5	6	7	8	9	10	11	12	13	14	15	16	17
Genetic screening[1]	▓																	
Lifestyle improvements	▓																	
Make prenatal appointment						▓	▓	▓	▓									
First prenatal visit									▓	▓	▓							
Routine prenatal tests									▓	▓	▓	▓						
Optional prenatal tests[2]										▓	▓	▓	▓					
Ultrasound exam[3]																		
Glucose test[4]																		
Group B strep test																		
Childbirth classes																		
Look for child care[5]														▓	▓	▓	▓	
Getting ready: Breast or bottle? Disposable or cloth?																		
Buying baby gear: car seats, cribs, supplies, and more																		
Birth plan																		
Preparations for labor and childbirth																		

The shading represents the period of time when the test or activity is most likely to occur.

1 Genetic screening can be done at any point in pregnancy but is ideally done before conception.

2 Screening and diagnostic tests to check for abnormalities, see Chapter 21.

3 Timing varies. Most commonly performed between weeks 18 and 20.

4 Done earlier if you're at high risk of gestational diabetes.

5 Depends on availability of infant care in your area.

18	19	20	21	22	23	24	25	26	27	28	29	30	31	32	33	34	35	36	37	38	39	40

HOW TO RESPOND

Here's a guide to possibly troublesome signs and symptoms you may experience throughout your pregnancy and when you should notify your care provider. When in doubt, it's better to be safe than sorry.

Signs or symptoms	When to contact your care provider
Vaginal bleeding, spotting or discharge	
Slight spotting that goes away within a day	Within 24 hours during months 1-3; same day during months 4-7; immediately during months 8-10
Any bleeding that lasts longer than a day	Within 24 hours during months 1-3; immediately during months 4-10 or if you're Rh negative
Moderate to heavy bleeding	Immediately
Any amount of bleeding accompanied by severe pain, fever or chills	Immediately
Passing of tissue	Immediately
Greenish or yellowish vaginal discharge with odor or with vulval redness or itching	Within 24 hours
Steady or heavy discharge of watery fluid from your vagina	Immediately
Pain	
Occasional pulling or pinching sensation on one or both sides of your abdomen	Next visit
Occasional mild headaches	Next visit
A moderate, bothersome headache that doesn't go away	Within 24 hours
A severe or persistent headache, especially with dizziness, faintness, nausea or vomiting, or visual disturbances	Immediately
Moderate to severe pelvic pain	Immediately
Any degree of pelvic pain that doesn't subside within 4 hours	Within 24 hours
Pain with fever or bleeding	Immediately
Leg pain with redness and swelling	Immediately
Uterine contractions, less than six each hour for 2 or more hours	Next visit
Uterine contractions, more than six each hour for 2 or more hours	Immediately

Signs or symptoms	When to contact your care provider
Vomiting	
Occasional or once daily	Next visit
More than three times daily with inability to eat or drink	Within 24 hours
Accompanied by pain or fever	Immediately
Other	
Fever lower than 102 F	Within 24 hours if fever persists
Fever of 102 F or higher	Immediately
Painful urination	Same day
Inability to urinate	Same day
Mild constipation	Next visit
Severe constipation, no bowel movement for 3 days	Same day
Consistently low mood, loss of pleasure	Next visit
Low mood, loss of pleasure, and thoughts of harming yourself or others	Immediately
Cravings for nonfood substances such as clay or dirt	Next visit
Sudden swelling of hands, face or feet	Same day
Sudden weight gain	Same day
Fainting or visual disturbances (blurring)	Immediately
Fatigue, weakness, shortness of breath, heart palpitations or lightheadedness	Next visit if occurring occasionally; same day if persistent
Severe shortness of breath	Immediately
Severe itching	Same day

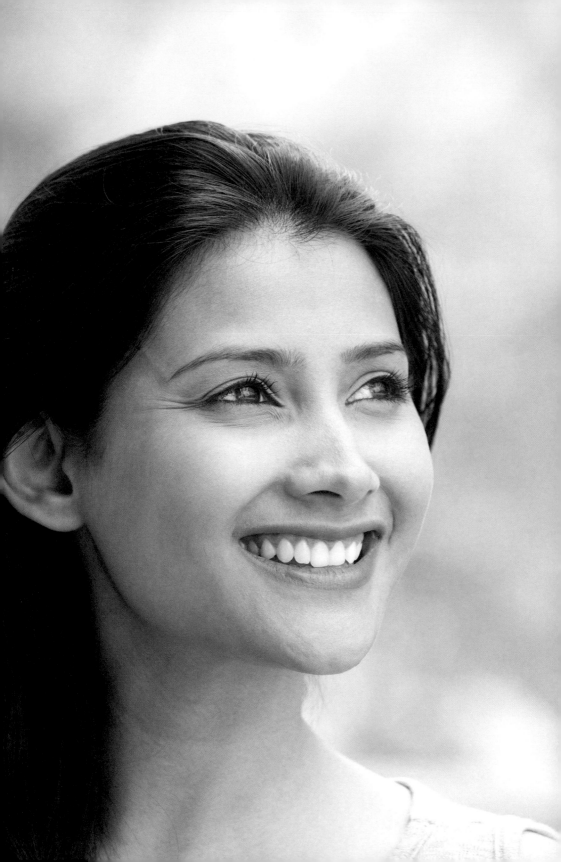

CHAPTER 4

Month 1: Weeks 1 to 4

My husband and I had been trying to conceive for almost a year. When my menstrual cycle was late, I was thrilled. My husband, ever cautious, took a wait-and-see attitude. After a few more days had passed, I bought a home pregnancy test. My husband waited in the living room while I took the test. Sure enough, a faint blue line appeared. I showed it to my husband, who said excitedly, "It's a maybe?" No maybe about it. We were expecting our first child!

— Paula

Congratulations! And welcome to pregnancy, one of life's most exciting adventures. Over the next 40 weeks, your body will undergo some amazing changes. You may be a bit nervous about what's in store, and that's perfectly normal. No doubt, you have lots of questions. What does my baby look like? How big is he or she? Is he or she going to be healthy? What do I need to do next?

To help answer some of these questions, and to calm those jitters and fears, we'll take you week-by-week through pregnancy in the following chapters, describing how your baby is constantly developing and changing. We'll also explain some of the changes taking place within your body, so you know what to expect and can prepare for what's ahead.

Pregnancy can be a wild ride. Try to relax, and enjoy the adventure to its fullest!

BABY'S GROWTH

The way care providers calculate the first month of pregnancy may seem a bit confusing. You don't actually become pregnant until halfway through the month, when conception occurs. Prior to that, your body is getting prepared.

Weeks 1 and 2 It may seem a bit strange, but the first week of your pregnancy is actually the beginning of your last menstrual period before you become pregnant. Why is that? Doctors and other health care professionals calculate your due date by counting 40 weeks from the start of your last cycle. That means they count your period as part of your pregnancy, even though your baby hasn't been conceived yet. Conception typically occurs about two weeks after the start of your last menstrual period.

Preconception During menstruation your body begins producing a hormone called follicle-stimulating hormone, which fosters development of an egg in your ovary. The egg matures within a small cavity in your ovary called a follicle. A few days later, after menstruation has ended, your body produces a hormone called luteinizing hormone. It causes the follicle to swell and burst through the wall of your ovary, releasing the egg. This is called ovulation. You have two ovaries, but in any given cycle, ovulation occurs from just one of them.

As the egg moves into your fallopian tube, which connects your ovary and uterus, it awaits a fertilizing sperm. Finger-like structures at the junction between your ovary and fallopian tube, called fimbriae, catch the egg when ovulation occurs, keeping it on the proper course.

If you have intercourse before or during this time, you can become pregnant. If fertilization doesn't occur, for whatever reason, the egg and the lining of your uterus will be shed through your menstrual period.

Fertilization This is when it all begins. Your egg and your partner's sperm unite to form a single cell — the starting point for an extraordinary chain of events. That microscopic cell will divide again and again, and in about 38 weeks, it will have grown into a new person made up of more than 2 trillion cells — your beautiful new baby girl or boy.

The process begins when you and your partner have sexual intercourse. When he ejaculates, your partner releases into your vagina semen containing up to 1 billion sperm cells. Each sperm has a long, whip-like tail that propels it toward your egg.

Hundreds of millions of these sperm swim up through your reproductive tract. They travel from your vagina, up through the lower opening of your uterus (cervix), through your uterus and into your fallopian tube. Many sperm are lost along the way with only a fraction of the sperm reaching the fallopian tube. Fertilization occurs when a single sperm makes this journey successfully and penetrates the wall of your egg.

Your egg has a covering of nutrient cells called the corona radiata and a gelatinous shell called the zona pellucida. To fertilize your egg, your partner's sperm must penetrate this covering. At this point, your egg is about $1/200$ of an inch in diameter, too small to be seen.

Up to 100 sperm may try to penetrate the wall of your egg, and several may begin to enter the outer egg capsule. But in the end, only one succeeds and enters the egg itself. After that, the membrane of the egg changes and all other sperm are locked out.

Occasionally, more than one follicle in an ovary matures and more than one egg is released into the fallopian tube. This can result in multiple births if each of the eggs is fertilized by a sperm.

As the sperm penetrates to the center of your egg, the two cells merge to become a one-celled entity called a zygote. The zygote has 46 chromosomes — 23 from you and 23 from your partner. These chromosomes contain many thousands of genes. This genetic material is like a blueprint, determining your baby's sex, eye color, hair color, body size, facial fea-

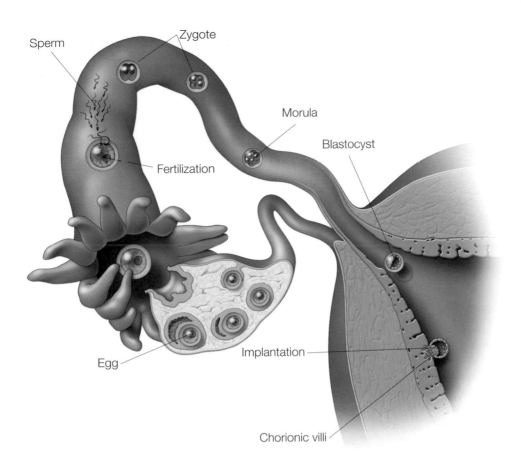

Sperm

Zygote

Morula

Blastocyst

Fertilization

Egg

Implantation

Chorionic villi

tures and — at least to some extent — intelligence and personality. Fertilization is now complete.

Weeks 3 and 4 Once your baby is conceived, he or she gets to work right away. The next step in the process is cell division. Within about 12 hours after fertilization, your one-celled zygote divides into two cells, and then those two each split into two, and so on, with the number of cells doubling every 12 hours. The cells continue to divide as the zygote moves through your fallopian tube to your uterus. Within about three days after fertilization, it becomes a cluster of 13 to 32 nonspecialized cells resembling a tiny raspberry. At this stage, your developing

baby is called a morula. It now leaves the fallopian tube to enter your uterus.

Within four to five days after fertilization, your developing baby — now made up of about 500 cells — reaches its destination inside your uterus. By this time, it has changed from a solid mass of cells to a group of cells arranged around a fluid-filled cavity, and is called a blastocyst. The inner section of the blastocyst is a compact mass of cells that will develop into your baby. The outer layer of cells, called the trophoblast, will become the placenta, which will provide nourishment to your baby as it grows.

After arriving in your uterus, the blastocyst clings to the uterine surface for a time. It then releases enzymes that

X AND Y

Will it be a boy, or a girl? As soon as many couples learn they're going to be parents, this is one of the first questions they have.

Your baby's sex is determined at the moment he or she is conceived. Of the 46 chromosomes that make up your baby's genetic material, two chromosomes called sex chromosomes — one from your egg and one from your partner's sperm — determine your baby's sex. A woman's eggs contain only X sex chromosomes. A man's sperm, however, may contain either an X or Y sex chromosome.

If, at fertilization, a sperm with an X sex chromosome meets your egg, which also has an X sex chromosome, your baby will be a girl (XX). If a sperm containing a Y sex chromosome joins up with your egg, your baby will be a boy (XY). It's always the father's genetic contribution that determines the sex of the baby.

dissolve the top surface lining of your uterus, allowing the blastocyst to embed itself there. This typically happens about a week after fertilization. By the 12th day after fertilization, the blastocyst is firmly embedded in its new home. It adheres tightly to the lining of your uterus, called the endometrium, where it receives nourishment from your bloodstream.

Also within about 12 days after fertilization, the placenta begins to form. At first, tiny projections sprout from the wall of the blastocyst. From these sprouts, wavy masses of tiny blood-vessel-filled tissue develop. Called chorionic villi, these masses grow amid the capillaries of your uterus and ultimately cover most of the placenta.

At 14 days after conception, four weeks since your last menstrual period, your baby is about 1/25 of an inch long. It is divided into three different layers, from which all tissues and organs will eventually develop:

▶ *Ectoderm.* This top layer will give rise to a groove along the midline of your baby's body, called the neural tube. Your baby's brain, spinal cord, spinal nerves and backbone will develop here.

- *Mesoderm.* This middle layer of cells will form the beginnings of your baby's heart and a primitive circulatory system — blood vessels, blood cells and lymph vessels. The foundations for bones, muscles, kidneys, and ovaries or testicles also will develop here.
- *Endoderm.* This inner layer of cells will become a simple tube lined with mucous membranes. It's from this tube that your baby's lungs, intestines and urinary bladder will develop.

YOUR BODY CHANGES

During this first month, you may not feel much different from normal. That's because early pregnancy symptoms often don't begin until midway through the second month.

What's happening and where Even though you may not feel pregnant yet, there are many changes taking place in your body!

Week 1 In the time leading up to conception, it's important to make lifestyle choices that prepare your body for pregnancy and motherhood and give your baby-to-be the best possible start in life. As you prepare for pregnancy, don't smoke, drink alcohol or use drugs. If you take prescription medications, ask your care provider for advice regarding their use during pregnancy.

It's also a good idea to take a daily vitamin supplement containing at least 400 micrograms of folic acid. Adequate folic acid will reduce your baby's risk of developing defects in the neural tube, the component of the embryo that gives rise to the brain, spinal cord, spinal nerves and backbone. Spina bifida, a spinal de-

fect that results in failure of your baby's vertebrae to fuse together, is an example of a neural tube defect that can be largely avoided with adequate folic acid.

Weeks 2 and 3 As you ovulate and an egg is released into your fallopian tube, the hormones involved in the process — estrogen and progesterone — cause a slight increase in your body temperature and a change in secretions from your cervical glands.

Immediately after fertilization, the corpus luteum — a small structure that surrounds your developing baby — starts to grow and produce small amounts of progesterone. This helps support your pregnancy and keeps your uterus from contracting. Progesterone also promotes growth of blood vessels in the uterine wall, essential for baby's nourishment.

Roughly four days after fertilization, finger-like projections that will become the placenta begin producing large amounts of a hormone called human chorionic gonadotropin (HCG). This hormone stimulates the ovaries to keep producing estrogen and progesterone, which cause changes in your uterus, endometrium, cervix, vagina and breasts. Eventually, placental tissue will become responsible for the production of estrogen and progesterone.

The hormone HCG is first detected in your blood and shortly thereafter in your urine. Home pregnancy tests can detect it in a sample of your urine about six to 12 days after fertilization occurs. These tests are usually about 97 percent accurate, although if you test within the first few days of your missed period, it's not uncommon to get a negative result when you're actually pregnant. To get the most reliable results, it's best to wait about a week after your period is due

ESTIMATING YOUR DUE DATE

Use this chart to determine milestones during your pregnancy. For example, if the first day of your last menstrual period was March 27, your estimated due date is January 1.

If the first day of your last menstrual period isn't listed, use the closest listed date and adjust the other dates accordingly. Let's say the first day of your last menstrual period was April 4 (one day past the listed date of April 3). Your estimated due date is then January 9 (one day past the listed due date of January 8).

Week 1	Week 3	Weeks 5-10		Week 12	Week 23	Week 40
If the first day of your last menstrual period was:	Conception likely occurred around:	Period of greatest risk of birth defects		Risk of miscarriage decreases	Some preemies can now survive	(full term) Estimated due date
		Beginning of organ formation	Major organs have formed			
Jan 2	Jan 16	Feb 6	Mar 13	Mar 27	Jun 12	Oct 9
Jan 9	Jan 23	Feb 13	Mar 20	Apr 3	Jun 19	Oct 16
Jan 16	Jan 30	Feb 20	Mar 27	Apr 10	Jun 26	Oct 23
Jan 23	Feb 6	Feb 27	Apr 3	Apr 17	Jul 3	Oct 30
Jan 30	Feb 13	Mar 6	Apr 10	Apr 24	Jul 10	Nov 6
Feb 6	Feb 20	Mar 13	Apr 17	May 1	Jul 17	Nov 13
Feb 13	Feb 27	Mar 20	Apr 24	May 8	Jul 24	Nov 20
Feb 20	Mar 6	Mar 27	May 1	May 15	Jul 31	Nov 27
Feb 27	Mar 13	Apr 3	May 8	May 22	Aug 7	Dec 4
Mar 6	Mar 20	Apr 10	May 15	May 29	Aug 14	Dec 11
Mar 13	Mar 27	Apr 17	May 22	Jun 5	Aug 21	Dec 18
Mar 20	Apr 3	Apr 24	May 29	Jun 12	Aug 28	Dec 25
Mar 27	Apr 10	May 1	Jun 5	Jun 19	Sep 4	Jan 1
Apr 3	Apr 17	May 8	Jun 12	Jun 26	Sep 11	Jan 8
Apr 10	Apr 24	May 15	Jun 19	Jul 3	Sep 18	Jan 15
Apr 17	May 1	May 22	Jun 26	Jul 10	Sep 25	Jan 22
Apr 24	May 8	May 29	Jul 3	Jul 17	Oct 2	Jan 29
May 1	May 15	Jun 5	Jul 10	Jul 24	Oct 9	Feb 5
May 8	May 22	Jun 12	Jul 17	Jul 31	Oct 16	Feb 12
May 15	May 29	Jun 19	Jul 24	Aug 7	Oct 23	Feb 19
May 22	Jun 5	Jun 26	Jul 31	Aug 14	Oct 30	Feb 26
May 29	Jun 12	Jul 3	Aug 7	Aug 21	Nov 6	Mar 5

Week 1	Week 3	Weeks 5-10		Week 12	Week 23	Week 40
If the first day of your last menstrual period was:	Conception likely occurred around:	Period of greatest risk of birth defects		Risk of miscarriage decreases	Some preemies can now survive	(full term) Estimated due date
		Beginning of organ formation	Major organs have formed			
Jun 5	Jun 19	Jul 10	Aug 14	Aug 28	Nov 13	Mar 12
Jun 12	Jun 26	Jul 17	Aug 21	Sep 4	Nov 20	Mar 19
Jun 19	Jul 3	Jul 24	Aug 28	Sep 11	Nov 27	Mar 26
Jun 26	Jul 10	Jul 31	Sep 4	Sep 18	Dec 4	Apr 2
Jul 3	Jul 17	Aug 7	Sep 11	Sep 26	Dec 11	Apr 9
Jul 10	Jul 24	Aug 14	Sep 18	Oct 2	Dec 18	Apr 16
Jul 17	Jul 31	Aug 21	Sep 25	Oct 9	Dec 25	Apr 23
Jul 24	Aug 7	Aug 28	Oct 2	Oct 16	Jan 1	Apr 30
Jul 31	Aug 14	Sep 4	Oct 9	Oct 23	Jan 8	May 7
Aug 7	Aug 21	Sep 11	Oct 16	Oct 30	Jan 15	May 14
Aug 14	Aug 28	Sep 18	Oct 23	Nov 6	Jan 22	May 21
Aug 21	Sep 4	Sep 25	Oct 30	Nov 13	Jan 29	May 28
Aug 28	Sep 11	Oct 2	Nov 6	Nov 20	Feb 5	Jun 4
Sep 4	Sep 18	Oct 9	Nov 13	Nov 27	Feb 12	Jun 11
Sep 11	Sep 25	Oct 16	Nov 20	Dec 4	Feb 19	Jun 18
Sep 18	Oct 2	Oct 23	Nov 27	Dec 11	Feb 26	Jun 25
Sep 25	Oct 9	Oct 30	Dec 4	Dec 18	Mar 5	Jul 2
Oct 2	Oct 16	Nov 6	Dec 11	Dec 25	Mar 12	Jul 9
Oct 9	Oct 23	Nov 13	Dec 18	Jan 1	Mar 19	Jul 16
Oct 16	Oct 30	Nov 20	Dec 25	Jan 8	Mar 26	Jul 23
Oct 23	Nov 6	Nov 27	Jan 1	Jan 15	Apr 2	Jul 30
Oct 30	Nov 13	Dec 4	Jan 8	Jan 22	Apr 9	Aug 6
Nov 6	Nov 20	Dec 11	Jan 15	Jan 29	Apr 16	Aug 13
Nov 13	Nov 27	Dec 18	Jan 22	Feb 5	Apr 23	Aug 20
Nov 20	Dec 4	Dec 25	Jan 29	Feb 12	Apr 30	Aug 27
Nov 27	Dec 11	Jan 1	Feb 5	Feb 19	May 7	Sep 3
Dec 4	Dec 18	Jan 8	Feb 12	Feb 26	May 14	Sep 10
Dec 11	Dec 25	Jan 15	Feb 19	Mar 5	May 21	Sep 17
Dec 18	Jan 1	Jan 22	Feb 26	Mar 12	May 28	Sep 24
Dec 25	Jan 8	Jan 29	Mar 5	Mar 19	Jun 4	Oct 1

before testing. This allows more HCG to build up in your body. See page 25 for more on using a home pregnancy test.

By the time your developing embryo travels through your fallopian tube and implants itself in the lining of your uterus — about a week after fertilization — your endometrium has grown thick enough to support it.

As the embryo implants, you may notice spotting, a very light menstrual flow or yellowish vaginal discharge. You may mistake it for the start of your normal menstrual period. This spotting comes from the small amount of bleeding that can occur upon implantation. At this point you are officially pregnant, though it's still too early for you to have missed a period.

In these first days after fertilization, miscarriage is common — often happening before a woman even knows she's pregnant. Scientists estimate that half of all pregnancies are lost before the

first period is missed. In the first week to 10 days after conception, infections or exposure to harmful environmental factors, such as drugs, alcohol, medications and chemicals, can interfere with the implantation process. Most of the time, however, miscarriage is due to unknown factors beyond anyone's control.

Week 4 Even this early in your pregnancy — just days after conception — your body is already undergoing significant physical changes.

Heart and circulatory system. Your body immediately begins producing more blood to carry oxygen and nutrients to your baby. The increase is greatest in the first 12 weeks, when pregnancy makes enormous demands on your circulation.

By the end of your pregnancy, your blood volume will have increased 30 to 50 percent. To accommodate the increased blood flow, your heart begins to

BABY'S SEX: CAN PARENTS CHOOSE?

Is there any way to increase your odds for having a boy or girl?

The short answer is no. There's not much the average couple can do to affect a baby's sex. Countless old wives' tales suggest that everything from a woman's diet to sexual position during conception can affect a baby's sex, but these theories remain unproved. Likewise, researchers have found that timing sex in relation to ovulation — such as having sex days before ovulation to conceive a boy or closer to ovulation to conceive a girl — doesn't work.

Rarely, couples face the agonizing problem of knowing they could pass a genetic trait to a child of a specific sex, usually a boy. Under those special circumstances couples may use in vitro fertilization with preimplantation genetic testing to prevent transmitting a serious genetic disorder. Using these techniques, embryos are tested for specific genetic conditions and sex before they're placed in a woman's uterus.

Despite the feasibility of these techniques, they're rarely used in circumstances where choosing a baby's sex for personal reasons is the only motivation.

pump harder and faster, and your pulse may quicken by as much as 15 beats a minute. These changes are a big reason why you feel so tired early in your pregnancy. Don't be surprised if you find that you're ready for bed right after the evening meal, or that you need to nap during the day.

Breasts. One of the first physical changes of pregnancy is a change in the way your breasts feel. They may feel tender, tingly or sore, or they may feel fuller and heavier. You may think that your breasts and nipples are already starting to enlarge, and it's possible they could be. These changes are stimulated by an increased production of the hormones estrogen and progesterone.

You may also notice that the areolas, the rings of brown or reddish-brown skin around your nipples, begin to enlarge and darken. This is the result of increased blood circulation and growth of pigmented cells, and it could be a permanent change to your body.

In addition, bumps, called Montgomery's tubercles, appear on the areolas. These bumps secrete lubricating and anti-infection substances that protect the nipples and areolas during breastfeeding.

Uterus. Not surprisingly, your uterus is rapidly changing. Its lining is thickening, and the blood vessels in the lining are beginning to enlarge to nourish your growing baby.

Cervix. Your cervix, the opening in your uterus through which your baby will emerge, already begins to soften and change color at this early stage. Your care provider may look for this change as confirmation of your pregnancy during your first examination.

YOUR EMOTIONS

Expect your emotions to be all over the place, because they will be. Pregnancy can be exciting, boring, satisfying and nerve-racking — sometimes all at once. You're also likely experiencing new and unexpected emotions — some of them comforting and others unsettling.

Mixed feelings Whether your pregnancy was planned or unplanned, you may have conflicting feelings about it. Even if you're thrilled about being pregnant, you may worry about whether your baby will be healthy and how you'll adjust to motherhood. You may also have concerns about the increased financial demands of raising a child. Don't beat yourself up for feeling this way. These concerns are natural and normal.

Mood swings As you adjust to being pregnant and prepare for new responsibilities you may be upbeat one day and feel down the next. Your emotions may range from exhilaration to exhaustion, delight to depression. Your moods can also change considerably over the course of a single day. Some of these mood swings may result from the physical stresses pregnancy is placing on your body. Some may simply be the result of fatigue. Your change in moods may also be due, in part, to certain hormones and changes in your metabolism.

To meet the demands of your growing baby, different hormones are produced at different levels throughout your pregnancy. Though the mechanisms aren't well-understood, the changes — sudden fluctuations in progesterone, estrogen and other hormones — likely contribute to mood swings during pregnancy. The effects of hormones from the thyroid and adrenal glands also may play a role.

There's also no doubt your moods are strongly influenced by the support you receive from your partner and family. Let them know how they can support you as you go through pregnancy.

Your partner's reaction If you have mixed feelings about being pregnant, chances are your partner does, too. He or she may be exhilarated by the anticipation of a loving relationship with a daughter or son. But, like you, your partner may worry about financial challenges or may fear that a baby will forever change your lifestyle. These feelings are normal. Encourage your partner to identify his or her doubts and worries and be honest about what he or she is feeling, both the good and the bad.

Your relationship with your partner Becoming a mother-to-be can take time away from your other roles and relationships. There may be times when your partner is interested in sexual activity and you aren't. In truth, you're probably just tired, sad or worried. Misunderstanding and conflicts between you and your partner are inevitable and normal during pregnancy, just like any other time in your relationship.

Understanding and communication are the keys to preventing or minimizing conflicts. It's important to talk openly and honestly with your partner so that you can anticipate and help minimize stress in your relationship.

SCHEDULING A PRENATAL CHECKUP

You've taken a home pregnancy test, and it says you're pregnant. Now's the time to set up your first appointment with the person you've chosen to provide your obstetric care during your pregnancy. Whether you've chosen a family physician, obstetrician-gynecologist or nurse-midwife, that person will treat, educate and reassure you throughout your pregnancy. Developing a strong relationship with your care provider starts now, at the very beginning of your pregnancy. Care providers enjoy the celebration inherent in pregnancy and birth and want to enhance your celebration of it, too. For more information on choosing a care provider who's right for you, see page 26.

Your first visit to your care provider will focus mainly on assessing your overall health, identifying any risk factors for you or baby and determining how far along you are in your pregnancy.

Getting yourself prepped At your first appointment, your care provider will review your past and current health, including any chronic medical conditions you have and problems that you may have encountered during past pregnancies.

In the time before your first appointment, you may want to write down details regarding your menstrual cycles, contraceptive use, family medical history, work environment and lifestyle. Some care providers make the first part of this appointment a one-on-one conversation with just you — the mom-to-be — and later invite your partner to join you. This gives you an opportunity to privately discuss any health and social issues from your past that you may want to keep private.

This first visit is also an opportunity for you to ask questions. Make it easy on yourself by jotting down your questions as you think of them. It's easier to collect your thoughts before your appointment than to do so during your visit.

EXERCISE OF THE MONTH

Seated trunk twist

This exercise helps to loosen and strengthen the back muscles and may help to relieve back pain in pregnancy.

1. Sit on the floor with your legs crossed.
2. Hold your right foot or leg with your left hand and slowly twist your upper torso to the right. Hold for several seconds.
3. Switch hands and repeat to the left.
4. Do this five to 10 times.

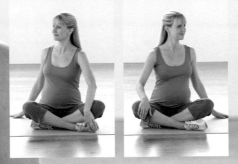

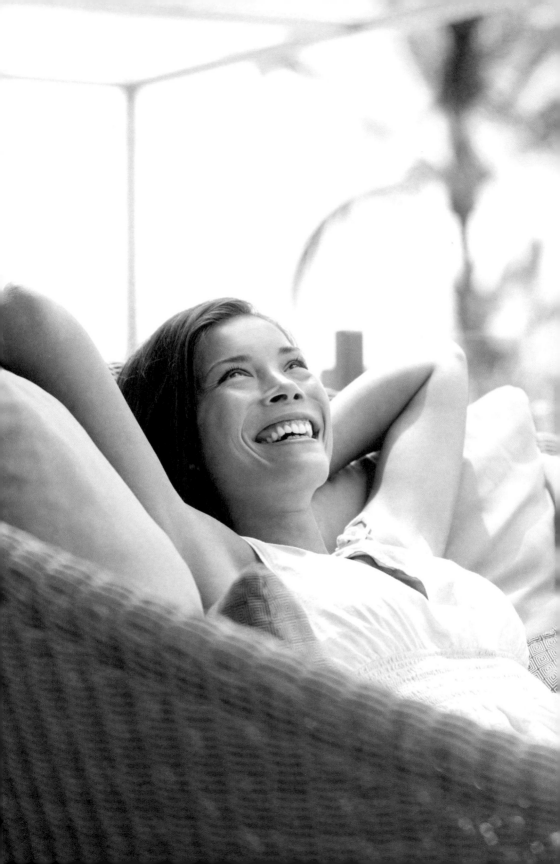

CHAPTER 5

Month 2: Weeks 5 to 8

It's probably a cliché, but when it happens to you, inside you, it feels like a miracle. I keep thinking, how does it know how to do all this? That tiny embryo knows how to grow and feed, how to multiply and divide itself to form a heart, lungs, arms, legs, and so on. I just keep living my life happily clueless, while this supercomplex miracle is happening right inside my belly.

— Lilli

OK, the first couple weeks of your pregnancy were pretty much a breeze. Or if you've been trying for a while, maybe they were difficult to get through because you were on high alert for early signs and couldn't wait to find out whether you were pregnant! Well, get ready: This month things are going to change. You'll soon begin to "feel" pregnant.

Month two is when most women experience extreme tiredness and fatigue. You also may find yourself making countless trips to the bathroom and walking around all day with that nauseated feeling.

BABY'S GROWTH

During weeks five through eight of your pregnancy, your baby's cells multiply rapidly and they begin to perform specific functions. This process of specialization is called differentiation. It's necessary to produce all the different cells that make up a human being. As a result of differentiation, your baby's main external features also will begin to take shape.

Week 5 No longer just a mass of cells, your baby — now officially called an embryo — is starting to take on a distinct form. The embryo has divided into three layers. In the top layer, a groove develops and then closes to form the neural tube, which will eventually develop into your baby's brain, spinal cord, spinal nerves and backbone. This groove runs along the midline of the body, from the top to the bottom of the embryo. The closure of the neural tube begins in the embryo's midsection and proceeds upward and downward from there. The top portion thickens to begin forming the brain.

From the embryo's middle layer of cells, the heart and the circulatory system are taking shape. A bulge at the center of the embryo will develop into your baby's heart. By week's end, the earliest blood elements and blood vessels have formed, both in the embryo and the developing placenta. Your baby's first heartbeats occur at 21 to 22 days after conception. You and your care provider can't hear them yet, but it may be possible to see the beating motion on an ultrasound. With these changes, circulation begins, making the circulatory system the first functioning organ system.

Your baby also has an inner layer of cells, from which lungs, intestines and the urinary bladder will develop. During week five, not much is happening in the inner cell layer. It will be awhile yet before those areas take shape.

At the moment of conception, your baby was a single-celled zygote and was microscopic in size. By the end of your fifth week of pregnancy, three weeks after conception, your baby is about 1/16 of an inch long, about the size of the tip of a pen.

Week 6 Growth is rapid during the sixth week, during which your baby will triple in size. Formation of baby's facial features is in the early stages. Optic vesicles, which later form the eyes, are beginning to develop. Passageways that will make up the inner ear also are beginning to form. An opening for the mouth is formed as cells migrate and grow into the forehead and nose and around the sides of the face. Below the mouth are small folds that ultimately will become your baby's lower jaw and neck.

By the sixth week of your pregnancy, the neural tube along your baby's back has closed over. The brain is growing rapidly to fill the now-formed, enlarging head. Your baby's brain is also developing distinct regions.

In the front of the chest, your baby's heart is pumping fetal blood through the

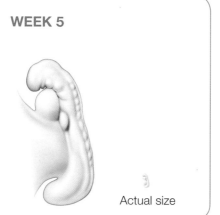

WEEK 5

Actual size

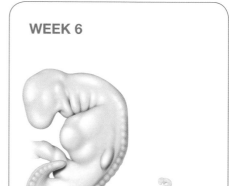

WEEK 6

Actual size

main blood vessels and beating at a regular rhythm. The beginnings of the digestive and respiratory systems are forming. In addition, small blocks of tissue are developing in pairs down your baby's midline. These will form the connective tissue, ribs and muscles of your baby's back and sides. Small buds that will grow into your baby's arms and legs are now visible.

By six weeks into your pregnancy, four weeks after conception, your baby is about 3/16 of an inch long.

Week 7 This week the umbilical cord, the vital link between your baby and your placenta, is clearly visible starting near the site where your baby implanted in your uterus. The umbilical cord contains two arteries and one large vein. Nutrients

CAN STRESS CAUSE MISCARRIAGE?

Are you stressed about stress in your life possibly causing a miscarriage? Relax. Although it's a common concern, evidence hasn't shown a connection. An estimated 10 to 20 percent of known pregnancies end in miscarriage. Typically, early miscarriage is caused by a fetal chromosomal abnormality or another problem in the development of the embryo. Other causes of repeated miscarriage may include:

‣ Chromosomal abnormalities in either parent
‣ Blood-clotting problems
‣ Abnormalities of the uterus or cervix
‣ Hormone imbalances
‣ Immune responses that disrupt implantation

If you're concerned about early miscarriage, concentrate on taking good care of yourself and your baby and avoid known risk factors for miscarriage — such as smoking and drinking alcohol.

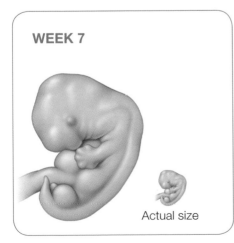

WEEK 7

Actual size

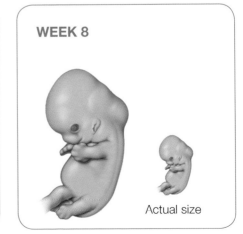

WEEK 8

Actual size

and oxygen-rich blood pass from your placenta to your baby by way of the single vein and then back to your placenta through the two arteries.

In addition, your baby's brain is becoming more complex. Passages necessary for circulation of spinal fluid have formed. Your baby's growing skull is still transparent. If you were able to get a look at it under a magnifying glass, you might see the smooth surface of your baby's tiny, developing brain.

Baby's face is taking on more definition this week. A mouth perforation, tiny nostrils, ear indentations and color in the irises of the eyes are now visible. The

WHAT TO AVOID

Your developing baby is most vulnerable during weeks five through 10 of your pregnancy. During this time, all of baby's major organs are forming, and injury to the embryo could result in a major birth defect. Things that have the potential to cause damage include:

▶ *Teratogens (substances that can cause birth defects).* Examples of these include alcohol, certain medications and recreational drugs. It's best simply to avoid them.

▶ *Infections.* Viruses and bacteria can potentially harm your baby in early pregnancy. A baby can only acquire infections through the mother, but you may not even feel ill with some of the conditions that can cause serious defects. Vaccination and natural immunity protects you against many potentially harmful infections. Still, it makes sense to take appropriate precautions to avoid exposure to illnesses such as chickenpox, measles, mumps, German measles (rubella), cytomegalovirus (CMV) or the Zika virus.

▶ *Radiation.* High doses of ionizing radiation, such as radiation therapy for cancer, can harm your baby. Low doses of radiation, on the other hand, such as those used in a diagnostic X-ray, generally don't pose a significant increase in the risk of birth defects. To be on the safe side, if an issue arises in which an X-ray could provide important information, talk with your care provider about his or her recommendations for X-ray during pregnancy. Unless they're very extensive, diagnostic X-rays may be more helpful than harmful, even in early pregnancy. If you had an X-ray before you knew you were pregnant, don't be alarmed. It's highly unlikely the fetus received enough radiation to cause any problems.

▶ *Poor nutrition.* Extremely poor eating habits during pregnancy can harm your baby. Eating too little of a specific nutrient may impact cell development. However, an early-stage embryo isn't likely to be harmed if mild nausea and vomiting limit your daily calories. Be sure to take a vitamin supplement daily that contains at least 400 micrograms of folic acid. This will reduce your baby's risk of developing spina bifida or other neural tube defects.

lenses of baby's eyes are forming and the middle portions of the ears are connecting the inner ear to the outer world.

Your baby's arms, legs, hands and feet are taking shape, though the beginnings of fingers and toes are about a week away. The arm bud that sprouted just last week has already developed into a shoulder portion and a hand portion, which looks like a tiny paddle.

At seven weeks into your pregnancy, your baby is 1/3 of an inch long, a little bigger than a pencil eraser.

Week 8 Your baby's fingers and toes begin to form this week, although they're still webbed. His or her tiny arms and legs are growing longer and more defined. Paddle-shaped foot and hand areas are evident. Wrists, elbows and ankles are clearly visible. Your baby may even be able to flex at the elbows and wrists.

The eyelids are also forming. Until they're done growing, your baby's eyes will appear open. This is also the week your baby's ears, upper lip and tip of the nose begin taking on recognizable form.

Your baby's digestive tract is continuing to grow, especially the intestines. Heart function and circulation are now more fully developed. Your baby's heart is pumping at about 150 beats a minute, about twice the adult rate.

At the eighth week of your pregnancy, your baby is just over 1/2 of an inch long.

YOUR BODY CHANGES

The second month of pregnancy brings enormous changes for your body. It's the time you're likely to experience the discomforts and annoyances of early pregnancy, such as nausea, heartburn, fatigue, insomnia and frequent urination. But don't let these symptoms get you down. Think of them as signs that your pregnancy is proceeding normally.

What's happening and where Hormones are the chemical messengers that regulate many aspects of your pregnancy, and this month your hormones kick into high gear. Hormones released throughout pregnancy have many important functions. Hormones influence the growth of your baby, and they trigger physiological changes in several of your body's systems. In fact, the hormonal changes of pregnancy affect nearly every part of your body.

Digestion Nausea and vomiting, commonly referred to as morning sickness, may be the most significant hormone-related change you'll experience this month. Exactly what causes the nausea and vomiting for morning sickness isn't known, but changes in your gastrointestinal system in response to high hormone levels almost certainly play a role. Increased estrogen and progesterone slow down the pace at which your food passes

SPOTTING

You may experience some vaginal bleeding during the first 12 weeks of your pregnancy. Statistics indicate that as many as 25 percent of pregnant women may have some bleeding (spotting). However, statistics also indicate that only about half these women will have miscarriages. For more information on spotting and vaginal bleeding, see page 424.

through your digestive tract. Therefore, your stomach empties somewhat more slowly, which may make you more likely to have nausea and vomiting. The hormone HCG also may play a role, as levels of HCG rise and peak along the same timeline as nausea and vomiting in the first trimester. But no direct link has been found between morning sickness and HCG either. See below for more discussion of morning sickness.

Heart and circulatory system Your body continues to produce more blood to carry oxygen and nutrients to your baby. This increase in blood production, which continues throughout your pregnancy, will be especially high this month and next, due to enormous demands on your circulation. Despite this effort, your blood vessels are dilating even more quickly and your circulation is just a bit short of blood volume. To accommodate these changes, your heart continues to pump harder and faster. These changes in blood circulation can cause signs and symptoms such as fatigue, dizziness and headaches.

Breasts Stimulated by increased production of estrogen and progesterone, your breasts continue to enlarge as the milk-producing glands inside them grow in size. You may also notice that the rings of brown or reddish-brown skin around your nipples (areolas) are starting to enlarge and darken. This is the result of increased blood circulation. Your breasts may feel tender, tingly or sore. Or they may feel fuller and heavier.

Uterus If this is your first pregnancy, your uterus has previously been about the size of a pear. Now it's starting to expand. By the time you deliver your baby, it will have expanded in volume to about 500 times its original size. Through this month and the next, your uterus will still fit inside your pelvis. However, its increasing size may cause you to feel the need to urinate more often. You may also leak urine when you sneeze, cough or laugh. This is a simple matter of crowding. During the first few months of pregnancy, your bladder lies directly in front and slightly under your uterus. As your uterus grows, your bladder gets crunched.

The placenta also is continuing to grow and secure its attachment to the uterus. Sometimes this results in minor bleeding. While not typically a cause for concern, if this does happen, let your care provider know.

Cervix This month, your cervix turns a bluish tinge and continues to soften. Over the course of your pregnancy, your cervix will gradually become softer as it prepares for the thinning (effacement) and opening (dilation) necessary for childbirth. By the seventh week of pregnancy, the mucous plug is well-established in your cervix. This structure blocks the cervical canal during pregnancy, to help prevent germs from getting into your uterus. The plug loosens and passes late in pregnancy, typically when your cervix starts to thin out and open in preparation for labor.

COPING WITH MORNING SICKNESS

Morning sickness is one of the dreaded aspects of pregnancy. Some women are lucky enough to escape it, but most women experience some level of nausea during pregnancy. The term *morning sickness* is a misnomer, however, because

EXERCISE OF THE MONTH

Backward stretch

When your lower back or your shoulders (or both) start to feel tight, try this move to relieve tension.

1. Kneel on your hands and knees with your arms straight and your hands directly beneath your shoulders.
2. Curl backward slowly, tucking your head toward your knees and keeping your arms extended.
3. Hold for several seconds, then slowly return to all fours. Repeat five to 10 times.

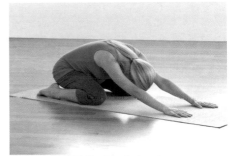

the condition isn't limited to mornings. It can strike at any time, day or night.

Morning sickness affects an estimated 50 to 80 percent of pregnant women. It's most common during the first trimester and is characterized by nausea with or without vomiting. Signs and symptoms typically start at five to eight weeks, sometimes beginning as early as two weeks after conception. They often subside by weeks 13 to 14; however, some women experience morning sickness well beyond the first trimester.

Treatment isn't usually needed for morning sickness. However, home remedies such as snacking throughout the day and sipping ginger ale or ginger tea can help relieve nausea. Rarely, morning sickness is so severe that it's classified as hyperemesis gravidarum, which can require hospitalization and treatment with intravenous (IV) fluids and medications.

Hormones and more What causes morning sickness isn't entirely clear, but the hormonal changes of pregnancy are thought to play a significant role. The condition can affect any pregnant person, but you might be more likely to experience morning sickness if:

▶ You experienced nausea or vomiting from motion sickness, migraines, certain smells or tastes, or exposure to estrogen (in birth control pills, for example) before pregnancy

▶ You experienced morning sickness during a previous pregnancy

▶ You're pregnant with twins or other multiples

On the positive side, studies suggest that women who experience morning sickness are less likely to have early pregnancy loss. However, this doesn't mean that if you don't experience morning sickness you're at risk of miscarriage. Some women simply seem to be more immune to the nauseating effects of early pregnancy.

How to ease the queasiness To help relieve morning sickness:

▶ *Choose foods carefully.* Opt for foods that are bland or dry, easy to digest, and lower in fat. Some research suggests that protein-based foods may relieve nausea better than foods rich

---

THE 'WARMED-UP' EFFECT

If you've been pregnant once before, you may notice that you're bigger than you were at the same time during your last pregnancy. You may also notice that side effects seem to be happening earlier this time.

You could call this the warmed-up effect. Like a balloon that's easier to blow up the second or third time around, your uterus may expand more quickly and easily once it has been through one pregnancy. Your abdominal muscles and ligaments have already been stretched once, so they give more easily as your uterus expands on the second go-round.

The downside is that because your uterus is getting bigger faster, you may experience symptoms such as pelvic pressure and back pain sooner in this pregnancy than you did in your first pregnancy.

in carbohydrates. Salty snacks are sometimes helpful, as are foods that contain ginger — such as ginger lollipops. Avoid greasy, spicy and fatty foods.

- *Snack often.* Before getting out of bed in the morning, eat a few soda crackers or a piece of dry toast. Nibble throughout the day, rather than eating three larger meals. An empty stomach may aggravate nausea.
- *Drink plenty of fluids.* Sip water or ginger ale. It may also help to suck on hard candy, ice chips or ice pops.
- *Pay attention to triggers.* Avoid foods or smells that seem to make your nausea worse. Keep rooms well-ventilated and free of cooking odors, which can aggravate nausea.
- *Get plenty of fresh air.* Weather permitting, open the windows in your home or workplace. Take a daily walk outdoors.
- *Take care with prenatal vitamins.* If you feel queasy after taking prenatal vitamins, take the vitamins at night or with a snack. It may also help to chew gum or suck on hard candy after taking your prenatal vitamin. If these steps don't help, ask your care provider if it might be possible to switch to a type of prenatal vitamin that doesn't contain iron.
- *Experiment with acupressure and acupuncture.* Although they haven't been proved to be effective, some women find these therapies to be helpful in relieving morning sickness. Acupressure involves stimulating certain points on the body with pressure. Acupressure wristbands, available in pharmacies without a prescription, are designed to stimulate a certain point on the wrist. This action is thought to reduce nausea. Acupuncture involves inserting hair-thin nee-

dles into your skin. Some women find it helpful, but it requires an appointment with a licensed acupuncturist.

YOUR EMOTIONS

Pregnancy is a psychological journey as well as a biological one. You're the child of your parents, yet soon you'll be the mother of your own child. You'll have a new role to play and a new identity. The emotions you're feeling in the face of this reality can be both overwhelmingly positive and distressingly negative.

Anticipation Anticipation is a normal part of making the transition to parenthood. Beginning early in pregnancy, you start collecting information about how to be a good mother, based on the parenting

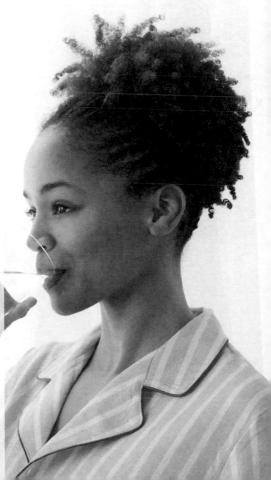

you received as a child and your observations of other families you've encountered. The memories of how you were raised, along with your personal ideals of parenting, serve as a bank of images that you can draw from as you think ahead to what your own parenting style will be.

During this time of anticipation, you'll probably have dreams and fantasies about what your baby will be like. These visualizations are the beginnings of your emotional bond with your baby.

Worries and concerns During your second month of pregnancy, the excitement you felt when you learned you were pregnant may be dampened by fear.

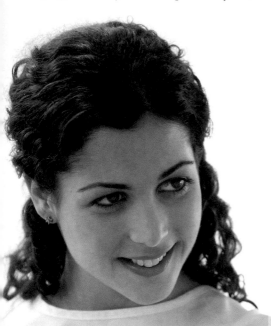

What if you might have done something to harm your baby before you knew you were pregnant? What about that aspirin you took for a headache? Or that glass of wine you had with dinner? Or that bout of the flu? If you have concerns, share them with your care provider. Doing so may help put your mind at ease.

You may also be worried about other things. How will you cope with your pregnancy? Will you have problems at your job? What about arranging for child care? Can you handle the pain of labor and delivery? Will your baby be healthy? Discuss these worries with your partner. If you hide them, worries can cause tension in your relationship. They can create a sense of distance between you and your partner at a time when you both need the warmth and assurance of a close, loving relationship.

Some women experience disturbing, anxiety-provoking dreams or feelings during early pregnancy. These thoughts may seem irrational, yet they're normal and very common. For most new parents, such thoughts usually pass. However, if troubling thoughts and feelings persist and you find them disturbing, consider talking to your care provider, who may refer you to a therapist or counselor to help you manage this anxiety.

PRENATAL CHECKUP

The time is finally here to see your care provider. Your first prenatal checkup is an exciting time. This will likely be your longest and most comprehensive checkup. Therefore, allow plenty of time in your schedule — up to three hours — so that you won't feel rushed. You'll probably meet several different people, including nurses and office staff.

Your first prenatal checkup with your care provider is an opportunity to review your general health and lifestyle and talk about being pregnant and giving birth. To get the most out of your first visit, keep the following tips in mind:

▶ *Be proactive.* Discuss ways you might improve your lifestyle to ensure the healthiest possible pregnancy. Possible topics to cover include your diet, exercise, smoking and alcohol use.

▶ *Don't hold back.* Raise any concerns or fears you may have about your pregnancy and childbirth. The sooner these fears and concerns are addressed, the sooner you can have peace of mind.

▶ *Be honest.* Tell the truth when talking with your care provider. The quality of care you receive depends in large part on the quality of the information you provide.

What's going to happen? Most women have prenatal visits every four to six weeks until their eighth month. Then the visits become more frequent. If you have a chronic health problem, such as diabetes or high blood pressure, you may need more-frequent visits to monitor your health and your baby's health.

Medical history Gathering as much information as possible about your past

---

FIRST APPOINTMENT CHECKLIST

Discussion of your medical history at your first appointment with your care provider will likely cover the following topics:

○ Details of any previous pregnancies
○ The typical length of time between your periods
○ The first day of your last period
○ Your use of contraceptives
○ Prescription or over-the-counter medications you're taking
○ Allergies you have
○ Medical conditions or diseases you have had or now have
○ Past surgeries, if any
○ Your work environment
○ Your lifestyle behaviors, such as exercise, diet, smoking or exposure to secondhand smoke, and use of alcoholic beverages or recreational drugs
○ Risk factors for sexually transmitted infections — such as you or your partner having more than one sexual partner
○ Past or present medical problems, such as diabetes, high blood pressure (hypertension), lupus or depression, in your or your partner's immediate family — father, mother, siblings
○ Family histories, on both sides, of babies with congenital abnormalities or genetic diseases
○ Details on your home environment, such as whether you feel safe and supported at home

and present health is one of your care provider's biggest goals during your first visit. He or she will review your past and current health, including any chronic medical conditions you have and problems you've had during past pregnancies. Come to your appointment prepared to answer questions about many aspects of your health and lifestyle.

While discussing your medical history, you'll also have a chance to ask questions you may have about your pregnancy. If you've been keeping a running list of questions, bring the list to your first appointment.

Physical exam The physical examination will likely include weight, height and blood pressure measurements, as well as an overall assessment of your general health. A pelvic exam also may be part of this evaluation. If you are due for a Pap test, the pelvic exam will include a speculum examination. A speculum is placed in the vagina so that your care provider can check your vagina and the opening to your uterus (cervix). Changes in your cervix and in the size of your uterus help your care provider determine how far along you are in your pregnancy.

With the speculum in place, your care provider may gently collect some cells and mucus from your cervix to perform a Pap test and to screen for infections. The Pap test helps detect abnormalities that indicate precancer or cancer of the cervix. Infections of the cervix, including sexually transmitted infections such as gonorrhea and chlamydia, can affect your pregnancy and the health of your baby.

After removing the speculum, your care provider may insert two gloved fingers into your vagina to check your cervix and, with the other hand on top of your abdomen, check the size of your uterus and ovaries.

Many women are apprehensive about having a pelvic exam. During the exam, try to relax as much as you can. If you tense up, your muscles can tighten, which can make the exam more uncomfortable. Keep in mind that a typical pelvic exam takes only a couple of minutes.

Expect that you may have some vaginal bleeding after your pelvic exam and Pap test, especially within 24 hours of your visit. The bleeding may be just some light spotting, or it may be a little heavier. It usually goes away within a day. This happens because the cervix, which has already begun to soften due to pregnancy, is more inclined to bleed after a Pap test. The bleeding is from the outside of your cervix and isn't a risk to your baby. If you're concerned about it, talk to your care provider.

Lab tests Routine laboratory tests during your first prenatal visit include blood tests to determine your blood type (A, B, AB or O) and rhesus (Rh) factor — Rh positive or Rh negative — and to determine if you still have immunity to certain diseases from previous vaccinations, such as German measles (rubella) or hepatitis B.

Your blood is also screened for red blood cell antibodies — most commonly, Rh antibodies. These types of antibodies can increase your baby's risk of developing anemia and jaundice after birth.

In addition, you will be tested for HIV, the virus that causes AIDS, and for syphilis, chlamydia and gonorrhea. If you have any of these sexually transmitted infections, treatment during pregnancy will reduce the risk of transmission to your baby. Tests for immunity to chickenpox, measles, mumps and toxoplasmosis may be done as well. Some women may be screened for thyroid problems. It typically takes just one needle stick and one blood sample to run all of these tests.

You may also be asked to provide a urine sample. An analysis of your urine can determine whether you have a bladder or kidney infection, which would require treatment. The urine sample can also be tested for increased sugar, indicating diabetes, and protein, indicating possible kidney disease.

An ultrasound exam may be performed at your first prenatal checkup to verify your due date, to check that the pregnancy is within the uterus (ruling out ectopic pregnancy — see page 484), or to determine if you may be carrying multiples.

TWINS, TRIPLETS AND MORE

You're ready for one baby, but what about two or three? For some women, this month's prenatal visit may bring surprising news that they're expecting twins, triplets or, in rare cases, even more, called multiple gestations.

Multiple babies are generally discovered at the time of your first ultrasound. The stage of pregnancy at which you may receive your first ultrasound varies from one medical center to another. In some practices, an ultrasound is done at the first prenatal visit, while in others it may not happen until the second or third visit. How early in your pregnancy you see your care provider also is a factor.

If your care provider performs an ultrasound at your first visit and you're more than a couple of weeks into your pregnancy, it's possible you may find out very early that you're carrying multiples. An ultrasound can detect most multiples by the eighth week of pregnancy, possibly sooner. During an ultrasound examination, sound waves create an image of your uterus and your baby — or babies.

Physical signs of a multiple pregnancy include a uterus that's larger than normal or extreme fatigue and nausea. If your care provider suspects that you're carrying multiple babies, he or she may perform an ultrasound exam to confirm these suspicions.

Older moms and individuals who have undergone infertility treatment to achieve pregnancy are at increased risk of having multiples.

How multiples are made There are two types of twins: identical and fraternal. Identical twins occur when a single fertilized egg splits and develops into two fetuses. Genetically, the two babies are identical. They will be the same sex and look exactly alike. Fraternal twins occur when two separate eggs are fertilized by two different sperm. In this case, the twins can be two girls, two boys, or a boy and a girl. Genetically, the twins are no more alike than are any other siblings.

Early in pregnancy it's often possible to determine if twins are identical or fraternal with an ultrasound exam. The appearance of the placenta and membranes are key to making this determination.

Triplets can occur in several ways. In most cases, three separate eggs are produced by the mother and fertilized by three separate sperm. Another possibility is for a single fertilized egg to divide two ways, creating identical twins, with a second egg fertilized by a second sperm, resulting in a fraternal third baby. It's also possible for a single fertilized egg to divide three ways, resulting in three identical babies, although this is extremely rare.

Quads and greater numbers of multiples most often result from four or more eggs being fertilized by separate sperm. Use of fertility drugs or assisted reproductive techniques is generally involved.

FRATERNAL VS. IDENTICAL

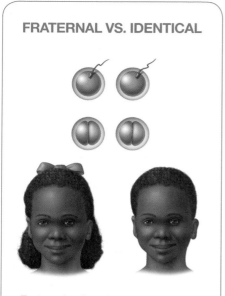

Fraternal twins, the most common kind, occur when two different eggs are fertilized by two different sperm.

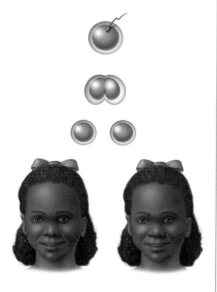

Identical twins occur when a single fertilized egg splits and develops into two fetuses that have identical genetic makeups.

What it means for you If you're carrying multiples, some side effects of pregnancy may be a bit more unpleasant. Nausea and vomiting, heartburn, insomnia, and fatigue can be problematic. Because of the increased space required by your growing babies, you may also have abdominal pain and shortness of breath. Later in your pregnancy, you may feel pressure on your pubic bone, the structure located over the lowest part of the front of your pelvis.

Carrying multiple babies means you'll probably be seeing your care provider more often. Special care is often essential in multiple pregnancies. Your care provider may want to more closely track the growth of your babies and more closely monitor your health, anticipating potential problems before they occur.

With more than one baby to nourish, nutrition and weight gain also become more important. If you're carrying twins, your care provider may recommend that you take in about 300 more calories a day. The American College of Obstetricians and Gynecologists recommends a weight gain of 37 to 54 pounds for twins. However, if you were overweight before becoming pregnant, your recommended weight gain will be less. For additional multiples, the recommended weight gain will be higher, depending on the number of babies you're carrying and your weight when you became pregnant.

A lowered blood cell count (anemia) is more likely with multiples. Therefore, your care provider may recommend that you take a supplement with 60 to 100 milligrams of elemental iron. You may also be asked to limit some of your activities, such as work, travel and exercise.

Possible complications Carrying more than one baby can increase your chances of some pregnancy complications. In most situations, multiple babies are born healthy, especially if the multiples are twins. The more babies you carry, the greater the potential for complications. These may include:

Preterm labor When contractions begin to open the cervix before the 37th week of pregnancy, this is known as preterm labor. Nearly 60 percent of twins and more than 90 percent of triplets are born before the 37th week of pregnancy. The average gestational age of twins is 35 weeks. Triplets frequently arrive by 32 weeks, sometimes earlier. Almost all larger numbers of multiples come earlier.

Babies that arrive early have a greater chance of having low birth weights (less than 5½ pounds) and having other health complications. For that reason, your care provider will likely monitor you closely for signs of preterm labor. You'll want to do the same. For more on preterm labor, see page 168.

Preeclampsia Preeclampsia is a condition that can develop during pregnancy, which includes elevated blood pressure. Preeclampsia is more common in mothers of multiples. Signs and symptoms of preeclampsia include rapid weight gain, headaches, abdominal pain, vision problems, and swelling of your hands and feet. It's important to contact your care provider if you experience any of these problems.

Cesarean birth The chance of needing a cesarean section is higher with multiples. However, you may still be able to have a vaginal delivery, depending on the position of the babies and other factors. If you're carrying more than two babies, your care provider likely will recommend a cesarean section as the safest delivery method for the babies.

Twin-twin transfusion This condition usually occurs only in identical twins. It can happen when a blood vessel in the placenta connects the circulatory systems of the two babies, and one twin receives too much blood flow and the other too little. A baby receiving too much may grow larger and develop an overload of blood in its circulatory system. The other twin may be smaller, grow more slowly and become anemic.

In such circumstances, early delivery of the twins may be necessary. Certain treatments also may help. Draining off excess fluid through amniocentesis may be beneficial. At some specialized hospitals, laser surgery is used to seal off the connection between the blood vessels.

Conjoined twins This occurs very rarely. Conjoined twins result from an incomplete division of identical twins. In the past, babies with this condition were commonly referred to as Siamese twins. Conjoined twins may be joined at the chest, head or pelvis. In some cases, the twins may share one or more internal organs. Surgery may be performed after birth to separate conjoined twins. The complexity of the operation depends in part on where the twins are joined and how many organs they share.

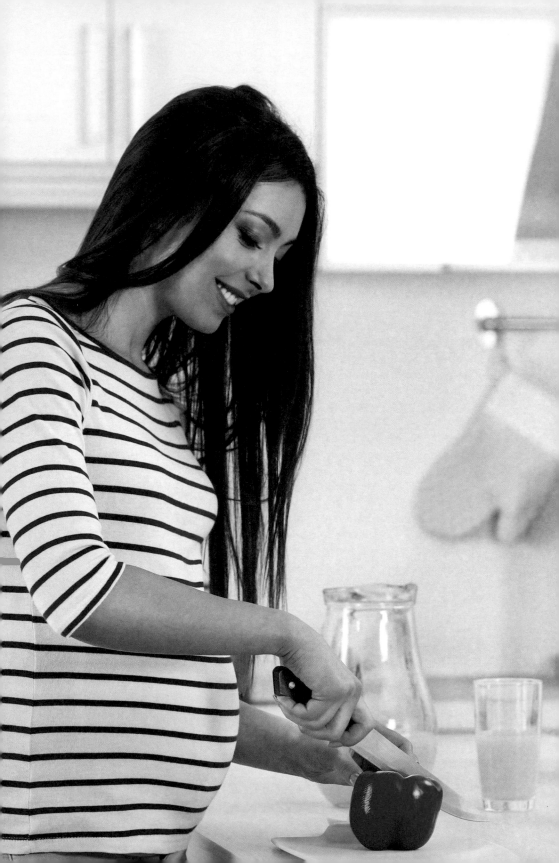

CHAPTER 6

Month 3: Weeks 9 to 12

I feel like my body is preparing me for motherhood by reminding me what it's like to be a child. I eat every three hours, want things I don't need, cry because I'm tired and I've become a bit of a narcissist.

— Yumna

Hang in there — you will start to feel better soon! As you enter the last month of your first trimester, the signs and symptoms of early pregnancy — fatigue, hunger, nausea, increased urination — are at their peak, and they may be getting the best of you. Things should start to improve in a few weeks. For many women, the first is the worst. Once they get past the first trimester, the remainder of their pregnancy is fairly comfortable.

BABY'S GROWTH

Your baby is still very small at this point in time — only about an inch long — but changing rapidly. During the third month, he or she begins to take on a much more human shape.

Week 9 This week your baby is looking less like a tadpole and more like a person. The embryonic tail at the bottom of the spinal cord is shrinking and disappearing, and the face is more rounded. Compared with the rest of the body, your baby's head is quite large and is tucked down onto the chest. The hands and feet are continuing to form fingers and toes, and elbows are more pronounced. Nipples and hair follicles are forming.

Your baby's pancreas, bile ducts, gallbladder and anus have formed, and the intestines are growing longer. Internal reproductive organs, such as testes or ovaries, start to develop this week, but the external genitals don't yet have noticeable male or female characteristics.

Your baby may start making some movements this week, but you won't be able to feel them for several more weeks. At nine weeks into your pregnancy, seven weeks since conception, your baby still weighs only about ⅛ of an ounce.

Week 10 By week 10, all of your baby's vital organs have begun to form. The embryonic tail has disappeared completely, and baby's fingers and toes are fully separated. The bones of the skeleton are now forming. Your baby's eyelids are more developed and are in the process of closing. The outer ears are starting to assume their final form. Your baby is also starting to develop buds for teeth. His or her brain is now growing more quickly. This week almost 250,000 new neurons are being produced every minute. If your baby is a boy, his testes will start producing the male hormone testosterone.

Week 11 From now until the time your baby is full term, he or she is officially described as a fetus. With all organ systems in place, growth becomes more rapid. From week 11 until week 20 of pregnancy — the halfway mark — your baby will about triple in length and grow to nearly 8 or 9 times its current weight. To accommodate this development, blood vessels in your placenta are growing larger and more numerous to keep up the supply of nutrients to your baby. His or her ears are moving up and to the side of the head this week, and his or her reproductive organs are developing quickly, too. What was a tiny tissue bud of external genitalia has begun to develop into either a penis or a clitoris and labia majora, which will soon be recognizable.

Week 12 Your baby's face takes on further definition this week, as the chin and nose become more refined. This week also marks the arrival of fingernails and toenails. Your baby's heart rate may speed up a few beats per minute. By the 12th week of your pregnancy, your baby is nearing 3 inches long and weighs about 2 ounces. The end of this week marks the end of your first trimester.

YOUR BODY CHANGES

The third month of pregnancy is the last month of your first trimester. Some of the discomforts and annoyances of early pregnancy, such as morning sickness, fatigue and frequent urination, may be particularly troublesome this month. But the

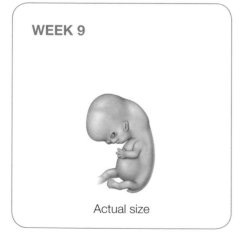

WEEK 9

Actual size

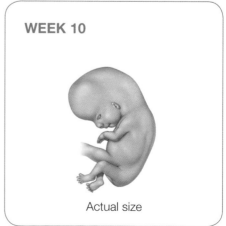

WEEK 10

Actual size

end is in sight — at least for a while. For most women, the side effects of early pregnancy will greatly diminish in the second trimester.

What's happening and where Hormone production continues to increase this month, but a shift is taking place. By the end of your 12th week of pregnancy, your baby and placenta will be producing more of the hormones estrogen and progesterone than your ovaries do.

This continued increase in hormone production may continue to cause you to experience unpleasant signs and symptoms, such as nausea and vomiting, breast soreness, headaches, dizziness, increased urination, insomnia, and vivid dreams. Nausea and vomiting may be especially bothersome. If you have morning sickness, it may last this entire month. For many women, though, morning sickness begins to subside midway into the next month.

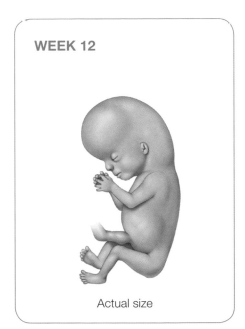

WEEK 12

Actual size

Heart and circulatory system Increased blood production will continue throughout your pregnancy, but at the end of this month it will slow. To accommodate this change, your heart is continuing to pump harder. It's also pumping faster. These changes in your circulatory system may be continuing to cause unwelcome physical signs and symptoms, such as fatigue, dizziness and headaches.

Eyes While you're pregnant, your body retains extra fluid, which causes the outer layer of your eye (cornea) to thicken. This change often becomes obvious by about the 10th week of your pregnancy, lasting until about six weeks after your baby is born. At the same time, the pressure of fluid within your eyes, called intraocular pressure, decreases about 10 percent during pregnancy. Because of these two events, you may notice slightly blurred vision. Your eyes will return to normal after you give birth.

Breasts Your breasts and the milk-producing glands inside them continue to grow, stimulated by increased production of estrogen and progesterone. The areolas, the rings of brown or reddish-brown skin around your nipples, may become larger and darker. Your breasts may continue to feel tender or sore, though the soreness is probably easing a bit. Your breasts may also feel fuller and heavier.

Uterus Up to your 12th week of pregnancy, the uterus fits inside your pelvis. It's probably hard for anyone to tell you're pregnant just by looking at you. Even so, you'll likely have pregnancy-related signs and symptoms. Throughout this month, due to your uterus' increasing size and proximity to your bladder, you'll probably continue to need to urinate more often. By the end of the month, your uterus will have expanded out of your pelvic cavity, so the pressure on your bladder won't be as great.

Bones, muscles and joints You may continue to feel some twinges, cramps or pulling in your lower abdomen. The ligaments supporting your uterus are stretching to accommodate its growth. Those twinges may soon develop into sharp pain on one side or the other, early in the second trimester, usually provoked by a sudden movement. This pain results from stretching of the round ligament that tethers the uterus to the abdominal wall. It isn't harmful, but it can hurt.

Weight When you add everything up — your baby's weight, the placenta, the amniotic fluid, the increased amount of blood your body has produced, the fluid that's accumulated in your body tissues, and your bigger uterus and breasts — you'll probably have gained 1 to 4 pounds by the end of your 12th week of pregnancy. If you've struggled with morning sickness, you might have stayed at the same weight or even lost a pound. But don't worry. Most of your weight gain will occur in the second half of your pregnancy.

YOUR EMOTIONS

For the past couple of months, your emotions have centered around news of your pregnancy and all of the changes in store. Now that reality has sunk in — at least somewhat — your emotions may change course a bit. This month, as you start developing a small potbelly, you may become more focused on how your own body is changing in shape. While some women love the physical changes of pregnancy, others struggle with them.

Dealing with body image Changes in your body's shape and function can affect the way you feel. During the first trimester, your body forms fat stores, most of it below the waist. In addition, your breasts will put on almost a pound each. During this time, your body may not look and feel like your own. Given the cultural emphasis on being slim, you may be bothered by changes in your body image, especially if this is your first pregnancy. Simply put, you may feel fat. Try to remember that your body is changing for the important work of growing and nurturing your baby.

If you struggle with the changes taking place in your body, you may be having

---

THAT PREGNANCY GLOW

Ready for some good news about your body's changes this month? Your increased blood volume and increased production of the hormone human chorionic gonadotropin (HCG) are working together to give you that pregnancy glow. Greater blood volume is bringing more blood to your blood vessels, resulting in skin that looks slightly flushed and plump. In addition, the hormones HCG and progesterone, which are causing the skin glands on your face to secrete more oil, are helping make your skin look smoother and slightly shinier. However, if you commonly experienced acne breakouts during your menstrual period before you were pregnant, this extra oil may be making you more prone to acne.

trouble enjoying or even wanting to have sex with your partner. If you're feeling this way, keep a couple of things in mind. For most women, while interest in intercourse continues during pregnancy, it may decrease a bit. This is perfectly normal. Also, though it may be hard for you to believe, you partner may be excited about the changes to your body that come with pregnancy.

PRENATAL CHECKUP

You'll likely have your second prenatal visit with your care provider this month. This visit may include many of the same things that occurred at your first visit, but it should be shorter.

If your second visit occurs around the 12th week of your pregnancy, your care provider may try to listen for your baby's heartbeat. If a heartbeat isn't there, don't panic. It may still be too soon. Your provider may also verify the baby's heartbeat with an ultrasound.

Prenatal tests: Yes, no, not sure?
At this month's prenatal checkup, your care provider may talk with you about prenatal testing for fetal abnormalities. Prenatal tests are performed to assess the health of your baby, generally by way of a blood test or ultrasound exam. Some prenatal tests are optional while others are highly recommended or required. In certain states, some tests are mandated by state law, such as tests for HIV or other sexually transmitted infections.

Many women have questions about prenatal testing, and that's perfectly normal. Your prenatal checkup is a good time to discuss your concerns with your care provider, so that when the time comes to make decisions about prenatal testing,

you will be informed. You may also want to check on which tests your insurance will cover, as coverage varies for tests that are considered optional. Prenatal tests are generally performed between the 10th and 20th weeks of pregnancy, depending on the tests. Certain genetic screening tests need to be performed at a very specific time.

Some women want to have all of the tests performed, and others opt for just some, mainly those tests that are required or recommended. To help you learn more about prenatal genetic tests, see Chapter 21. If your care provider doesn't discuss the risks and benefits with you, don't be afraid to ask.

Boy or girl: Do you want to know?
In the coming weeks, you may be able to find out the sex of your little one — if you want to. Many parents find out the big news of baby's sex from a standard ultrasound done around 18 to 20 weeks.

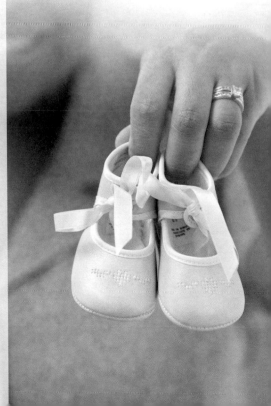

EXERCISE OF THE MONTH

Side plank

This exercise will help strengthen your core muscles, which are key in supporting your growing belly throughout pregnancy.

1. Lie on your left side and raise yourself onto your left forearm, with your left shoulder directly above your left elbow. Rest your right arm alongside your body.

2. Hold this position for several seconds and then lower yourself to the floor. Do this five to 10 times.

3. Repeat on the other side.

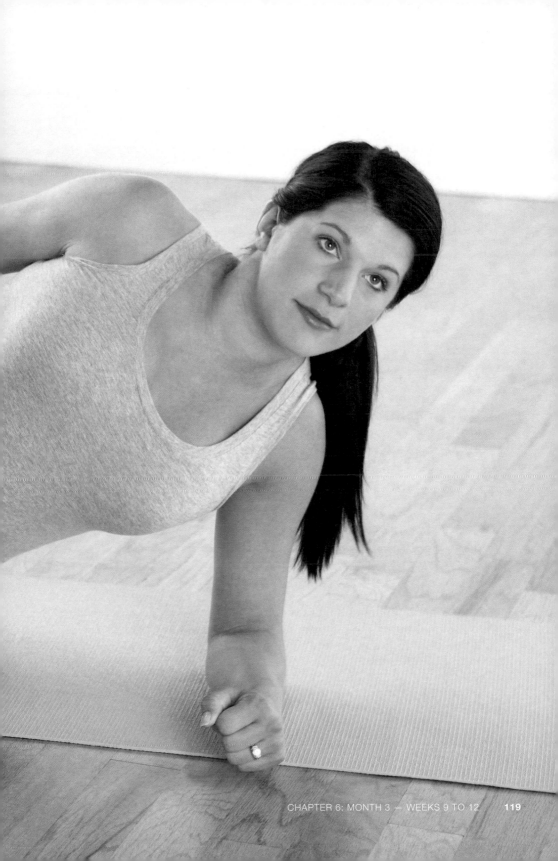

SEX DURING PREGNANCY

Has pregnancy spiked your interest in sex? Or is sex the last thing on your mind? Either way, here's what you need to know about sex during pregnancy.

Is sex OK during pregnancy? As long as your pregnancy is proceeding normally, you can have sex as often as you like — but you may not always want to. At first, hormonal fluctuations, fatigue and nausea may sap your sexual desire. During the second trimester, increased blood flow to your sexual organs and breasts may rekindle your desire for sex. But by the third trimester, weight gain, back pain and other symptoms may once again dampen your enthusiasm.

Can sex during pregnancy cause a miscarriage? Many couples worry that sex during pregnancy will cause a miscarriage, especially in the first trimester. But sex isn't a concern. Early miscarriages are usually related to chromosomal abnormalities or other problems in the developing baby — not to anything you do or don't do.

Does sex during pregnancy harm the baby? Your developing baby is protected by the amniotic fluid in your uterus, as well as the mucous plug that blocks the cervix throughout most of pregnancy. Sexual activity won't affect your baby.

What are the best sexual positions during pregnancy? As long as you're comfortable, most sexual positions are OK during pregnancy. As your pregnancy progresses, experiment to find what works best. Rather than lying on your back, you might want to lie next to your partner sideways or position yourself on top of your partner or in front of your partner.

Can orgasms trigger premature labor? Orgasms can cause uterine contractions, but these contractions are different from the contractions you'll feel during labor. If you have a normal pregnancy, orgasms — with or without intercourse — don't seem to increase the risk of premature labor or premature birth. Likewise, sex isn't likely to trigger labor even as your due date approaches.

Are there times when sex should be avoided? Although most women can safely have sex throughout pregnancy, sometimes it's best to be cautious. Your health care provider may recommend avoiding sex if:
- You're at risk of preterm labor
- You have unexplained vaginal bleeding
- You're leaking amniotic fluid
- Your cervix begins to open prematurely (cervical incompetence)
- Your placenta partly or completely covers your cervical opening (placenta previa)

As early as 10 weeks into your pregnancy, you may be able to learn the sex of your baby through cell-free fetal DNA (cfDNA) screening, one type of prenatal testing. However, this test is used to screen for genetic problems, such as Down syndrome. Thus, it's not recommended for the primary purpose of learning the baby's sex. (See chapter 21 to learn more about prenatal testing.) If you do have a cfDNA test done, make sure you and your partner are prepared for all of the information it may provide. Likewise, invasive genetic testing may be an option if there are complications with your pregnancy or genetic concerns. These tests can also tell your baby's sex.

The question is, Do you want to know? Discuss with your partner whether you want to find out the sex of your baby during your pregnancy or if you prefer to wait until delivery. Some parents prefer to know right away for practical reasons, while others simply cannot stand the suspense! On the other hand, many prefer the excitement of not knowing whether their child is a boy or girl until it's born. There is no right or wrong answer when it comes to this decision.

If you want to keep your baby's sex a secret, let your health care team know so that they don't let the information slip during an ultrasound or while discussing test results. Results from cfDNA screening or invasive testing will include information about the sex of your baby, but you can ask your provider not to reveal it.

If you do decide to find out early, keep in mind that cfDNA screening and prenatal ultrasound don't have perfect accuracy. There's a chance the information about baby's sex from one may conflict with results of the other, or may be flat-out wrong. You may get a surprise after all!

ALTERNATIVE PRENATAL CARE MODELS

In some clinics and hospitals, a program called centering pregnancy is offered as an alternative to traditional prenatal care visits. In this care model, a group of women with similar due dates gather regularly throughout pregnancy. Partners are encouraged to come, too.

At each centering pregnancy meeting, participants measure their weight and blood pressure. Then each participant gets one-on-one time with the nurse midwife or other care provider to address any personal questions or concerns, check the baby's growth, and listen to the baby's heartbeat. After this individual time, the group joins together for discussion or a guest speaker.

The primary focus of each meeting is interaction with other participants, women at the same point in their pregnancies who are dealing with the same issues and joys. The group learns from everyone's questions and experiences.

Unlike traditional classes or lectures, group prenatal care helps provide a sense of community. After all the babies are born, the centering group will often stay in touch and continue to meet.

Other alternative prenatal care programs are becoming available as well, such as OB Nest at Mayo Clinic. In this care model, women are scheduled for fewer office visits but are provided with equipment to monitor their own blood pressure and the fetal heart rate at home. Each woman is assigned a specific nurse as their point of contact. The women can also take part in an online community.

These programs can be empowering alternatives to traditional prenatal care for women with low-risk pregnancies. If you're comfortable with a more relaxed approach, one of these may be a good fit.

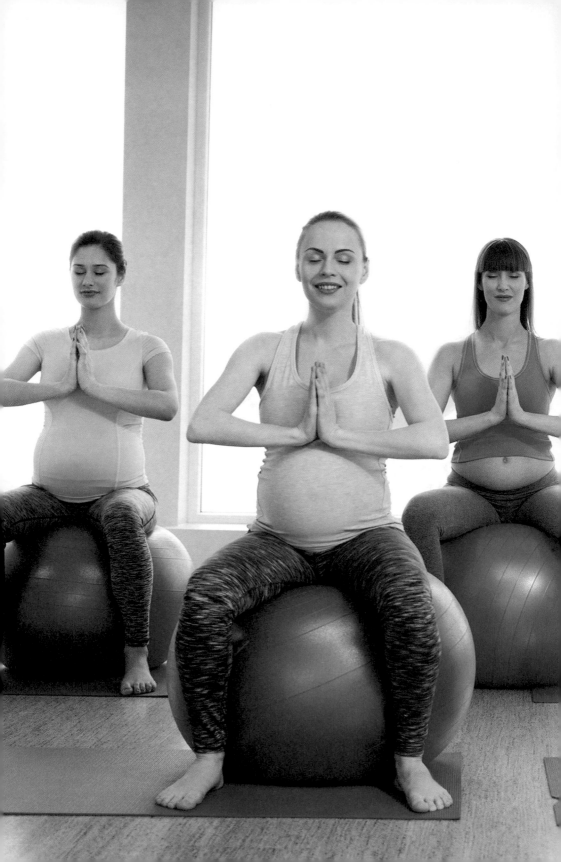

CHAPTER 7

Month 4: Weeks 13 to 16

We made it through the first trimester. What a relief! My husband and I now feel more comfortable telling people that we're expecting a baby. My tummy is already starting to show a little, too, which is fun. And I feel better. I have more energy, and I'm not so nauseated and dizzy.

— Amy

One down and two to go! The beginning of the second trimester is generally a time of relief for most pregnant women. You've made it past the first three months — the stage of pregnancy when pregnancy loss is most common. You're also at the point when the fatigue and nausea of early pregnancy should start subsiding.

The second trimester is often considered the easiest stage of pregnancy because this is when most women feel their best. So, enjoy this time. Get out and do the things you love. You might even want to take a vacation or plan some outings. Face it, you've earned it — and baby will be here before you know it.

BABY'S GROWTH

As you enter the second trimester, all of your baby's organs, nerves and muscles have taken basic form and are beginning to function together. Growth continues at a rapid pace, but baby is still small — just 2 to 3 ounces as this month kicks off.

Week 13 Your baby's eyes and ears are now clearly identifiable, although the eyelids are fused together to protect the developing eyes. They won't reopen until around weeks 28 to 30. Tissue that will become bone is developing around your baby's head and within the arms and legs. If you were able to sneak a peek at your baby this week, you might see some tiny ribs.

Your baby is now moving his or her body in a jerky fashion, flexing the arms and kicking the legs. But you won't be able to feel these movements until your baby grows a bit larger. Your baby may be able to reach a thumb to his or her mouth, and sucking may begin within a few weeks.

Week 14 Your baby's reproductive system is the site of most of the action this week. If you're having a boy, his prostate gland is developing. If you're having a girl, her ovaries are moving down her abdomen into her pelvis. In addition, because the thyroid gland is now functioning, your baby starts producing hormones this week. By the end of this week, the roof of your baby's mouth (palate) will be completely formed.

Week 15 Eyebrows and hair on your baby's scalp are starting to appear this week. If your baby is going to have dark hair, the hair follicles may begin making the pigment that will give the hair its dark color.

Your baby's eyes and ears now have a baby-like appearance, and the ears have almost reached their final position, although they're still riding a little low on the head. Your baby's skin is adding hair follicles and accessory glands, but it is still very thin.

The bone and marrow that make up baby's skeletal system continue to develop this week. Muscle development is continuing, too. By the end of the week, your baby will be able to make a fist.

Week 16 The skeletal and nervous systems have made enough connections to signal movements of the limbs and body. In addition, your baby's facial muscles are now well-enough developed to allow for a variety of expressions. Inside your uterus, your baby may be squinting or frowning at you, although these movements aren't conscious expressions of emotions.

Your baby's skeletal system continues to develop as more calcium is deposited on the bones. If you're having a girl, millions of eggs are forming in her ovaries this week. Beginning at 16 weeks, your baby's eyes are sensitive to light.

Although you probably don't even know it, your baby may be having frequent bouts of the hiccups. Hiccups often develop before your baby performs lung movements associated with breathing. Because your baby's trachea is filled with fluid rather than air, the hiccups don't make that characteristic hiccup sound.

At 16 weeks into your pregnancy, your baby is between 4 and 5 inches long and weighs a little more than 4 ounces.

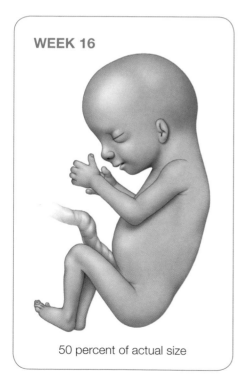

WEEK 16

50 percent of actual size

YOUR BODY CHANGES

This week begins what's sometimes called the golden period of pregnancy. The nausea and fatigue of early pregnancy have lessened, and the discomforts of the third trimester haven't yet begun. Plus, your risk of miscarriage is now greatly reduced. New sensations also are common during this time.

What's happening and where The changes that began in your first weeks of pregnancy are increasing and accelerating — and becoming more obvious to others. Your hormone levels continue to increase this month, influencing the growth of your baby and affecting every organ system in your body. Here's an overview of what's happening.

Heart and circulatory system Your circulatory system continues to expand rapidly, and the result is a lowering of your blood pressure. During the first 24 weeks of your pregnancy, your systolic blood pressure (top number) and diastolic blood pressure (bottom number) will both probably drop by five to 10 points. During the third trimester, they may gradually return to pre-pregnancy levels. Be aware that you may experience dizziness or faintness during hot weather or when you're taking a hot bath or shower. This happens because heat makes the tiny blood vessels in your skin dilate, temporarily reducing your blood pressure further and slowing the blood returning to your heart.

Your body continues to make more blood this month. Right now, the extra blood you're producing is mostly the fluid portion of blood (plasma). During the first 20 weeks of pregnancy, you produce plasma more quickly than you produce red blood cells. Until your red blood cells have a chance to catch up, they're outnumbered, resulting in lower concentrations.

If you don't get the iron you need this month to help your body make more red blood cells, you may become anemic. Anemia results when you don't have enough red blood cells in your blood and, therefore, not enough of the protein hemoglobin to carry oxygen to your body's tissues. Anemia can make you tired and more susceptible to illness, but unless the anemia is severe, it's unlikely to hurt your baby. During pregnancy, the body is programmed so that even if you're not getting enough iron, your baby is.

Respiratory system Stimulated by the hormone progesterone, your lungs are already taking in more air by the second trimester. In fact, with each breath, you're inhaling and exhaling up to 30 to 40 percent more air than before. These changes

CONGESTION PROBLEMS

The increased blood flow throughout your body may be causing some new unpleasant side effects in your nose and gums — congestion troubles resulting from extra blood flowing through your veins and arteries.

Your nasal tissues may be swollen and fragile. And your nasal membranes may be producing more mucus, resulting in nasal stuffiness. You may also experience nosebleeds, even if you never did before. And don't be surprised to find your gums bleed when you brush your teeth. Many pregnant women experience gum softening or bleeding (see page 403). None of these problems will harm you or your baby.

are allowing your blood to carry large quantities of oxygen to your placenta and baby. In addition, they're allowing your blood to remove more carbon dioxide from your body than normal.

You may notice that you're breathing slightly faster these days than before you became pregnant. You may also start experiencing shortness of breath. Two-thirds of all pregnant women do, usually beginning around the 13th week of pregnancy. This likely occurs because your brain is decreasing the carbon dioxide level in your blood in order to make it easier to transfer more carbon dioxide from your baby to you. To do this, the brain adjusts your breathing volume and rate.

To accommodate your increased lung capacity, your rib cage will enlarge over the course of your pregnancy, by 2 to 3 inches in circumference.

Digestive system Increased amounts of the hormones progesterone and estrogen tend to relax smooth muscles in your body, including your digestive tract. The result is a slowing down of your digestive system. The movements that push swallowed food from your esophagus down into your stomach are slower, and your intestinal tract also takes longer to empty.

This slowdown allows nutrients more time to be absorbed into your bloodstream and reach your baby. Unfortunately, when you combine the slowdown with an expanding uterus that's crowding out other abdominal organs, the result often is heartburn and constipation, two of the most common and uncomfortable side effects of pregnancy. You may begin experiencing these side effects this month. Up to half of all pregnant women experience heartburn. The story is much the same with constipation, which also affects as many as half of all pregnant women.

Breasts Your breasts and the milk-producing glands inside them continue to grow in size this month, stimulated by increased production of estrogen and progesterone. Darkening of the skin around your nipples (areolas) may be especially noticeable now. Although some of this increased pigmentation will fade after you've given birth, these areas are likely to remain darker than they were before you were pregnant. Expect your breasts to feel tender or sore and fuller and heavier.

Uterus Now that you're in your second trimester, your uterus is positioned higher and more forward, which is changing your center of gravity. Without even knowing it, you may be starting to adjust your posture and the ways you stand, move and walk. You may at times feel as if you're going to tip over. This is normal. You'll return to your more graceful self after your baby is born.

As your uterus is becoming too big to fit within your pelvis, your internal organs are being pushed out of their usual places. Greater tension is also being placed on your surrounding muscles and ligaments. All this growth may cause some aches and pains.

You may also experience some pain in your lower abdomen this month. This is probably related to the stretching of ligaments and muscles around your expanding uterus. The stretching doesn't pose a threat to you or your baby.

Because of the pressure your uterus is placing on the veins in your legs, you may experience leg cramps, especially at night. You may also notice that your navel is starting to protrude. This, too, is the result of pressure from your growing uterus. After you deliver your baby, your navel will almost certainly return to its normal shape.

EXERCISE OF THE MONTH

Back press

This small movement strengthens your core to support good posture in pregnancy.

1. Stand with your back against a wall and your feet shoulder-width apart a few inches from the wall.
2. Press the small of your back against the wall. Hold for several seconds.
3. Repeat five to 10 times.

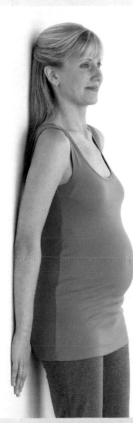

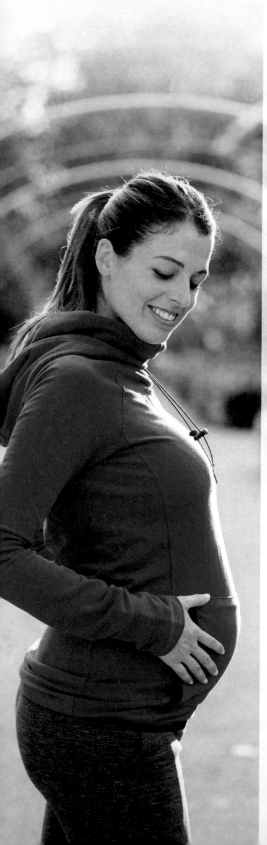

Urinary tract The hormone progesterone is relaxing the muscles of your ureters, the tubes that carry urine from your kidneys to your bladder, slowing your flow of urine. In addition, your expanding uterus is further impeding your urine flow. These changes, combined with a tendency to excrete more glucose in your urine, can make you more prone to bladder and kidney infections.

If you're urinating even more often than normal, feeling burning during urination or experiencing a fever, you may have a urinary tract infection. Report these signs and symptoms to your care provider. Abdominal pain and backache also may signal a urinary tract infection. Recognizing and treating urinary tract infections are especially important during pregnancy. Left untreated, these infections can be a cause of preterm labor later in pregnancy.

Bones, muscles and joints Your bones, joints and muscles are adapting to the stresses of carrying your baby. The ligaments supporting your abdomen are becoming more elastic, and the joints between your pelvic bones are beginning to soften and loosen. Ultimately, these changes will make it easier for your pelvis to expand during labor and childbirth so that your baby can pass through. But for now, the changes may cause some back pain.

The lower portion of your spine may start to curve backward to compensate for the shift in your center of gravity caused by your growing baby. This change in your posture also can strain your back muscles and ligaments and cause some back pain.

Vagina You may notice more vaginal discharge this month, caused by turnover of the rapidly growing cells in the vagina.

These cells combine with normal vaginal moisture to form a thin, white discharge. Its high acidity is thought to play a role in suppressing the growth of potentially harmful bacteria.

The hormone changes of pregnancy can disrupt the normal balance of organisms in the vagina, causing one type of organism to grow faster than the others. This can cause a vaginal infection. If you have vaginal discharge that's greenish or yellowish, strong smelling, or accompanied by redness, itching and irritation of the vulva, contact your care provider. But don't be too alarmed. Vaginal infections are common in pregnancy and can be easily and successfully treated.

Don't use an over-the-counter yeast infection medication without talking to your care provider first. Because other types of vaginal infections can cause signs and symptoms similar to those caused by yeast infections, it's best for your care provider to determine what type of vaginal infection you have before you start treatment.

Skin A common occurrence of pregnancy is skin darkening. This is thought to be a result of increased hormone production, although the exact cause isn't known. You may be noticing darker areas of skin on or around your nipples, in the area between your vulva and anus (perineum), and on your armpits and inner thighs. It's also common to see a darker line, called the linea nigra, form down the middle of your abdomen. These changes may be more pronounced if you have dark skin. Skin darkening almost always fades after delivery, but some areas are likely to remain darker than before you were pregnant.

You may notice mild skin darkening on your face, too. This condition, called chloasma, or the mask of pregnancy,

affects up to 70 percent of all pregnant women. It usually appears on the forehead, temples, cheeks, chin and nose. It may not be as intense as other changes in pigmentation, and it generally fades completely after delivery. When you're outside, it's important to use sunscreen, especially on your face. Sun exposure may increase normal skin darkening.

You may also notice redness on the palms of your hands. In addition, some women experience bluish, blotchy patches on their legs and feet, especially when they're cold. These skin changes usually disappear after your baby is born.

Weight gain You'll probably gain about half a pound a week or a little more this month, for a total of about 2 to 3 pounds. Don't be surprised if your weight gain varies somewhat, with more weight gained some weeks than others.

YOUR EMOTIONS

Now that you're growing out of your jeans and you've been able to hear your baby's heartbeat, your baby may seem more real to you. Chances are, you also feel better and have more energy. This is all good!

Feeling productive While your mood and energy are up, jump on your to-do list and start taking care of the "housekeeping" details of pregnancy. If you're interested in childbirth classes, now is the time to investigate your options. Now may also be a good time to familiarize yourself with maternity and paternity leave policies.

And, if you haven't already, this is a good time to start thinking about child care for when you go back to work. You may think it's too soon, but openings for infant care in some regions and cities can be difficult to find, so it's best to start looking early.

As you take care of these details, you may find it a little difficult to concentrate. You may even feel a little scatterbrained or forgetful. This is normal, no matter how organized you were (or weren't) before pregnancy. Take these foggy moments in stride. You'll be back to your usual self in a few months.

TIME TO GO SHOPPING

As your belly begins to grow in size, you'll find that many of your clothes no longer fit or they don't fit well. You may be able to get by for a few months by wearing your looser-fitting clothes, but soon you'll need maternity clothes. The good news is, it's a great time to be pregnant. Today's maternity clothes offer a wide range of flattering on-trend and classic styles, so you shouldn't have to sacrifice your personal style to stay comfortable.

Here are some points to keep in mind when you're ready to expand your wardrobe:

▶ *Your tummy is just beginning to expand.* Don't buy too much right now. You may want to purchase more clothes later on if you outgrow the first batch! Or if you want to be able to wear an item throughout your pregnancy, make sure to buy it in a big enough size.
▶ *You're not limited to maternity clothes.* You may find that regular clothes in larger sizes will work just as well.
▶ *New may not be necessary.* Consignment maternity clothes or a friend's hand-me-downs are often gently used and still in style.

PRENATAL CHECKUP

Your visit to your care provider this month will include tracking your baby's growth, confirming your due date if that wasn't done at an earlier visit and watching for any problems with your health.

Your care provider may measure the size of your uterus to help determine the baby's age. This is done by checking what's called the fundal height — the distance from the top, or far end (fundus), of your uterus to your pubic bone. To find the top of your uterus, your care provider may gently tap and press on your abdomen and measure from that point down along the front of your abdomen to your pubic bone.

In addition to performing the fundal height check, he or she may check your weight and blood pressure and ask you about any symptoms you've been experiencing. If you haven't done so already, you may get to hear your baby's heartbeat using a Doppler ultrasound machine.

THINKING AHEAD TO CHILD CARE

A very difficult decision for many working women is what they will do once the baby is born. Like many parents, you may grapple over whether you want to return to work or stay home. And if you do go back, should you work full time or part time? If you're the primary breadwinner, or a co-breadwinner, is your partner interested in scaling back on work or becoming a stay-at-home parent?

If you know that you and your partner will both be returning to work after your child is born, begin looking for child care as early as possible. If you're not sure if you're going back, it's probably best to explore your options while you make your decision. Consider these factors:

- *Your budget.* Know the cost of child care and how it'll affect your budget. If the expense is prohibitive, get creative. Perhaps you or your partner could adjust work hours or schedules to reduce the need for child care.
- *Your expectations.* Be open and honest with any prospective child care provider about your preferences and expectations, from discipline to diapers. For example, do you prefer disposable diapers or cloth? If you choose cloth, can the provider accommodate that? What other things are especially important to you?
- *Your family dynamics.* If a loved one offers to care for your baby, give the offer serious thought. It could be a great financial help, but be prepared for the emotions that can accompany such an arrangement. Your family member may also offer you plenty of advice along with those child care hours — more advice than you'd like! You don't want the arrangement to cause a rift in family relations.

Child care options Child care options vary. For example, some larger companies provide child care on-site for their employees. For most women, though, their options include the following:

In-home care Under this arrangement, someone comes to your home to provide child care. The person may live with you, depending on your agreement. Some examples of in-home caregivers are relatives, nannies and au pairs. Au pairs typically come to the United States on student exchange visas and provide child care in exchange for room and board and usually a small salary. The advantages of hiring an in-home caregiver are that your

child can stay at home, you set your own standards, and you have more flexibility. But you also have certain legal and financial obligations as an employer.

Family child care Many people provide care in their homes for small groups of children. Homes that offer child care usually have to meet state or local safety and cleanliness standards. Family child care allows your child to be in a home setting with other children, often at a lower cost than that of an in-home caregiver or a child care center. Quality varies, so it's important that you visit the home and get references from current or previous clients.

Child care centers Child care centers are organized facilities with staff members who are trained to care for groups of children. These centers are typically required to meet state or local standards. Some of the advantages of child care centers include socialization with other children, a large selection of toys and activities, and

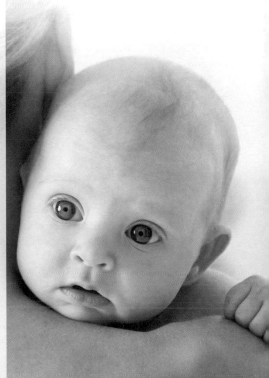

a full staff of caregivers, which can relieve worries about finding backup care. Depending on where you live, you also may have options of centers with a specific approach, such as the Montessori method or language immersion. However, child care centers may not let you bring your child if he or she is mildly ill, and they usually require you to be fairly punctual. When considering a center, check the ratio of children to caregiver. If one adult has too many children to care for, your child may not get as much individual attention as you want.

Making your decision Consider all of your options, and don't be afraid to ask questions or go back for a second visit, and maybe even a third.

Once you've found child care you feel comfortable with, you can return to work with confidence knowing that your child is in good hands. Often, when mothers first return to work after the baby is born, they feel guilty for leaving the child. Or they're anxious that the child may bond more with the caregiver than with them. But don't worry, you'll still have time to spend with your child. The bond between parent and child is unique and can't be replaced.

Work and family balance Research supports the positive effect of a loving, nurturing relationship between parent and child. The most influential factor in parenting is probably not the sheer quantity of time you spend with your child. Even stay-at-home parents don't spend all of their time interacting with their children. They have errands to run, dishes to wash, clothes to fold and other duties that come with running a household.

Whatever your choice, if you feel happy and fulfilled, it will affect your child. If you resent your arrangement or feel cheated by it, you may pass on these feelings to your child.

If you're still uncertain whether you want to return to work after your baby is born, here are some things to think about. Keep in mind, there is no right or wrong in this decision, but there's probably a choice that's best for you. Talk it over with your partner and friends and family who have made different choices. Then make the best decision for you and your family. You may also find that over time, your choice may change, as your circumstances change.

Your financial needs Although money isn't everything, it is necessary to provide basic care for your family. If you need the income, spending some time away from your child is probably preferable to enduring chronic stress over money issues.

If you or your partner makes enough income to sustain your family, you may not feel the need to have both of you split your time between work and home. Many stay-at-home parents take a break from working because the cost of child care can be nearly equal to an income. If the loss of income is more stressful than imagined, however, a stay-at-home parent might consider a part-time job or a job that can be done at home.

Your desire to maintain a career Women who've worked hard to attain a certain position or whose occupation is meaningful to them often feel reluctant to give it up. You may desire and enjoy the intellectual challenges and adult interaction that come from working outside the home. You may also be considering whether a break in your career could have a long-term impact on your professional advancement and your earning potential.

When your intellectual and social needs are being met at work, you may feel more prepared to function at home. If you're happy at work, chances are good you'll be happy at home.

Your desire to be a full-time parent Just the opposite, perhaps being your child's primary caregiver is more important to you than keeping your job. If your real desire is to stay at home with your children, see if you can make it work. Many full-time parents become part of a strong community with other local parents and kids, allowing for plenty of social interaction for their children — and themselves — through play dates and other activities.

Your ability to manage stress It takes energy to handle the juggling act of parenthood and working outside the home. Some people manage the stress that comes with these dual roles just fine. Others struggle with it.

Consider how well you can handle multiple roles and responsibilities. If you work, can you provide your children with the sort of attention you'd like them to have? Will your performance at work and at home decline? Will you have the support of friends and family to help you through some of the more difficult days?

Whatever you decide, strive for an arrangement in which you feel successful and engaged — and remember to go easy on yourself. Parents who are fulfilled in their parenting and career roles will provide positive role models for their kids.

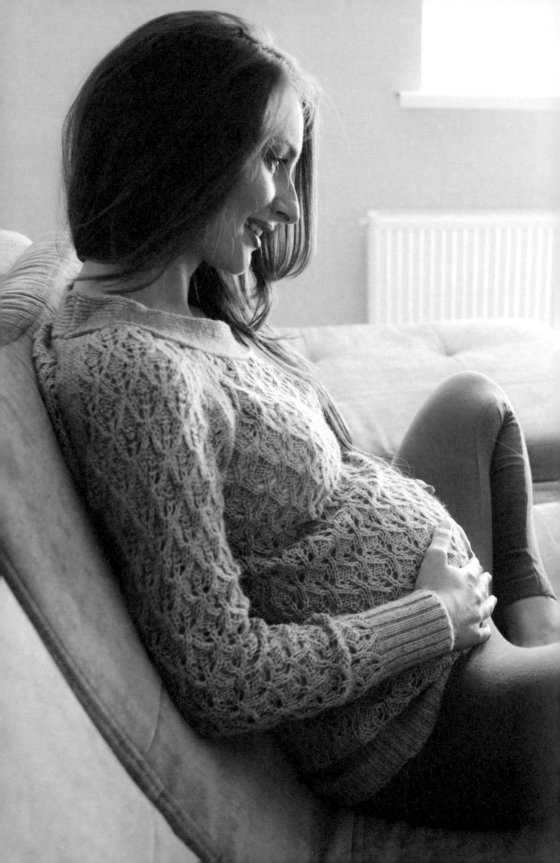

CHAPTER 8

Month 5: Weeks 17 to 20

It is the most amazing feeling — it feels like someone is tickling me lightly from the inside. All of a sudden I feel this movement, and then it disappears before I can put my hand on my abdomen. These little touches are the joy of my day. I'm feeling my baby move.

— Kelly

The fifth month often brings another joy of pregnancy. For many moms, it marks the first time they're able to feel baby move inside. This movement often is greeted with relief — feeling baby move is an indication that all is well. Now, not only is your tummy getting bigger, but baby is becoming interactive!

BABY'S GROWTH

During the fifth month, your little boy or girl will start to fill out more. Gradually, he or she is beginning to look more like the child you imagine holding in your arms. Baby is still very small, though. As you near the halfway point of your pregnancy, the child inside still weighs less than a pound!

Week 17 Eyebrows and the hair on your baby's scalp continue to appear. Baby's toenails are growing more this week, too. His or her fingernails are even further along in development.

Your little one is becoming more active in the amniotic sac, rolling and flipping. Baby also continues to experience bouts of the hiccups. Although you aren't able to hear them, you may begin to feel them, especially if this isn't your first baby.

Week 18 During week 18 your baby's bones begin to harden, a process called ossification. Your baby's leg bones, collarbone and inner ear are among the first to ossify. With the bones in the inner ear now developed enough to function and the nerve endings from your baby's brain now hooked up to the ears, your baby can hear sounds. He or she may hear your heart beating or your stomach rumbling. Your baby may even become startled by loud noises.

Your little one can also now swallow. Inside your uterus, your baby may be swallowing a good dose of amniotic fluid every day. Scientists think this helps with the development of baby's gut and lungs, and it also keeps your amniotic fluid at the appropriate, constant level.

Week 19 During week 19 your baby's skin becomes covered with a slippery, white, fatty coating called *vernix caseosa*, or vernix for short. Vernix helps protect baby's delicate skin, keeping it from becoming chapped or scratched. Under the vernix, fine, down-like hair called *lanugo* covers your baby's skin.

In addition, brown fat starts to develop under your baby's skin. This will help keep your baby warm after birth, when the temperature change from your uterus to the outside world will be quite stark. Your baby will add more layers of fat in the later months of your pregnancy.

Your baby's kidneys are now developed enough to make urine. The urine is excreted into your amniotic sac, the bag of waters inside your uterus that contains your baby and your amniotic fluid. Unlike your urine, your baby's urine is completely sterile because he or she is living in a sterile environment. Therefore, when your baby swallows amniotic fluid containing urine, it is not a problem.

His or her hearing is now well-developed. Baby is probably hearing lots of different sounds, maybe even your conversations. Mom's voice is by far the most prominent in any conversation. If you sing or talk to your baby, it's reasonable to think he or she might notice. It's less clear whether your baby is able to recognize particular sounds.

Your baby's brain continues to develop millions of motor neurons, nerves that help the muscles and brain communicate. As a result, baby now may make conscious muscle movements, such as sucking a thumb or moving his or her head, as well as involuntary movements. You may or may not be able to feel these movements yet. If you haven't, you will soon.

Week 20 Baby's skin is thickening and developing layers this week, under the protection of the vernix. Skin layers include the epidermis, the outermost layer of skin; the dermis, the middle layer, which makes up 90 percent of the skin; and the subcutis, the deepest layer of skin, made up mostly of fat.

Your baby's hair and nails continue to grow. If you could sneak a peek at your baby this week, it would look remarkably

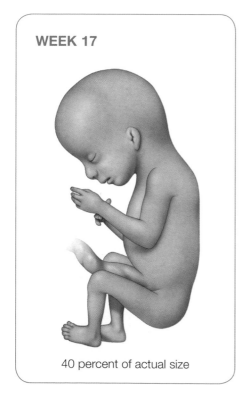

WEEK 17

40 percent of actual size

baby-like, with thin eyebrows, hair on the scalp and rather well-developed limbs.

Now at the halfway point of your pregnancy, you've probably begun to feel your baby's movements. Make a note of the date, and tell your care provider at your next visit. Your baby is now about 6 inches long or a little more, and he or she weighs about 10 to 14 ounces.

YOUR BODY CHANGES

As you reach the midway point of pregnancy, your uterus will expand to your navel. Unless you are very tall, your pregnancy now is probably quite obvious.

At first, you may not recognize your baby's movements. Some women describe the movements as feeling like "butterflies" in your stomach or a growling stomach. These early movements will be erratic. They'll become more regular later in your pregnancy.

What's happening and where As with previous months, your hormone levels continue to increase this month, influencing baby's growth and affecting all of your organ systems.

Heart and circulatory system Your circulatory system continues to expand rapidly. As a result, your blood pressure will probably stay lower than normal this month and the next.

Your body also continues to make more blood. The extra blood you're producing is mostly plasma (fluid). Later, your body will increase production of red blood cells — provided you're getting enough iron. Iron deficiency anemia, a condition marked by a decline in red blood cells, can result if you don't get the iron you need each day to fuel increased

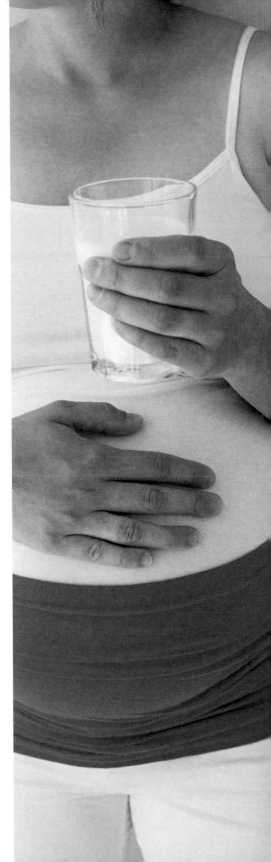

production of red blood cells. The condition most often develops after 20 weeks of pregnancy and can make you tired and more susceptible to illness. But unless it's severe, it's unlikely to hurt your baby.

You may continue to experience some annoying side effects such as nasal congestion, nosebleeds and bleeding gums when you brush your teeth. These changes are the result of increased blood flow to your nasal passages and gums.

Respiratory system Stimulated by the hormone progesterone, changes in your lungs continue this month. With each breath, you inhale and exhale up to 40 percent more air than before, which pulls about 20 percent more oxygen into your system. Still, many women become aware of some shortness of breath.

Digestive system Under the influence of pregnancy hormones, your digestive system remains sluggish. Because of this and your expanding uterus, heartburn and constipation may continue. You're not alone, if that helps. As many as half of all women experience heartburn or constipation during pregnancy.

Breasts Changes in your breasts may be especially noticeable this month. With more blood flowing to them and the milk-producing glands inside growing in size, they now may be almost two cup sizes larger than before you were pregnant. Veins in your breasts may be more visible now, too.

Uterus It goes without saying that your uterus is expanding. By your 20th week, it will reach your navel. When it reaches its full size, it will extend from your pubic area to the bottom of your rib cage. By now your expanding uterus is almost certainly affecting your center of gravity

and, therefore, how you stand, move and walk. You may feel especially clumsy, and you may also experience continued aches and pains, especially in your back and lower abdomen.

Around the 20th week of pregnancy, you may feel a pulling or stabbing pain in your groin or a sharp cramp down your side, especially after making a sudden move or reaching for something. This pain results from stretching your round ligament, one of several ligaments that hold your uterus (see page 417). The pain usually lasts several minutes before going away, but it's not harmful. It's a good idea, however, to discuss any continuous pain with your care provider.

Urinary tract Because your urine flow remains slow, you remain at continued risk of developing a urinary tract infection. You are urinating more often than normal because of your pregnancy. But if increased urination is accompanied by a burning sensation, pain, fever or a backache, you may have a urinary tract infection. Contact your care provider.

Bones, muscles and joints The ligaments supporting your abdomen are becoming more elastic, and the joints between your pelvic bones continue to soften and loosen. In addition, your lower spine is probably now curving backward to help balance your extra weight in the front. Together, these changes may cause you to experience some back pain.

Back pain can begin at any time during pregnancy, but it most commonly starts between the fifth and seventh months. You may find the pain to be a mere annoyance. However, if you had back problems before you became pregnant, the pain may be more severe and interfere with your daily activities. For more on back pain, see page 388.

EXERCISE OF THE MONTH

Wall slide with ball

Strengthen your lower body as well as your core for a solid, stable base throughout your pregnancy — and after, when you're chasing around a speedy baby.

1. Stand up straight with a fitness ball behind your back and against the wall and your feet shoulder-width apart.
2. Slide down the wall until you reach a 90-degree angle — a sitting position.
3. Slowly slide back up.
4. Repeat five to 10 times.

Vagina Vaginal discharge continues. The thin, white discharge is caused by the effects of hormones on the glands in your cervix and the skin of your vagina. It's normal in pregnancy and isn't a cause for concern. Contact your care provider, though, if you have vaginal discharge that's greenish or yellowish, strong-smelling, or accompanied by redness, itching and irritation of the vulva. These are signs and symptoms of a vaginal infection. Also contact your care provider if discharge is blood-tinged or associated with vaginal bleeding.

Skin You may continue to experience mild skin darkening on your face and around your nipples. Most of these changes are nothing to worry about. Moles may also change during pregnancy. However, if you have a new mole or a mole that has changed considerably in size, shape or appearance, contact your care provider.

Weight gain You'll probably gain about a pound a week this month, for a total of about 4 pounds. By the time you reach your 20th week, you may have gained about 10 pounds.

YOUR EMOTIONS

The fifth month may bring a sense of reality. Not only is your tummy continuing to grow in size, you can now feel baby move. That's really your child in there!

Baby on the move! Feeling your baby flip, kick or punch for the first time — usually by the 20th week of pregnancy — is a great source of wonder and reassurance for most women. Experiencing these movements is also a more pleasant reminder of being pregnant than the nausea and fatigue of early pregnancy. In time, your partner will be able to feel

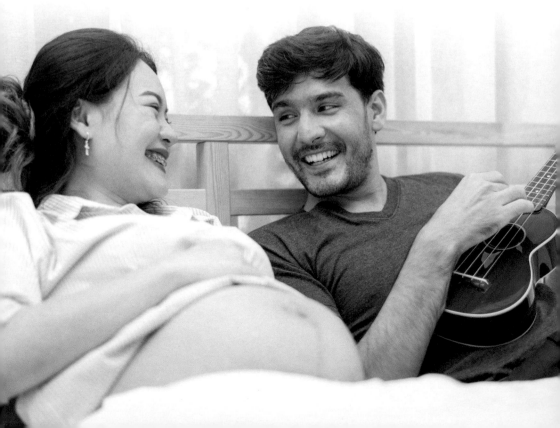

baby's movements, too, by placing a hand on your abdomen.

You may be wondering if you can communicate with your baby at this point. That's hard to know. But it certainly can't hurt to talk to your baby, or even introduce your favorite music (softly). As the baby's hearing continues to develop, he or she will become familiar with the voices heard most over the next few months.

PRENATAL CHECKUP

Your visit to your care provider this month will again focus on tracking baby's growth and watching for any problems with your own health. The usual steps will take place — checking your weight and blood pressure and measuring your fundal height. Your provider may also ask if you're feeling the baby move yet.

If your checkup is between 18 and 20 weeks, it will likely also include an ultrasound. This is an exciting benchmark for many parents, as your provider may be able to tell the baby's sex, depending on baby's position during the scan. (If you want to keep that information a surprise, remember to give your care team a heads-up!) During the ultrasound, your provider will also evaluate the baby's anatomy overall, the amount of amniotic fluid and baby's heart rate.

If your checkup is earlier this month, your provider may wait until early next month for the ultrasound.

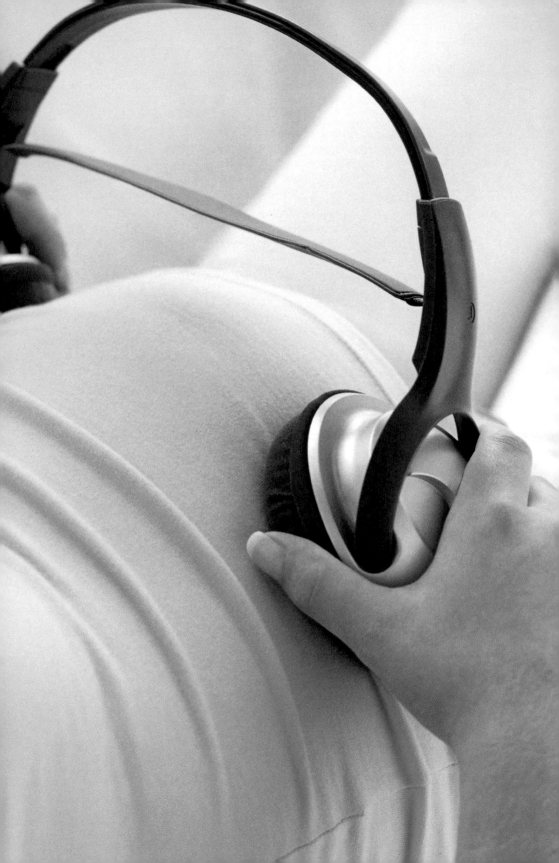

CHAPTER 9

Month 6: Weeks 21 to 24

My baby bump is now pretty evident to everyone, which is a nice change from people not knowing whether it's a baby or just general weight gain. It's always been important to me to stay in shape, so I'm trying to eat well and exercise and gain weight within a healthy range. Some days go better than others. I think the fact that I feel better now helps. I'm starting to get really excited, and I wonder a lot about what the baby will look like.

— Tessa

Two down and one to go — almost! This month marks the last full month of your second trimester. That means you're almost two-thirds of the way there. Your baby's growth is continuing at a more rapid pace than early in your pregnancy, as has been the case for the previous couple of months. In fact, if your little one was born at the end of this month, he or she would have about a 50 percent chance of survival. The odds get better with each passing week as baby's lungs and other organs continue crucial development.

BABY'S GROWTH

While most of baby's organs are structurally developed or nearing development, baby is still quite small. But by the end of this month, he or she will finally pass the 1-pound mark!

Week 21 Your baby's digestive system is more developed this week and is functioning at a basic level. As baby swallows amniotic fluid each day, the digestive tract can now absorb small amounts of sugar from the fluid passing through. Any processing of the sugars, however, is only done as practice. Baby is still completely dependent on the placenta for his or her nourishment.

Also by this point, your baby's bone marrow is making blood cells. The fetal liver and spleen work along with the bone marrow to form the cells for baby's blood supply.

Week 22 The senses of taste and touch advance this week. Taste buds have been developing on your baby's tongue, and his or her brain and nerve endings are now mature enough to process the sensation of touch. If you could sneak a peek at your baby this week, you might see him or her experimenting with this newfound sense of touch — feeling his or her face, sucking a thumb, or touching other body parts.

Your baby's reproductive system is continuing to develop, too. If you're having a boy, this week his testes begin to descend from the abdomen down to the scrotum. If you're having a girl, her uterus and ovaries are now in place, and her vagina is developed. Your baby girl has already made all of the eggs she'll need for her own reproductive life.

By 22 weeks into your pregnancy, baby is about 7½ inches long from head to rump and weighs about 1 pound.

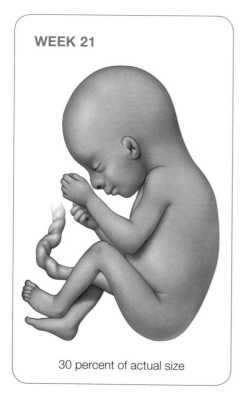

WEEK 21

30 percent of actual size

Week 23 Over the next few weeks, your baby's lungs develop rapidly, beginning preparation for life on the outside. The lungs are just beginning to produce a substance that lines the air sacs called surfactant. This substance allows the air sacs to inflate easily. It also keeps them from collapsing and sticking together when they deflate.

If your baby was born before this time, the lungs would have had little chance of working. Now it's possible that the lungs could function to some degree outside the womb. However, your baby would need a lot more surfactant to handle breathing air without help.

In addition, the blood vessels in your baby's lungs are growing and developing in preparation for breathing. He or she is making breathing movements, but these are just trial runs. Your baby is still receiving oxygen through your placenta. There's no air in the lungs until after birth.

Although your baby now looks like a baby, he or she is still slender and delicate looking, with little body fat and thin, nearly translucent skin. Later in your pregnancy, when fat production catches up to skin development, your baby will grow into this skin and will look more like an infant.

Babies born at 23 weeks can sometimes survive if they receive the appropriate medical care in a neonatal intensive care unit. But complications are common and usually serious. On the bright side, the long-term outlook for premature babies is improving each year as knowledge in the field of neonatal medicine continues to expand. But there's no doubt that at this age, baby is far better off staying in the uterus, if at all possible.

Week 24 This week your baby is beginning to get a sense of whether he or she is upside down or right-side up inside your uterus. That's because your baby's inner ear, which controls balance in the body, is now developed.

By the 24th week of your pregnancy, your baby is around 8½ inches long and weighs about 1½ pounds. Babies born at 24 weeks have a greater than 50-50 chance of survival, and the odds get better with every passing week. Still, complications are frequent and serious.

YOUR BODY CHANGES

This month, baby's kicks may be much stronger than the fluttery, butterflies-in-the-stomach feeling of last month.

What's happening and where During the first five months of your pregnancy, the level of the hormone progesterone was slightly higher than the level of estrogen. This month your estrogen level is catching up. At 21 or 22 weeks, the two hormones will be at about the same level.

Your heart and circulatory system Your blood pressure will probably continue to stay lower than normal this month. After your 24th week, it will begin to return to where it was before you were pregnant. This is because your body continues to make more blood this month, filling your very relaxed blood vessels. Production of red blood cells should be catching up to production of plasma.

You may continue to experience nasal congestion, nosebleeds and bleeding gums, due to increased blood flow to your nasal passages and gums.

Your respiratory system To accommodate your increasing lung capacity, your rib cage is enlarging. By the time your baby is born, the distance around your rib cage will have expanded by 2 to 3 inches. After your child is born, it will return to its pre-pregnancy size.

Baby is also pushing up on your diaphragm. However, the expansion of your chest diameter has more than compensated for this compression. You may still breathe slightly faster, but any shortness of breath has probably lessened.

Breasts Your breasts may now be ready to produce milk. You may see tiny droplets of watery or yellowish fluid appearing on your nipples, even this early. This early milk is called colostrum and is loaded with active, infection-fighting antibodies from your body. If you breast-feed, colostrum will be your baby's food for the first few days after birth.

Blood vessels in your breasts continue to become more visible, too, showing through your skin as pink or blue lines.

Uterus This month, perhaps around your 22nd week of pregnancy, your uterus may begin practicing for labor and delivery. It starts exercising its muscle mass to build strength for the big job ahead. These warm-up contractions are called Braxton Hicks contractions. They're occasional, painless contractions that feel like a squeezing sensation near the top of your uterus or in your lower abdomen and groin.

Braxton Hicks contractions are also called false labor. That's because they're very different from the contractions involved in true labor. Braxton Hicks contractions are irregular in frequency and vary in length and intensity. True labor contractions follow a pattern, growing longer, stronger and closer together.

That said, it can be easy to mistake Braxton Hicks contractions for the real thing. Contact your care provider if you're having contractions that concern you, especially if they become painful or if you have more than six in an hour. The biggest difference between true labor and Braxton Hicks contractions is the effect on your cervix. With Braxton Hicks contractions, your cervix doesn't change. With true labor, the cervix begins to open (dilate) and thin out (efface). You may need to see your care provider to determine whether the contractions are the real thing.

For more information on Braxton Hicks contractions see page 394.

Urinary tract You continue to be at risk of developing a urinary tract infection. Slowed urine flow is caused by your growing uterus and flabbier muscle tone in the ureters, which carry urine from your kidneys to your bladder. If you think you may have a urinary tract infection, contact your care provider.

Bones, muscles and joints The ligaments supporting your abdomen continue to stretch, and the joints between your pelvic bones continue to soften and loosen in preparation for childbirth. In addition, your lower spine is curving backward to help you balance the weight of your growing baby. Together, these changes can cause back and hip pain.

Vagina You may still experience thin, white vaginal discharge with little or no odor. If your vaginal discharge is greenish or yellowish, strong-smelling or accompanied by redness, itching or irritation of the vulva, you may have a vaginal infection. Contact your care provider.

Weight gain You'll probably gain about a pound a week this month, for a total of about 4 pounds. You may gain 1½ pounds one week and only half a pound the next,

IS IT FALSE LABOR OR TRUE LABOR?

Contraction characteristic	False labor (Braxton Hicks contractions)	True labor
Frequency of contractions	• Irregular • Do not become closer together	• Regular pattern • Grow closer together
Length and intensity of contractions	• Vary • Usually weak • Don't get stronger	• At least 30 seconds long at onset • Become longer • Become stronger
How contractions change with activity	• Usually stop if you walk, rest or change positions	• Won't go away no matter what • May grow stronger with activity, such as walking
Location of contractions	• Centered in lower abdomen and groin	• Wrap around from back to abdomen • Radiate throughout your lower back and high on abdomen

Pelvic tilt with ball

This version of a pelvic tilt is a safe way to strengthen your abdominal muscles in pregnancy.

1. Sit on the floor with your back leaning against a fitness ball, your feet on the floor and your arms at your sides.
2. Push the small of your back upward and hold for several seconds. Return to the starting position.
3. Repeat five to 10 times.

but that's not cause for concern. As long as your weight gain is remaining relatively stable, without any sudden increases or decreases, you're doing great.

YOUR EMOTIONS

You may find (or your partner may tell you!) that your mood swings are improving. This may be because hormone production is occurring at a more even pace. You're also becoming more accustomed to the changes occurring inside you. However, as your due date looms a little closer, you may start to experience new fears.

Confronting your fears This month you may begin to worry about the process of giving birth. In fact, you may have

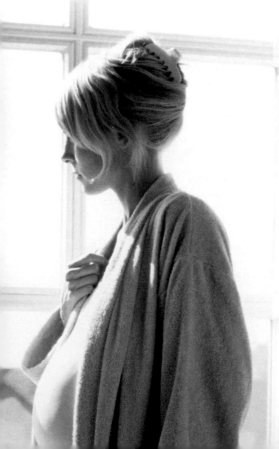

been having these fears for a while: "What if I don't make it to the hospital in time? How will I cope with baring myself in front of strangers? What if I lose control during labor? What if there's something wrong with the baby?"

Your partner is probably pondering some of these same questions. Often, parents-to-be have the same concerns as their partners but don't admit it. Each may think he or she must be strong for the other. Your partner may also be worried about something happening to you during labor and delivery.

Take time to sit down and make a list of your fears, and ask your partner to do the same. Then compare lists and share these concerns with your care provider. Sharing helps. When you share your fears, they have less power over you.

Being intimate If you're like many women, you may be more interested in sex now than you were earlier in your pregnancy. You may even be more interested in sex now than you were before you became pregnant. This may be because you feel better, are sleeping better and you have more energy. Enjoy this feeling while it lasts — and before your baby arrives, which will likely affect your sex life. This heightened sexuality is by no means universal, and it's possible you may not feel it at all. As you enter the final months of pregnancy, you may find your desire for sex waning again.

PRENATAL CHECKUP

By now, your visits are probably starting to get pretty routine, but that's OK. Routine visits often mean everything is going well and progressing on schedule. As during your last visit, your care provider will likely check the size of your uterus by determining the fundal height — the distance from the top (fundus) of your uterus to your pubic bone. This month your fundal height will probably be about 21 to 24 centimeters — roughly equal to the number of weeks of your pregnancy.

In addition to performing the fundal height test, your care provider will check your weight and blood pressure and evaluate your baby's heart rate. Your care provider may also ask you about any signs and symptoms you may be experiencing. And if you didn't have a standard or anatomy ultrasound late last month, you'll likely have one in the first week or two of this month.

CHILDBIRTH CLASSES

If this is your first pregnancy, you may get a little nervous — maybe even scared — when you start thinking ahead to labor and delivery. That's natural. After all, you've never been through it before!

So how do you help calm those nerves? Go to class. If you haven't signed up yet for childbirth classes, it's a good time to do so. Childbirth classes help you and your partner prepare for labor and childbirth. Such classes are available at most hospitals and birthing centers, so ask about them at one of your prenatal visits. Typically, the classes are offered as one- to two-hour sessions over the course of several weeks or as full-day sessions that take place over one or two weekends.

You'll likely learn about signs of labor, pain relief options during labor, birthing positions, postnatal care and care of a newborn, including information on breast-feeding. At these classes you'll also learn about what will happen to your body during labor and birth, which can help you feel positive rather than fearful about the process. Especially if you're a first-time parent, you may find that childbirth classes help calm your fears and answer many of your questions.

In addition, as part of your classes, you may be given a tour of the facility where you will have your baby, so when the big day arrives, you'll know where to go and have a better idea of what will happen. You'll also likely meet other expectant couples who have questions and concerns similar to yours, which can be comforting. If you plan to have your partner or another loved one (other than a doula) act as a labor coach during labor and delivery, consider having him or her attend childbirth classes with you.

Different types Some childbirth education classes cover specific types of births, such as C-section birth, vaginal birth after C-section (VBAC) and multiple births. Refresher courses are also available for parents who simply want to review the basics.

Other classes are more general in nature, or they focus on specific methods of childbirth. For example:

▶ *Lamaze.* The goal of Lamaze is to increase confidence in your ability to give birth. Lamaze classes help you understand how to cope with pain in ways that both facilitate labor and promote comfort — including focused breathing, movement and massage. This method is based on the idea that a woman's inner wisdom guides her through childbirth.

▶ *Bradley.* The Bradley Method emphasizes that birth is a natural process. You're encouraged to trust your body, focusing on diet and exercise throughout pregnancy. You're taught to manage labor through deep breathing, a variety

THINKING AHEAD: FINDING A CARE PROVIDER FOR YOUR BABY

It's a good idea to decide who you want to provide health care to your baby before your child is born. You'll have someone you can call with any questions regarding newborn care — and most first-time parents have questions. If you don't already have a care provider in mind, ask for recommendations from friends or family members with children. Your own care provider also may be an excellent referral source.

Types of providers Family physicians, pediatricians, pediatric nurse practitioners, and pediatric physician assistants are all qualified to provide health care for children.

Family physicians Family physicians provide health care to people of all ages, including children. They are trained in adult and pediatric medicine. A family physician can see your child from babyhood all the way through adulthood. Family physicians take care of most medical problems. Also, if the rest of your family sees the same physician, your doctor will gain an overall perspective of your family. If you already have a family doctor you trust, ask whether he or she will see infants.

Pediatricians Many parents choose a pediatrician for their child's health. Pediatricians specialize in the care of children from infancy through adolescence. After medical school, they go through a three-year residency program. Some pediatricians receive further training in subspecialties such as allergies, infectious disease, cardiology and psychiatry. A pediatrician can be particularly helpful if your child has a health condition or needs special medical attention.

Nurse practitioners and physician assistants Nurse practitioners are registered nurses with advanced training in a specialized area of medicine, such as pediatrics or family health. After nursing school, a nurse practitioner must go through a formal education program in his or her specialty field. A physician assistant must complete a master's level physician assistant program and may pursue additional, specialized training through a postgraduate fellowship or residency. A pediatric nurse practitioner or physician assistant focuses on caring for infants, children and teens. Most of these midlevel care providers can prescribe medications and order medical tests. They work closely with physicians and medical specialists.

Issues to consider No matter what type of provider you choose, it's important that you feel comfortable with that person. You may wish to meet with several care providers before having your baby. Factors you may wish to explore include:
- What are the provider's qualifications?
- Do you like his or her bedside manner?
- Did the individual answer your questions to your satisfaction?
- How accessible is your care provider, either by phone or by appointment?
- If you're in a managed care plan, is the provider part of the plan's network?

of relaxation techniques, and the support of your partner or labor coach.

▶ *Mindfulness-Based Childbirth and Parenting (MBCP).* As the name implies, this newer method is driven by the concept of mindfulness — paying attention in the present moment without judgment. MBCP reframes childbirth as a transformation, teaching you to notice the sensations of labor pain apart from its effects on your outlook and to notice the calm moments among the unpleasant ones. Recent research found that this method may help women cope with labor pain more effectively than traditional methods not involving mindfulness, with lower use of some pain medications. It could possibly even help to prevent postpartum depression. An intensive, shorter childbirth-focused class based on the MBCP method may also be available, called Mind in Labor.

Many other classes borrow elements from these methods. In addition, you may find classes on other alternative approaches to childbirth, including hypnotherapy and water birth.

What to look for Look for a class taught by a certified childbirth educator. This may be a nurse, midwife or other certified professional. The classes should be small, with no more than eight to 10 couples, to facilitate discussion and allow for personalized instruction. The classes should also be comprehensive, addressing all aspects of labor and delivery, as well as newborn care. Be sure to ask about the cost as well. Childbirth education classes are often recommended near the sixth or seventh month of pregnancy — but anytime before you go into labor is helpful.

In addition, first time parents may want to look for separate classes or clinics that offer more-detailed information on topics that will be helpful after baby arrives. Check for classes near you on baby-care basics, breast-feeding, and car seat safety and installation.

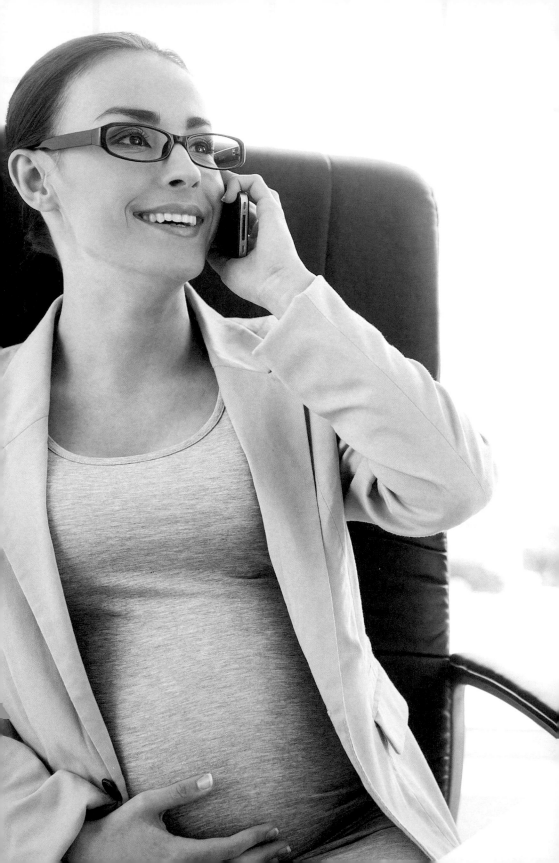

CHAPTER 10

Month 7: Weeks 25 to 28

During our pregnancy, we knew virtually nothing about babies. So we studied. A lot. I memorized a chart describing different baby cries, so I would know when baby was hungry, had a dirty diaper or was just plain bored. I could tell you the difference between types of diaper rashes before I even changed a diaper. Also, what brand of stroller I had really mattered to me. All the hip moms had it, and I wanted one. But it turns out, your child doesn't care about your hip stroller or your funky, awesome changing pad. If you want to get them, fine. But they're for you. Your baby only needs to be comfortable, well-fed and, most of all, loved.

— Patty

You are now in the homestretch of your pregnancy — the word *stretch* being the key! Over the next three to four months, your baby will do most of his or her growing in size before entering the outside world. And, yes, your tummy will continue to stretch as baby makes things even more crowded in there.

BABY'S GROWTH

This month, your little boy or girl will add more body fat, which will make his or her skin look more smooth and less wrinkled. The skin will also begin to take on a little more color.

Week 25 At this time, your baby's hands are now fully developed, complete with miniature fingernails and the ability to curl his or her fingers into a tiny fist. This week, he or she is probably using these hands to discover different body parts. Your little one is exploring the environment and structures inside your uterus, including the umbilical cord. The nerve connections to your baby's hands have a long way to go, though. She or he won't yet be able to grasp a big toe, except by accident.

Week 26 Your baby's eyebrows and eyelashes are now well-formed, and the hair on his or her head is longer and more plentiful. Your baby still looks red and wrinkled, but more fat is accumulating under the skin with each passing day. As your baby continues to gain weight over the next few months, this wrinkly suit of skin will become a better fit.

Your baby's footprints and fingerprints are now formed. And all the components that make up the eyes have developed, but your baby probably won't open his or her eyes for about two more weeks. By 26 weeks, your baby weighs between 1½ and 2 pounds.

Week 27 By the 27th week, your baby looks like a thinner, smaller, redder version of what he or she will look like at birth. Baby's lungs, liver and immune system aren't yet fully mature, but they're getting close. If birth were to occur this week, your baby's chance of survival would be good — about 94 percent of babies born at this age survive. However, babies born this early may still face significant health problems, including difficulty breathing, heart conditions, anemia, and physical and intellectual disabilities.

Baby may start recognizing your voice this week, as well as your partner's. But it's probably hard to hear clearly, given that his or her ears are covered with vernix, the thick, fatty coating that protects the skin from becoming chapped or scratched. It's also hard for your baby to hear through the amniotic fluid in your uterus — similar to the difficulty in hearing under water.

At 27 weeks, baby is now three to four times as long as he or she was 12 weeks into your pregnancy.

Week 28 Your baby's eyes, which have been sealed shut for the last few months, may begin to open and close this week. If you could sneak a peek at your baby, you might now be able to determine the color of his or her eyes. But in many cases, baby's eyes change in color during the first six months of life, especially if his or her eyes are blue or gray-blue at birth. So, the color they are now may not reflect what they'll be later in life.

Your baby's brain also continues to develop and expand rapidly this week. In addition, he or she continues to accumulate layers of fat underneath the skin.

Your baby is now sleeping and waking on a regular schedule, but this schedule isn't like that of an adult or even of a newborn. Baby probably sleeps for only 20 to 30 minutes at a time. You're most likely to notice baby's movements when you're sitting or lying down.

By the 28th week of your pregnancy, the end of your seventh month, your baby is about 10 inches long, crown to rump, and weighs 2 to 3 pounds.

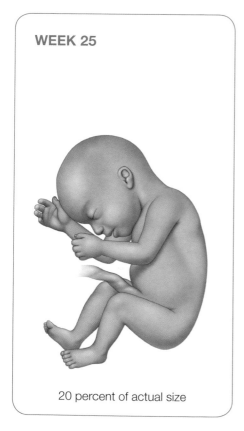

WEEK 25

20 percent of actual size

YOUR BODY CHANGES

As you watch your belly get bigger, you may wonder if there's any room left for your womb to grow more. Yes, there is — it's amazing what the body can do.

What's happening and where As your uterus expands further upward, your baby will become increasingly active, especially in the second half of the month.

Heart and circulatory system Your blood pressure may begin to increase, gradually returning to where it was before you became pregnant.

In addition, you may experience heart palpitations, episodes of fluttering or pounding in your chest — as if your heart has skipped a beat. As your uterus enlarges, it may impede the return of blood to your heart. This sensation may worry you, but it usually doesn't signify anything serious and it often lessens later in pregnancy. Still, if you experience this feeling, tell your care provider, especially if you also have chest pain or shortness of breath.

Respiratory system Your lung capacity continues to increase this month, stimulated by the hormone progesterone. This respiratory change allows your blood to carry in more oxygen and carry out more carbon dioxide than normal. As a result, you may continue to breathe slightly faster and experience some shortness of breath.

Digestive system The movement of food through your digestive system remains slow, and your expanding uterus is crowding and pressing on your intestines. As a result, you'll likely continue to experience heartburn or constipation or both.

Breasts You may notice the development of tiny, bump-like skin glands encircling your areolas. This is another way that your body is preparing for breast-feeding. When the time comes, these glands will secrete oils to moisturize and soften the skin around your nipples and areolas. This helps keep your nipples from cracking and chafing as you breast-feed.

Uterus This month your uterus will reach the midway point between your navel and breasts. Eventually, it will occupy the area from your pubic bone to the bottom of your rib cage.

Baby will likely become more active this month, particularly in the second half of the month. For many babies, their most active time is between 27 and 32 weeks. They are now big enough to pack a punch, and they still have room to do so. With the increased activity, you may have trouble distinguishing your baby's kicks and punches from false contractions or even true contractions. Remember a couple of things. False labor contractions (Braxton Hicks) have no predictable rhythm. They vary in length and strength and occur irregularly. True labor contractions follow a pattern — they get longer, stronger and closer together (see page 395). If you're having contractions that concern you, contact your care provider.

Urinary tract Your urine flow continues to be slow this month, due to your expanding uterus and relaxed muscles in the tubes carrying urine from the kidneys to the bladder (ureters). As a result, you're at continued risk of developing a urinary tract infection. Talk with your care provider if you're urinating more frequently and also experiencing burning, pain, fever, or a change in the odor or color of your urine.

Bones, muscles and joints The ligaments supporting your pelvic bones become even more elastic this month. Ultimately, this will make it easier for your pelvis to expand during childbirth so that your baby can pass through. Now, however, lack of usual support from these ligaments increases your risk of back strain. Joints in your pelvis may hurt with this newfound flexibility as well. You'll feel the pain in the middle-front of your pelvis or on either side of your back.

Vagina Vaginal discharge may increase. If it's thin and white with little or no odor, there's no cause for concern.

Weight gain This month you'll probably continue to gain around a pound a week. By this point, most of the weight you're gaining isn't fat. It stems from baby's weight gain, a growing placenta, additional amniotic fluid and fluid accumulation in your body tissues.

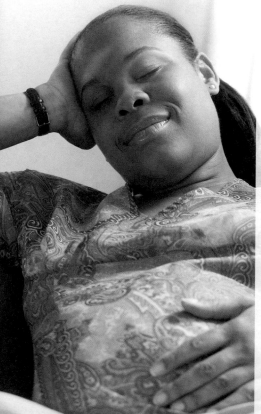

YOUR EMOTIONS

From now until the day your baby arrives is an exciting time, but it can also be a bit stressful. You may be busy purchasing supplies, finishing baby's room, attending childbirth classes and making more-frequent visits to your care provider. Plus, the last three months of pregnancy can bring new physical demands on your body.

Enjoy a little break Slow down, sit back and relax — while you can. Make an effort to enjoy this month of your pregnancy, before the craziness and discomforts of the final months begin. You might want to write down your thoughts in a journal, play soft music or talk soothingly to your baby. Take photos so that you can show your baby what you looked like when he or she was "under construction." Do whatever works for you to revel in the emotions and sensations of being pregnant.

PRENATAL CHECKUP

At this month's visit, your care provider may be able to tell you whether your baby is positioned headfirst or feet- or rump-first in your uterus. Babies in the feet- or rump-first position are in what's called the breech position. However, your baby still has lots of time to change position and probably will. So don't be worried if you hear your baby is lying breech.

At this point in your pregnancy, you need to be alert to the possibility of pre-term labor — contractions that begin opening (dilating) your cervix before the 37th week. Babies born this early usually have a low birth weight — less than 5½ pounds — which can put them at risk of

EXERCISE OF THE MONTH

Leg lift
Strengthen your lower body with this simple move.

1. Kneel on your hands and knees with your hands shoulder-width apart.
2. Lift your right knee and then straighten your right leg behind you so that it's parallel to the floor. Don't arch your back.
3. Repeat five to 10 times on both sides.

LOSING YOUR PERSONAL SPACE

An interesting thing seems to happen to you when you're pregnant — or, rather, it happens to everyone else around you. Personal boundaries seem to melt away. You have no more personal bubble. Your belly may become fair game for everyone, from relatives to complete strangers.

Remember: Pregnant or not, you get to determine who's allowed to touch your body. Maybe you're comfortable with extended family members reaching out to feel the baby kick. But many women cringe when people outside the family go in for a belly rub with no invitation (and no hesitation). You'll likely get very good at noticing the telltale signs: rapidly approaching, hands outstretched, the words "Oh, you don't mind," uttered with a smile after the stranger's hands are already patting your tummy. If you don't want the touch but aren't comfortable speaking up (or can't do it in time), you may try to cover your belly with your own hands first, as a gentle reminder that it's your own body.

Another common phenomenon is the loss of discretion or sensitivity for your feelings around body image. It can lead friends, family, neighbors and complete strangers to comment on how big you are or aren't. Some people might feel free to comment on the amount of weight they think you've gained. If it's a woman who has been pregnant before, she may think of it as a way to connect over the shared experience. Still, you have the right to keep that personal health information private.

A third part to this unique experience involves all the women you know telling you about difficult pregnancy, childbirth and postnatal experiences they or a friend of theirs had. However well-meaning the storyteller may be, don't mistake a tale of a 92-hour labor as a forecast for your personal experience. The same goes for stories of difficult breast-feeding experiences. Take everything with a grain of salt. If you have concerns about certain potential challenges or complications, talk with your care provider.

And after your pregnancy, keep in mind how these encounters made you feel. Another woman in the midst of the wonder and anxiety of pregnancy might really appreciate your sensitivity and a tale of a positive experience.

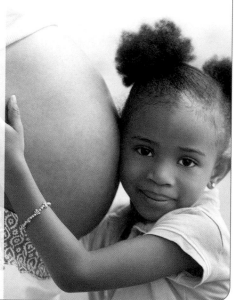

health problems. Signs and symptoms of preterm labor include:

- Uterine contractions that feel like abdominal tightening
- Contractions accompanied by low back pain or a feeling of heaviness in your lower pelvis and upper thighs
- Light spotting or bleeding, watery fluid leaking from your vagina, or thick discharge tinged with blood

At this month's checkup, you'll typically also have a glucose challenge test to check for gestational diabetes, a type of diabetes that develops in some women during pregnancy. In addition, if you're rhesus (Rh) factor negative, you'll likely be tested for Rh antibodies and may receive your first injection of Rh immune globulin (RhIg).

Glucose challenge testing This testing is usually done sometime during weeks 24 through 28 of your pregnancy, although your care provider may perform the test earlier if you have certain risk factors. If earlier testing had normal results, your provider may repeat the test this month. For the test, you drink a full glass of a sugary solution, and then after an hour, blood is drawn from a vein in your arm so that your blood glucose level can be checked. If the results are abnormal, you'll likely have to come back for a second test.

If you need the second test, you'll be asked to fast overnight. When you arrive at your care provider's office, you'll drink another, more concentrated glucose solution. Over the next three hours, your blood will be drawn hourly, yielding four different blood glucose measurements: fasting (before drinking the solution) and one, two and three hours after starting the test. Among women whose first glucose test result was abnormal, studies show that only a small percentage are

diagnosed with gestational diabetes after follow-up testing.

If you are diagnosed with gestational diabetes (see page 439), you'll need to carefully control your blood glucose for the remainder of your pregnancy. This will include daily blood sugar monitoring.

Rh antibodies testing Rh factor is a type of protein found on the surface of red blood cells. More than 85 percent of people have it and are known to be Rh positive. Those who don't have it are Rh negative. This is the "positive" or "negative" part of your blood type.

When you're not pregnant, your Rh status has no effect on your health unless you need a blood transfusion. During pregnancy, if you're Rh positive, there's no cause for concern. But if you're Rh negative and your baby is Rh positive — which can happen if your partner is Rh positive — Rh incompatibility may result. Your body sees the Rh protein from your baby's blood as a foreign substance and makes antibodies to destroy it. This can be more of a cause for concern in subsequent pregnancies. (See page 431.)

If you are Rh negative, this month you may receive an injection of Rh immune globulin (RhIg). The RhIg coats any Rh positive cells that are floating in your bloodstream, preventing them from being recognized as foreign, so antibodies won't form. Think of it as a pre-emptive strike against possible future complications.

Tdap vaccine booster The Centers for Disease Control and Prevention (CDC) recommends that women receive a tetanus, diphtheria and acellular pertussis (Tdap) booster vaccine between weeks 27 and 36 of each pregnancy. This vaccine can protect you from infection during and after pregnancy. Importantly, it also helps you pass protective antibodies to your

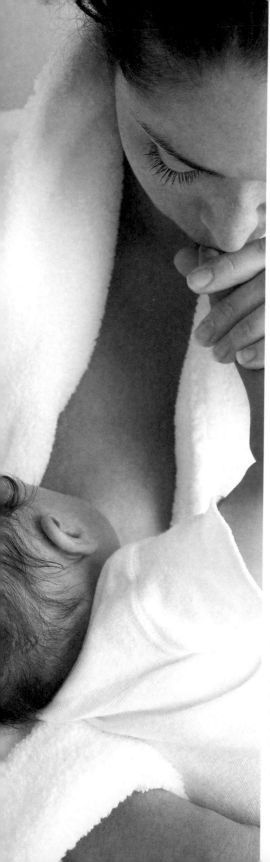

baby before birth. Whooping cough (pertussis) is particularly dangerous to newborns, who can't safely be vaccinated against the disease until two months of age. A booster shot in pregnancy can protect your baby during those first critical months of life.

THE BREAST OR BOTTLE QUESTION

If you haven't come to a decision already, it's probably time to think about how you plan to feed your baby, once he or she is born. Breast-feeding is the optimal way to nourish a newborn — it provides numerous benefits for both you and baby. And Mayo Clinic experts encourage you to breast-feed. However, depending on your circumstances, certain factors may lead you to consider formula-feeding.

A tough decision for some women
Some women know right from the start what they'll do — breast-feed or bottle-feed with formula — while others struggle with the decision. If you're one of those who aren't certain, start to do some research and explore your options. Even if you haven't made a final decision when baby arrives, it's better to be familiar with the health and lifestyle implications of each choice to help you make the call.

If you feel anxious about breast-feeding, you're certainly not alone. You might consider taking a prenatal class on the topic, taught by a lactation consultant or another trained provider. A focused class can help you learn about getting started, establishing your milk supply, and recognizing success or hunger cues. It will also typically address common issues.

If you think you prefer to formula-feed your baby, make sure you've learned

QUESTION & ANSWER

Are sagging breasts inevitable after breast-feeding? I'm worried about the toll breast-feeding may take on my breasts.

It's normal to wonder how breast-feeding will affect your breasts, but take heart. Research has shown that breast-feeding doesn't negatively affect breast shape or volume.

In fact, pregnancy itself may be the culprit. During pregnancy, the ligaments that support your breasts may stretch as your breasts get fuller and heavier. This stretching may contribute to sagging breasts after pregnancy — whether or not you breast-feed your baby. Sagging breasts may be more noticeable with each subsequent pregnancy, especially if you have large breasts. But other factors also contribute to sagging breasts, including aging and smoking — both of which reduce skin elasticity. Being overweight can have a similar effect.

Breast milk is the ideal food for most babies, so don't let a fear of sagging breasts stop you from breast-feeding. To maintain the appearance of your breasts at any stage of life, make healthy lifestyle choices. Include physical activity in your daily routine. Eat a healthy diet. And if you smoke, ask your doctor to help you quit.

about breast-feeding and its benefits before solidifying your decision. Chapter 22 of this book can help you learn more about your options. The chapter covers a variety of issues and topics related to breast-feeding. It also provides information on formula-feeding.

For some women who prefer formula-feeding, or who can't breast-feed for medical reasons, forgoing the breast for the bottle can bring tremendous feelings of conflict. They may feel that they're not being good mothers or putting the needs of their children first. If you're among this group, try to let go of these thoughts. Don't shower yourself in guilt. For those women deciding between methods of feeding, the best thing to do is learn about both, and then take comfort in knowing that you made an informed decision.

If after reading through Chapter 22, you're still undecided about what to do,

here's a suggestion: Give breast-feeding a try. Make it part of your birth plan so that you'll receive breast-feeding support after you deliver, and consider asking your care provider for a lactation consultant referral. This specialist may provide additional support if you need it after returning home. Try to breast-feed for a few weeks. If it doesn't work for you, you can always switch to a bottle, or even bottle-feed your baby with breast milk. This way, you'll have the satisfaction of knowing that you gave it a shot. And who knows, maybe the experience will be very different from what you imagined.

Breast-feeding is a wonderful way to bond with your baby, and it has been shown to enhance babies' well-being in numerous ways. Of course, you can lovingly bond with your baby without breast-feeding — it's just one more natural tool toward that end.

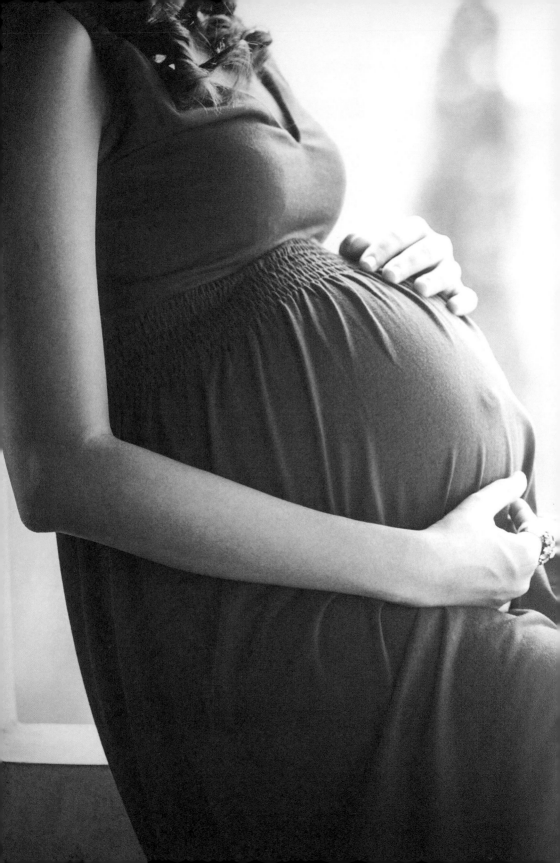

CHAPTER 11

Month 8: Weeks 29 to 32

At this stage in my pregnancy, I've been feeling pretty good. I usually have motivation and energy for about two days, but by the third day I'm finding that I need to slow down and take it easy or take a nap. I've also noticed lately that I feel very stretched and uncomfortable after I eat, even though I'm not full. I found out at a recent appointment that the baby likes to lie horizontally, and because baby is getting bigger and taking up more room, that may be contributing to the extra-stretched feeling.

— Lori

Now that your due date is getting closer, your pregnancy may start to get a little uncomfortable, if it hasn't already. During month eight you may experience leg cramps, pelvic pressure, increased back pain, swollen ankles and hemorrhoids — all common occurrences as baby starts growing at a more rapid rate. On the bright side, these aches and pains are an indication that you're soon going to see that little miracle.

BABY'S GROWTH

During these last couple of months, your baby is working on the finishing touches — the remaining steps that need to occur before he or she is fully developed.

Week 29 With the major body systems in place, your baby is now gaining weight more quickly. As space becomes tighter, you may not feel the baby's sharp jabs and punches as much as you did earlier. Baby is also developing a sleep and wake cycle. During periods of sleep, baby will be quiet.

Week 30 As baby gains weight, he or she is also adding layers of fat. From now until delivery, baby will gain about a half-pound a week. Baby may also begin practicing breathing movements this week by moving his or her diaphragm in a repeating rhythm. These movements may give your baby the hiccups. You may occasionally notice the hiccups as a slight twitching in your uterus. It may feel like little spasms.

At 30 weeks into your pregnancy, your baby weighs a little over 3 pounds and is about 10½ inches long, crown to rump.

Week 31 During week 31, baby's reproductive system continues to develop. If your baby is a boy, his testicles are moving from their location near the kidneys through the groin on their way into the scrotum. If your baby is a girl, her clitoris is now relatively prominent. The labia are still small, though, and don't yet cover it.

Your baby's lungs are now more developed, but they're not yet fully ready for life outside. If you go into preterm labor this early, or before 37 weeks of pregnancy, your care provider will likely give you a steroid injection to help baby's lungs mature. Babies that are born this week will still need care in a neonatal intensive care unit.

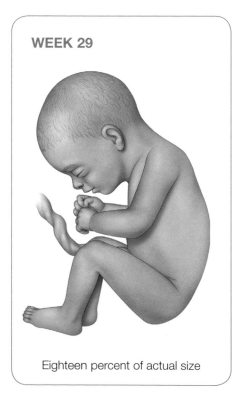

WEEK 29

Eighteen percent of actual size

Week 32 Lanugo, the layer of soft, downy hair on your baby's skin, starts to fall off this week. Baby will lose most of his or her lanugo over the next few weeks. Right after your baby's birth, you may see some remnants on his or her shoulders or back.

Some women may notice a change in baby's movements this week, now that he or she has grown to the point of being crowded inside your uterus. Although your baby is moving around just as much, kicks and other movements may seem less forceful. For many women, this change becomes more apparent about week 34.

You may want to check on your baby's movements from time to time, especially if you think you've noticed decreased activity. To do this, sit down and keep a tally of how often you feel your baby move. Your baby's kicks or movements may seem a little muffled, given the space constraints inside your uterus. If you notice fewer than 10 movements in two hours, contact your care provider.

By 32 weeks, your baby weighs about 4 pounds and is almost 11½ inches long, crown to rump. If you delivered at this point, the risk of your baby developing life-threatening complications would be much lower than in earlier weeks.

YOUR BODY CHANGES

This month, your uterus will continue its expansion toward the bottom of your rib cage, creating a new set of physical changes and signs and symptoms. You may also find that you tire more easily.

What's happening and where One thing you may notice this month is a change in your hair. It may seem fuller and healthier-looking. This is due to a change in your hair's growth cycle. Normally, hair on your scalp grows about a half-inch each month for two to seven years. It then goes into a resting phase, stops growing and eventually falls out. During pregnancy, thanks to hormonal changes, your hair tends to remain in the growing phase longer. Because fewer hairs fall out each day, you have a fuller head of hair.

Once your baby is born, many hair follicles will transition to the resting phase, and you'll lose hair each day. For a few months, your hair may even feel thinner. Usually, your hair will eventually return to normal.

Heart and circulatory system Your body is continuing to make more blood than normal, and your heart is pumping it faster. Unfortunately, the changes in your circulatory system that support your growing baby may be causing some new and uncomfortable side effects for you. As

CHANGES IN BABY'S MOVEMENT

Most pregnant women get to know their baby's patterns of movement and are attuned to changes in the frequency or intensity of those movements. You may notice a slight decrease in your baby's activity in the last few days before birth. In late pregnancy, the number of fetal movements you perceive often declines gradually. The baby has less room to move around in the uterus, especially after his or her head drops into the pelvis.

In addition, babies establish movement and sleep patterns as the pregnancy progresses, and you may notice times of increased or decreased activity for periods of one to three hours. Although a baby who isn't very active in the womb may be perfectly healthy, decreased fetal movement can be a sign that something is wrong. A significant drop in fetal activity in the last trimester of pregnancy may indicate a problem with the umbilical cord or placenta.

Self-care for decreased baby movement If you're concerned about the baby's activity, take a break from other activities. Sit down and drink a glass of juice or cold water. Concentrate on your baby's movements. In most cases, you'll find your baby is more active than you realized. Most babies will move at least four times each hour.

When to seek medical help Contact your care provider if you're worried about a decrease in your baby's movement. You may be asked when the last time was that you felt fetal movement or how many times you felt movement in the last couple of hours. Your care provider may want to check the condition of your baby.

Usually, everything is fine. If a problem is found, it's possible the baby may need to be delivered early, or other steps may need to be taken. Prompt action can prevent serious problems.

your veins become larger to accommodate your increased blood flow, they may protrude, and you may notice bluish or reddish lines beneath the surface of your skin, particularly on your legs and ankles.

Some pregnant women develop varicose veins, caused by weaknesses in the valves within the veins. They typically show up in the later months of pregnancy, when the veins in your legs have expanded and your uterus has grown to the point that it's putting increased pressure on the veins (see page 427). You may also develop spider veins. These tiny purplish or reddish spots with raised lines branching out from the center, like spider legs, are another consequence of increased blood circulation. You may notice them on your face, neck, upper chest or arms. They'll probably disappear a few weeks after your baby is born.

In addition, you may notice that your eyelids and face are becoming puffy, mostly in the morning. This, too, is the result of increased blood circulation.

One of the more unpleasant symptoms you may experience in pregnancy is hemorrhoids. These are varicose veins in your rectum that can be itchy and painful. They're caused by increased blood volume and increased pressure from your growing uterus. Constipation increases the risk. If you develop hemorrhoids, talk with your care provider. Eating a high-fiber diet, using over-the-counter topical products or applying an ice pack to the area may bring you relief.

Respiratory system Your diaphragm — the broad, flat muscle that lies under your lungs — is now pushed up and out of its normal place by your expanding uterus. As a result, you're probably feeling short of breath, as if you just can't get enough air. This may be a bit disconcerting for you, but there's no need to worry about your baby. Your lung capacity may be rearranged, but you're breathing more deeply. With each breath, you're still taking more air into your lungs than you did before you were pregnant.

Breasts Your breasts continue to grow this month, and they may begin to feel heavier. Over the course of your pregnancy, your growing breasts will account for about 1 to 3 pounds of the weight you gain. Only a small portion of this extra weight will be from fat. The majority of the weight you gain in your breasts will come from enlarged milk-producing glands and increased blood circulation.

Since you became pregnant, your pituitary gland has been making prolactin, one of the hormones that prepares and stimulates the production of milk from glands in your breasts. Over the next few weeks, you'll begin to make colostrum. This is the protein-laden milk that nourishes your baby during his or her first few days of life. If you haven't yet started to leak colostrum from your breasts, you may this month. However, some women don't leak any colostrum during pregnancy. It's not a sign of your body's ability to make milk for your baby.

Uterus Your uterus may continue to practice for labor and delivery by producing false labor (Braxton Hicks contractions). Remember, false labor contractions are sporadic, while true labor contractions follow a progressive pattern. True contractions get longer, stronger and closer together. If you're having contractions that concern you, contact your care provider, especially if they're painful or if you have six or more in an hour.

Urinary tract Given the increased pressure of your growing uterus on your bladder, don't be surprised if you leak

EXERCISE OF THE MONTH

Low back stretch

As your belly grows, this gentle stretch can help relieve tension from an arched lower back.

1. Get on your hands and knees with your head in line with your back.
2. Pull in your stomach, rounding your back slightly.
3. Hold the position for several seconds and then relax, keeping your back as flat as possible.
4. Repeat five to 10 times.

WATCHING OUT FOR PRETERM LABOR

The risk of preterm labor continues this month. Here's a reminder of the signs and symptoms to watch for:

- Uterine contractions — possibly painless — that feel like a tightening in your abdomen
- Contractions accompanied by low back pain or a feeling of heaviness in your lower pelvis and upper thighs
- Changes in vaginal discharge, such as light spotting or bleeding, watery fluid leaking from your vagina, or a thick discharge tinged with blood

If you notice at least six contractions in an hour (10 minutes apart or less), contact your care provider or your hospital, even if the contractions aren't painful. This is especially important if you have vaginal bleeding along with abdominal cramps or pain.

urine this month, especially when you laugh, cough or sneeze. This is one of the most annoying side effects of pregnancy, but it won't last forever. It generally disappears after baby is born.

You continue to be at risk of developing a urinary tract infection, too. If you're urinating more often than normal, experiencing burning on urination, or have a fever, abdominal pain or backache, contact your care provider. These could be signs and symptoms of a urinary tract infection and shouldn't be ignored.

Vagina If you have bright red bleeding from your vagina at any time this month, contact your care provider immediately. The bleeding could be a sign of placental abruption, a condition in which the placenta prematurely separates from the wall of the uterus before delivery. Bright red bleeding may also be a sign of an abnormal placenta location (placenta previa; usually diagnosed through ultrasound at 18 to 20 weeks), or the bleeding may be associated with preterm labor. These conditions all require emergency medical care.

Bones, muscles and joints In your pelvic area, the joints between the bones are becoming more relaxed. This is a necessary preparation for childbirth, but it may cause hip pain on one or both sides. Pain in your low back and pubic symphysis may be adding to your discomfort.

Your growing uterus may also be putting pressure on your two sciatic nerves, which run from your lower back down your legs to your feet. This may cause pain, tingling or numbness running down your buttocks, hips or thighs — a condition called sciatica. Sciatica is unpleasant, but it's generally temporary.

Skin The skin across your abdomen may be dry and itchy from all of the stretching and tightening. At least 20 percent of pregnant women have itchiness on their abdomens or all over their bodies. If your itching is severe and you have reddish, raised patches on your skin, you may have a condition called PUPPP, which stands for pruritic urticarial papules and plaques of pregnancy. PUPPP usually appears first on the abdomen and then spreads to the arms, legs, buttocks or thighs. Scientists aren't sure what causes PUPPP, but it's more common among women who are pregnant for the first time and women who are carrying twins or other multiples.

You may also notice pink, reddish or purplish indented streaks on the skin covering your breasts, abdomen or perhaps even upper arms, buttocks or thighs. These are stretch marks (see page 420). Contrary to popular belief, stretch marks aren't necessarily related to the amount of weight gain. They seem to be caused, quite literally, by a stretching of the skin, coupled with a hormone-related decrease in your skin's elasticity. Scientists think your genes play the biggest role in determining whether you'll get stretch marks.

Although various products may claim otherwise, there's no proven way to prevent stretch marks. Because stretch marks develop from deep within the connective tissue under your skin, applying creams or ointments generally won't keep them from appearing. With time, they should fade to light pink or grayish stripes, but it's unlikely that they'll completely disappear.

Weight gain You'll probably continue to gain about a pound a week this month.

As the month progresses, you may notice some burning, numbness, tingling or pain in your hands. These are symptoms of carpal tunnel syndrome, resulting from weight gain and swelling in pregnancy that presses on a nerve in the wrist.

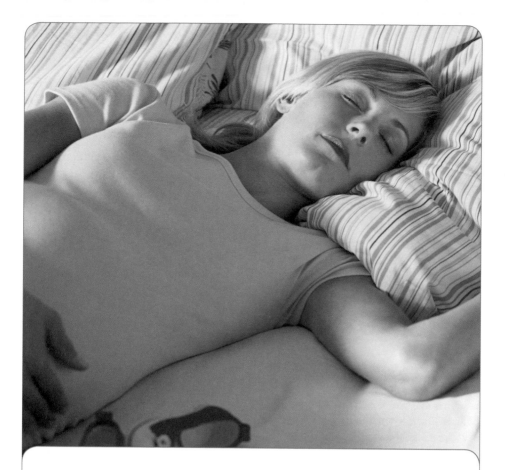

FINDING A COMFORTABLE SLEEP POSITION

As your belly continues to grow, you may find sleep becomes more difficult. In addition to heartburn and back pain, which can affect sleep, finding a comfortable sleep position gets tougher. Sleeping facedown is no longer possible. Sleeping on your back isn't comfortable either because all of the weight of your uterus rests on your spine and back muscles. In addition, lying on your back generally isn't recommended in later pregnancy because doing so may compress major blood vessels.

The best sleep position at this point is on your side. The left side is preferable to allow for maximum blood flow, but either side is fine. You may find the most comfortable position is to lie on your side with your knees bent and a pillow between your knees. Some women also like to place a pillow under their abdomen. Or, you might try a full-body pillow.

Few people remain in the same sleep position all night long, so if you wake up and find yourself lying on your back, don't panic. You haven't done anything to harm your baby. Just roll back onto your side and try to fall asleep.

Carpal tunnel symptoms will typically disappear after baby is born and any swelling resolves.

YOUR EMOTIONS

In just a few weeks, you'll be responsible for a new human being. As a result, you may feel more anxious than ever, especially if this is your first child.

Handling anxiety To help keep anxiety at bay, review some of the decisions that need to be made before your baby is born.

- Is your baby going to see a pediatrician or a family doctor?
- Are you going to breast-feed or use formula?
- If your baby is a boy, are you going to have him circumcised (see page 245)?

Taking stock of where you stand on these issues will help you feel more in control of the situation. Plus, it will make your new responsibilities seem less daunting once baby arrives.

In addition, the natural anticipation you're feeling about your baby's arrival may make it difficult for you to get to sleep or to sleep through the night. If you're feeling restless or anxious at night, try some of the relaxation exercises you learned in your childbirth classes. They may help you rest, and doing them now will be good practice for the big event.

PRENATAL CHECKUP

This will probably be the last time you go a whole month between prenatal checkups. Beginning next month, you'll likely see your care provider more frequently — every two weeks at first, and then once a week until your baby is born. During this month's prenatal visit, your care provider will again check your blood pressure and weight and ask you about any signs and symptoms you may be having. He or she may also ask you to describe your baby's movements and activity schedule — when baby is active and quiet. As with other prenatal appointments, your care provider will track baby's growth by measuring your uterus.

CORD BLOOD BANKING

One more decision to consider at this point in your pregnancy is whether you're interested in cord blood banking. In this procedure, blood is taken from your baby's umbilical cord following delivery, after the cord is clamped and cut. The blood within the cord is a rich source of stem cells, the cells from which all other cells are created, and it can be stored and preserved for possible future use in a stem cell transplant. Collecting a baby's cord blood poses few, if any, risks to either mother or baby. If the cord blood isn't collected for preservation or research, it's simply discarded.

Public vs. private There are two main ways to bank cord blood. The first is donating it to a public cord blood bank. Public banks collect and store cord blood for use by any individual who has a medical condition in which cord blood might provide a cure. The second type is a private bank. In this case, a baby's cord blood is stored for a fee, and the blood is saved for use by that family.

Some institutions may also collect umbilical cord blood for research studies. Your provider may inform you if studies involving cord blood collection are available at the hospital where you deliver. Cord blood collected for research will not be used to treat a medical condition.

Should you consider it? Donating cord blood to a public cord blood bank is an opportunity to help others. Cord blood transplants from unrelated donors can be used to treat many conditions, including leukemia, blood disorders, immune deficiencies and various metabolic problems. Public banks don't charge any fees to collect your baby's cord blood.

Donating cord blood to a private facility for possible personal use is controversial. It involves an up-front processing fee as well as a yearly storage fee, and the chance that your child will use his or her own banked cord blood in the future is remote. Also, should your child need a stem cell transplant to treat a condition, there's no guarantee that his or her banked cord blood would be suitable, as the blood's stem cells might carry the same genetic problems associated with the disease. However, if you have an older child in need of a stem cell transplant, privately banked healthy cord blood from within the family may be a solution.

The American Academy of Pediatrics (AAP) encourages donation to public cord blood banks but generally discourages private banking. According to the AAP, cord blood in public banks is used at a much higher rate than privately banked cord blood. It serves an increasing need as new uses for cord blood stem cells are developed. In recommending public donation over private, the AAP states: "It is important for parents to be aware that at this time, there are no scientific data to support the claim that autologous [one's own] cord blood is a tissue source proven to be of value for regenerative medical purposes, although researchers are examining this possibility."

If you're considering cord blood banking — whether it be a public or private donation facility — talk to your care provider. He or she can help answer any questions you may have and help you better understand the options to make an informed decision. Keep in mind that you must register for cord blood banking ahead of time so that a collection kit will be ready at your delivery.

BABY GEAR ESSENTIALS

You'll likely be making lots of nonmedical decisions around this month too, as it's time to go gear shopping. Chances are, you've already bought some things. The excitement of imagining your little one can make it hard to resist those tiny, adorable baby clothes and toys.

You'll want to give extra consideration to a few items, though, in deciding what to purchase. For these items especially, safety is key. Make sure that you're purchasing baby gear designed specifically to keep your baby as safe as possible.

Buying a car seat One of the most important pieces of baby equipment is a car seat, which you'll use right away on baby's first ride home from the hospital. Car seats are required by law in every state, and correct and consistent use of them is one of the best ways that parents can protect their children. It's never safe to hold an infant or child on your lap in a moving vehicle. And an infant must never ride in the front seat of a vehicle that has passenger air bags.

The safest place for all children to ride is in the back seat. And it's critical that the car seat be installed so that it's rear-facing, the only safe position for infants in cars. In a collision, a forward-facing baby is at greater risk of head and neck injuries because the head may be thrown forward.

Types of car seats There are three types of car seats available for infants: infant-only seats, convertible seats and 3-in-1 seats.

Infant-only seats. These car seats are designed for babies who weigh up to about 20 to 40 pounds, depending on the seat. They're best for newborns, and they may be the best fit for premature infants. Most models come with a detachable base that stays in the car. You can usually buy extra bases, too, to use in multiple vehicles. The car seat snaps easily into the base, allowing you to carry your baby in and out of the car in the car seat. This can be especially convenient if your child tends to fall asleep in the car.

Infant-only car seats typically come with a five-point harness, which provides the best protection, to secure your baby into the seat. The harness straps come over the infant's shoulders, across each hip and through the crotch area, and are buckled in place.

Convertible seats. These can be used for a baby or a toddler, until the child reaches 40 to 50 pounds or more. Convertible seats are bigger and heavier than infant-only seats and are designed for the whole seat to stay in the car. They should be installed rear-facing until your child is at least two years old or beyond the height or weight limit for the seat in that position. The seat can then be switched to a forward-facing seat and used until your child has outgrown the manufacturer's height or weight limit.

All convertible car seats manufactured today come with five-point

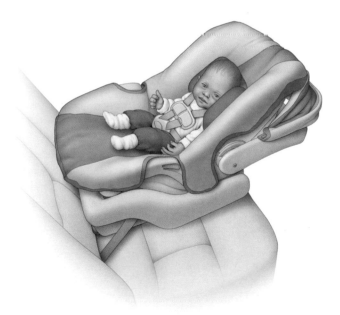

Infant-only seat

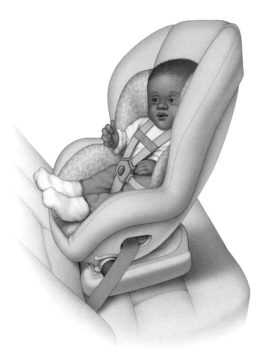

Convertible seat

harnesses. Although you'll save some money using a convertible seat, as your child can stay in it longer, an infant-only seat may be easier to use at first and may fit a newborn better.

3-in-1 seats. Also called all-in-one seats, these are similar to convertible seats in that they can be used both rear-facing and forward-facing. In addition, 3-in-1 seats can also be used as a booster seat after your child outgrows the height or weight limit for the forward-facing car seat. Some can be used for children weighing up to 100 pounds or more.

Choosing a car seat How do you know which car seat to buy? The best car seat is one that fits your child's age, weight and height, can be installed correctly, and is easy to use. Check to see if your hospital or clinic offers classes on car seats to help you learn more before you buy one.

When you're shopping, look at several different models. When you find a seat you like, try adjusting the harnesses and buckles. Be sure you understand how to use it. If possible, try installing the car seat in your vehicle before you buy it.

Keep in mind that babies are messy, so a car seat with easily removable, washable fabric will likely make your life easier. After baby's first diaper blowout in the car, you'll appreciate it.

Some other key features to look for when purchasing a car seat include:
- ▶ **Wide, twist-free straps.** A twisted strap is less effective in restraining a child in a crash.
- ▶ **Two-piece chest clips.** They help protect your child and are difficult for a child to detach.

- *Front-harness adjustments.* Some car seats have a mechanism in the front that adjusts the tightness of the harness.
- *Head-impact protection.* Most car seats have an added layer of foam or special plastic to improve head protection in case of an accident. The foam or plastic is recessed into the shell of the car seat around the head.

Avoiding common mistakes Here are some common mistakes that parents often make when it comes to car seat safety, and how to avoid them.

- *Buying a used car seat without researching its history.* If you're considering a used car seat, make sure the car seat meets current safety standards, comes with instructions, hasn't been recalled, hasn't been in an accident, and has no visible cracks or missing parts. If you don't know the car seat's history, don't use it. And whether new or used, check the car seat's expiration date, typically found in the manual or printed on a sticker on the seat. As the materials age, a car seat can become less safe for your child.
- *Placing the car seat in the wrong spot.* The safest place for your baby's car seat is the back seat, away from active air bags. If the air bag inflates, it could hit the back of a rear-facing car seat — right where your child's head is — and cause a serious or fatal injury. Placing a car seat next to a door with a side air bag may not be appropriate either. If you're only putting one car seat in the back seat, place the car seat in the center of the seat.
- *Incorrectly buckling up your child.* Before you install the seat, read the manufacturer's instructions. Make sure the seat is tightly secured — allowing no more than 1 inch of movement from side to side or front to back — and

facing the correct direction. Take time to secure your child in the seat correctly. Place the harness or chest clip even with your child's armpits — not at the abdomen or neck.
- *Improperly trying to keep your child upright.* Recline the car seat back according to the manufacturer's instructions, usually a 45-degree angle. This is so that your newborn's head doesn't flop forward on impact in case of an accident.
- *Moving to a forward-facing car seat too soon.* As your child gets older, resist the urge to place your child's car seat in the forward-facing position so that you can see his or her face in your rearview mirror. Riding rear-facing is recommended until a child is two years old or has outgrown the rear-facing height or weight limits for your seat.
- *Using the car seat as a replacement crib.* Remember that a car seat isn't a crib. Studies have shown that sitting upright in a car seat may compress a newborn's chest and can lead to reduced levels of oxygen. Although it's essential to buckle your child into a car seat during travel, don't let your child sleep in or relax in a car seat for long periods of time when you're out of the car.

Buying a crib Because your newborn will spend at least half of his or her time sleeping, where you put your son or daughter to sleep is no small matter. Accidents can happen if an infant is placed in an unsafe crib. When purchasing a crib, make sure that it meets current safety guidelines from the Consumer Product Safety Commission and the American Academy of Pediatrics.

In particular, if you're considering using a crib bought secondhand, borrowed or inherited, make sure it meets safety standards that were updated in 2011. These new standards banned drop-side rail cribs, which could trap and suffocate infants. The changes also required tougher testing, stronger slats and hardware, and more durable mattress supports. You'll also need to make sure your crib has no broken or missing parts, and that it comes with assembly instructions so you can be sure every part is installed correctly.

Some parents also purchase a play yard, with mesh or fabric walls, for traveling or for use around home. Keep in mind that these are subject to different federal safety requirements than permanent cribs or portable cribs. If you buy one, examine the unit carefully to make sure it is safe.

Crib safety Make sure your crib meets these requirements:

▶ The mattress should be firm and tightfitting so that baby can't get trapped between the mattress and the

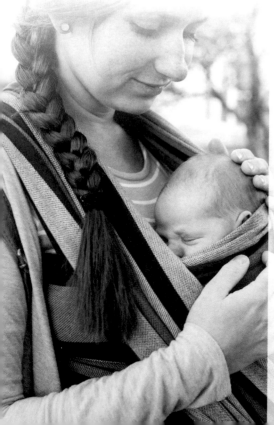

crib. If you can fit two fingers between the mattress and the side of the crib, the crib shouldn't be used. Use only a fitted bottom sheet made specifically for crib use.

▶ There should be no missing, loose, broken or improperly installed screws, brackets or other hardware.

▶ The crib's slats should be no more than $2^3/8$ inches apart — about the width of a soda can.

▶ The corner posts shouldn't be over $1/16$-inch high so a baby's clothing can't catch.

▶ There should be no cracked or peeling paint. All surfaces should be covered with lead-free paint.

▶ Use a baby sleeper, also called a wearable blanket, instead of a loose blanket.

▶ Don't put pillows, quilts, comforters, sheepskins, pillow-like bumper pads or pillow-like stuffed toys in the crib. They can lead to suffocation.

▶ Hanging crib toys should be out of the baby's reach.

▶ The crib should be away from cords for window blinds, curtains or drapes.

Buying a baby carrier Infant carriers allow you to keep your baby nestled close to your body while your hands are free for other activities. A variety of carriers are available, including front carriers, slings and back carriers. Front carriers and slings are especially useful the first several months. By the time your baby is 15 to 20 pounds, he or she may be too heavy to carry this way. Back carriers are best used when baby is older and better able to support himself or herself.

A front carrier consists of two shoulder straps supporting a deep fabric seat. A sling is a wide swath of fabric worn across your torso and supported by a shoulder strap. Some parents find slings to be cumbersome, while others love them.

Carrier safety When choosing a baby carrier, look for these features:

▶ You want a carrier that holds and supports your baby securely. Look for padded head support.

▶ Make sure the carrier is comfortable for both you and your baby. Look for wide padded shoulder straps, a padded waist or hip belt, adjustable straps, and leg holes that aren't too tight. Make sure a sling isn't so large that your baby gets lost in it.

▶ Is it easy to use? Make sure you can easily slip the carrier on and off.

▶ Select a carrier with a fabric that's durable and easy to clean. Cotton is a good choice because it is breathable, soft and washable.

▶ Choose a carrier that allows the baby to face both inward and outward.

▶ Look for a carrier with pockets or zippered compartments, which are handy for storing frequently used items.

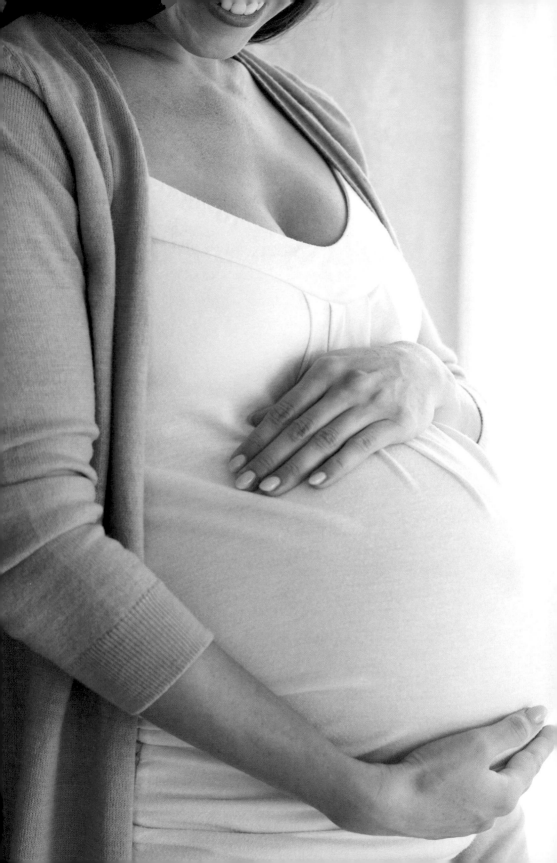

CHAPTER 12

Month 9: Weeks 33 to 36

My wife and I are having a baby quite late: I am 41 years old and she is 36. I worry about the physical changes my wife is going through, and I'm sorry that she has to endure the discomforts that come with the pregnancy. On the other hand, it's great to see via the ultrasounds that the baby is growing, or to feel the baby kicking with my hand on her belly. Things like that help me realize that this is for real. Perhaps it's good that the pregnancy lasts 10 months, because it gives us some time to get ready for the arrival of this new family member.

— Sylvaine

This can be a busy month as you prepare your home, your life and yourself for a new baby. It can also be a long month. The anticipation may be tormenting you — along with your back, feet and most everything else! The discomforts of late-stage pregnancy may now reach their peak. But keep in mind that your perseverance and patience are soon about to pay off.

BABY'S GROWTH

These days baby is gaining weight quickly, putting on about a half-pound a week.

Week 33 The next four weeks will be a period of extraordinary growth. At week 33, baby is almost fully developed. The pupils of his or her eyes can now constrict and dilate in response to light. Your baby's lungs are much more completely developed, which allows for greater optimism if he or she is born this week. There is still a higher risk of health problems compared with the risk at full-term, though. Most babies born at this age will need care in the neonatal intensive care unit.

Week 34 The white, waxy coating protecting your baby's skin (vernix) thickens this week. When your baby is born, you may see traces of vernix firsthand, especially under your baby's arms, behind the ears and in the groin area. Meanwhile, the soft, downy hair that covered the skin (lanugo) is now almost completely gone.

At 34 weeks into your pregnancy, your baby weighs about 4 to 6½ pounds and is about 12 inches long from his or her crown to rump.

Week 35 Baby continues to pack on the pounds, accumulating fat all over his or her body, especially around the shoulders. The crowded conditions inside your uterus may make it harder for this bigger, stronger baby to give you a punch, but you'll probably feel lots of stretches, rolls and wiggles.

Week 36 During week 36, your baby continues to add more fat underneath his or her skin. If you could sneak a peek at your baby this week, you'd see an infant you could almost describe as plump, with a fully rounded face. The fullness of your baby's face is the result of recent fat de-

posits and powerful sucking muscles that are fully developed and ready for action.

At 36 weeks into your pregnancy, the end of your ninth month, your baby weighs 5 to 7 pounds or a little more.

YOUR BODY CHANGES

Your growing baby may be disturbing your sleep these days. In addition, your muscles are sore from carrying this large bundle. Put these together, and you're probably feeling tired most of the time. If you're worn out, take a break. Rest and relax with your feet up. Fatigue is your body's way of telling you to slow down.

What's happening and where Your body is working hard this month to prepare for labor and delivery.

Respiratory system Because your diaphragm is pushed upward, you may continue to feel like you can't get enough air. If your baby drops lower into your uterus and pelvis this month, as some do, breathing may get a little easier.

Breasts The milk-producing glands inside your breasts continue to grow. Tiny oil-producing glands that moisturize the skin around your nipples and areolas may be more noticeable now.

Uterus This month, baby will settle into position inside your uterus, getting ready to make his or her grand entrance. If your baby is in the proper position, as most are — his or her head is down, with arms and legs pulled up tightly against the chest — you're ready to go.

You may actually feel your baby drop this month, settling deeper into your pelvis in preparation for delivery. This is

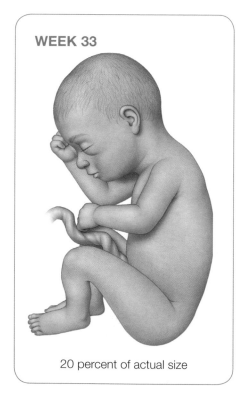

WEEK 33

20 percent of actual size

EXERCISE OF THE MONTH

Step-ups

This move helps to strengthen your lower body as your base of support.

1. Keeping your back straight, carefully step up onto a step stool with both feet on the center of the stool.
2. Step back down to your starting position.
3. Alternate your starting leg and repeat. Do this five to 10 times, or until you start to get tired.

also known as lightening, although that's a somewhat misleading term. While your upper abdomen may feel relief, that's usually more than compensated for by increased pressure in the pelvis, hips and bladder.

Some women, especially first-time moms, experience lightening several weeks before delivery. Others experience it the day labor begins. It's hard to say when your baby will drop in the pelvis or if you'll notice it when it happens.

Digestive system If your baby drops this month, you may notice an improvement in some of your gastrointestinal problems, such as heartburn or constipation. However, not all women experience lightening. As baby grows, he or she may continue to press under your rib cage as he or she descends down the birth canal.

Urinary tract Your urinary problems are likely to intensify if your baby drops this month. As your baby moves deeper into your pelvis, you'll feel more pressure on your bladder. Suffice it to say that you'll become very familiar with the bathroom. In the final weeks of your pregnancy, you may wake up several times a night just to urinate. This will most likely disappear soon after your baby is born.

Bones, muscles and joints The connective tissues in your body continue to soften and loosen in preparation for labor and delivery. This may be especially noticeable in your pelvic area. You may feel almost as if your legs are becoming detached from the rest of your body.

Don't give up your exercise program, but be careful while you're exercising this month. Given all the softening and loosening of connective tissues, it's easy to suffer a muscle or joint injury.

You may continue to have hip pain or low back pain caused by your growing uterus. You may also experience sciatic pain — tingling or numbness in your buttocks, hips or thighs caused by the pressure of your uterus on your sciatic nerves. As baby drops into the pelvis this pain may ease.

Vagina Your cervix may begin to soften this month, and some women will have both softening and dilation. This can begin weeks, days or hours before labor begins. Or your cervix might not soften or dilate at all before labor. Every person is different.

Late in pregnancy, some women feel a sharp pain in the vagina. If this happens to you, it doesn't mean that you're in labor. The cause of this pain isn't well-understood, but it doesn't pose a threat to you or your baby. Vaginal pain late in pregnancy usually isn't anything to be concerned about, but tell your care provider if you have a lot of discomfort.

You'll almost certainly have some contractions this month. It's possible they won't bother you at all, and you may not even notice them. If you do feel cramps at the same time as your uterus seems to tighten, pay attention to how regular and frequent the contractions are. False labor (Braxton Hicks) contractions are unpredictable, and even when frequent, they don't settle into a regular rhythm. The contractions of true labor are frequent — five minutes apart or closer — and are repeated at regular intervals.

Skin Some pregnancy-induced skin changes that may become more apparent this month include:

▶ Varicose veins, particularly on your legs and ankles
▶ Vascular spiders, especially on your face, neck, upper chest or arms

- Dryness and itchiness on your abdomen or all over your body
- Stretch marks on the skin covering your breasts, abdomen, upper arms, buttocks or thighs

Many of these changes will fade or disappear after your baby is born. Some evidence of stretch marks will likely remain, although the marks usually fade to grayish stripes.

Weight gain This is a weight-producing month. If your weight before pregnancy was in the normal range, you'll probably gain about a pound a week this month. But healthy weight gain in pregnancy is different for everyone. For some, your care provider may recommend watching your weight during this time.

PREPARING YOUR BODY FOR LABOR

In addition to your monthly exercises, here are a couple of other exercises that can help you prepare for labor. These exercises concentrate on the muscles that will receive the most stress during labor and delivery.

Kegel exercises The muscles in your pelvic floor help support your uterus, bladder and bowel. Toning them by doing Kegel exercises will help ease your discomfort during the last months of your pregnancy and may help minimize two common problems that can begin during pregnancy and continue afterward: leakage of urine and hemorrhoids. Strengthening your pelvic floor muscles appears to reduce your risk of developing urinary incontinence, both during and after pregnancy. Begin practicing Kegel exercises right away this month (or even

earlier in pregnancy) to strengthen the muscles by the time you deliver.

How to do them Identify your pelvic floor muscles — the muscles around your vagina and anus. To make sure you've found the right muscles, try to stop the flow of urine while you're going to the bathroom. If you stop it, you've found the right muscles. Don't make this a habit, though. Doing Kegel exercises while urinating or when your bladder is full can actually weaken the muscles. It can also lead to incomplete emptying of the bladder, which can increase your risk of developing a urinary tract infection.

If you're having trouble finding the right muscles, try a different technique. Place a finger inside your vagina and feel your vagina tighten when you squeeze. The muscles you squeezed are your pelvic floor muscles.

Once you've identified your pelvic floor muscles, empty your bladder and get into a sitting or standing position. Then firmly tense your pelvic floor muscles. Do this at frequent intervals for five seconds at a time, four or five times in a row. Work up to where you can keep the muscles contracted for 10 seconds at a time, relaxing for 10 seconds between contractions. Do three sets of 10 Kegel exercises throughout the day, and also do three sets of mini-Kegels. Count quickly to 10 or 20, contracting and relaxing your pelvic floor muscles each time you say a number.

While you're doing Kegel exercises, don't flex the muscles in your abdomen, thighs or buttocks. This can actually worsen the muscle tone of your pelvic floor muscles. And don't hold your breath. Just relax and focus on contracting the muscles around your vagina and anus.

Perineal massage Massaging the area between your vaginal opening and anus (perineum) in the last weeks before labor may help stretch these tissues in preparation for childbirth. This may lessen any stinging when your baby's head emerges from your vaginal opening. It may even help avoid the need for an incision in your perineum to enlarge your vaginal opening (episiotomy) as the baby's head is emerging. Nurse-midwives have long recommended perineal massage. There isn't yet definitive evidence that it prevents trauma to the perineum, but some studies have indicated promising results.

How to do it Wash your hands thoroughly with soap and hot water, and make sure your nails are trimmed. Then put a mild lubricant on your thumbs and insert them inside your vagina. Press downward toward the rectum, stretching the tissues. Repeat daily for about eight to 10 minutes. Your partner can help with this process, if you wish. You may experience a little burning or other discomfort as you massage your perineum. This is normal. However, stop if you begin to feel sharp pain.

A couple of additional points: You don't have to practice perineal massage if the idea of it makes you feel uncomfortable. And if you do it, it's no guarantee that you won't have an episiotomy. Certain birth situations, such as those involving a large baby or a baby in an abnormal position, may require an episiotomy.

YOUR EMOTIONS

You're probably thinking a lot this month about when labor will start and how your childbirth experience will go. Increasing anxiety during this time is understandable, as are worries about whether your baby will be healthy.

You may also be spending some time contemplating what the pain will be like during childbirth. How bad will it really be? How long will it last? How well will I cope?

Preparing yourself for labor It's to be expected that you may feel anxious about labor and childbirth, but realize that women go through labor and give birth every day. It's a natural process. To help you prepare, and stay calm:

▶ *Educate yourself.* Knowing what's going to happen to your body when you give birth will make you less tense and fearful as it actually takes place. With less fear and tension, your pain may be less, too. Childbirth classes are an excellent place to meet other moms-to-be and learn about the changes your body goes through in labor and childbirth. Also, make sure to read the chapters on labor and delivery in this book.

▶ *Talk with women who have had positive birth experiences.* Learn what techniques worked for them during the labor and childbirth process.

▶ *Tell yourself that you'll do the best you can.* How the process goes depends on the circumstances and your strengths. There's no right or wrong way to have a baby.

▶ *Familiarize yourself with the various pain relief options available to you during labor.* Read Chapter 23 to learn more about pain medications used during labor and natural childbirth techniques. But try not to develop fixed ideas about what you'll use and what you won't. Until you're actually in the moment, you won't know what your needs will be. It's best to be informed, but flexible.

PRENATAL CHECKUP

You'll probably see your care provider every other week this month, or even more often. As during previous visits, he or she will likely check your weight and blood pressure, as well as the activity of your baby. Your care provider will measure your uterus, which will probably measure between 33 and 34 centimeters in the first half of this month — roughly equal to the number of weeks of your pregnancy. Your care provider will also ask you about any signs or symptoms that may suggest labor, including regular contractions, leakage of fluid from the vagina or vaginal bleeding. Depending on your symptoms, your cervix may be checked for softening and dilation.

Strep test At this point in your pregnancy, your care provider may screen you for group B streptococcus (GBS), if he or she hasn't already done so. This test is commonly referred to as the group B strep test. A culture swabbed from just inside the vagina and the rectum is tested for the bacterium. GBS typically lives harmlessly in the body, and although it usually poses no risk to you, women who harbor it may pass the bacterium to their babies during labor and delivery. Newborns don't yet have the proper immunity to live with this bacterium without risk of complications. If group B strep is found, antibiotics will likely be given to you once you go into labor. This reduces the risk that your baby will acquire the bacterium.

Checking baby's position During your visits this month, your care provider will check baby's position. The position baby is in by the 33rd week of your pregnancy will likely be the position he or she will be in for delivery, whether it's head first, rump first or feet first. However, if

you've had several children, there's a greater possibility that your baby may change position in the final weeks.

To determine how baby is positioned inside your uterus, your care provider can check to see which part of your baby's body is farthest down in your pelvis, ready to be born first. This is called the presenting part. To check this, your provider will carefully press on the outside of your abdomen. If your care provider is still uncertain about the baby's position, an ultrasound may be performed.

If your baby is positioned head first, you're good to go. When the baby is positioned rump first or feet first, he or she is in what's called a breech position.

If a baby in breech position isn't already too far down in your pelvis, your care provider may suggest a procedure in which the baby is turned from breech to head first. This is called an external cephalic version. Your care provider applies pressure to your abdomen in certain spots to try to move your baby into the proper

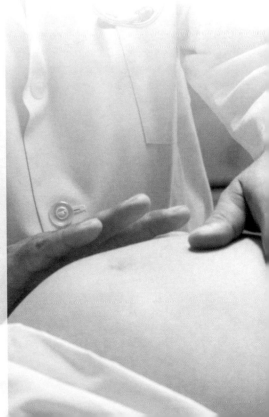

position. Medication is often used to relax the uterus for easier movement. The procedure is typically done in or near a delivery room, in case any complications arise and the baby needs to be delivered quickly. In addition, the baby is monitored before and after the procedure to check the heart rate. External cephalic version is generally tried at 37 weeks or later so that the baby is less likely to return to a breech position before birth.

YOUR BIRTH PLAN

If you haven't already started, now's the time for you to think about your options and preferences regarding labor, delivery and postpartum care. Creating a birth plan encourages you to consider all the decisions that may be involved, and it also gives you an opportunity to talk about your preferences with your care provider.

BIRTH PLAN CHECKLIST

Your birth plan may include details such as:
○ Concerns you may have regarding giving birth.
○ Things you look forward to during birth.
○ Your support person during labor and delivery, and anyone else you'd like present for the birth. Note that your hospital may limit the number of people allowed in the room.
○ Natural pain relief preferences — aromatherapy, shower, birthing ball, music, dim lights, walking, rocking chair.
○ Pain medication preferences — laughing gas (nitrous oxide), epidural or other.
○ Goals in terms of medication use — no medications, some medications, or wait and see.
○ Hydration preferences — do you wish to sip water during labor, have unrestricted access or have no oral intake?
○ Positions for pushing and delivery — sitting up, lying on your back and using stirrups, lying on your side, using a birthing chair or stool, or squatting.
○ Preferences regarding the delivery — do you want to observe with a mirror?
○ Preferences for photos or video — do you want your partner or another support person to take pictures or videos at the birth? (Your hospital may have restrictions on photos or recording, so check the hospital's policy.)
○ Preferences for what happens right after birth — do you want the baby handed directly to you or wrapped in a blanket and then handed to you?
○ Circumcision preference, if you have a boy.
○ How you plan to feed your baby.
○ Preferences regarding being present at the baby's first bath and exams.
○ Mom and baby follow-up care.
  In addition, you may inform your care providers about your preferences for procedures, such as avoiding episiotomy or cesarean birth. But ultimately, the clinical situation typically dictates what procedures are needed to keep you and baby safe. Your care team will ask for your consent before going forward with any procedure.

Keep in mind that your birth plan is not set in stone. No one can predict how birth will go, and things may change. For example, you may think that you don't want any pain relief medication, but you may change your mind during labor. But a plan does help ensure your experience will come as close to your expectations as reasonably possible.

Your care provider may ask you to fill out a form stating your preferences. Or you may create a birth plan of your own or as part of your childbirth classes. Be sure to communicate your wishes to your care provider.

Pain management If you haven't decided yet how you're going to manage the pain that accompanies childbirth, now is the time to do so. Yes, childbirth is painful — but you can deal with it in a number of ways. To help labor and delivery go as smoothly as possible, it's best to know what may help you handle the pain when it arrives.

Knowing your options There are various options for controlling labor-related pain. Some women take classes to learn breathing and relaxation techniques, and they rely on these techniques to manage the pain. Other women prefer to use pain-relieving medications. There are two main types: Analgesic medications lessen the pain, while anesthetic medications block the pain. You also may use a combination of options — breathing techniques and medication. You might choose to go unmedicated through the first part of labor — generally the easier part — and then use medication in the later part of labor when the pain may be more intense.

To figure out which approach is best for you, familiarize yourself with all of your options and then decide. If you have friends who've been through labor, ask what worked best for them. Most of all, remember that it's completely your choice.

For more information on the various pain relief options and what to expect with each, see Chapter 23.

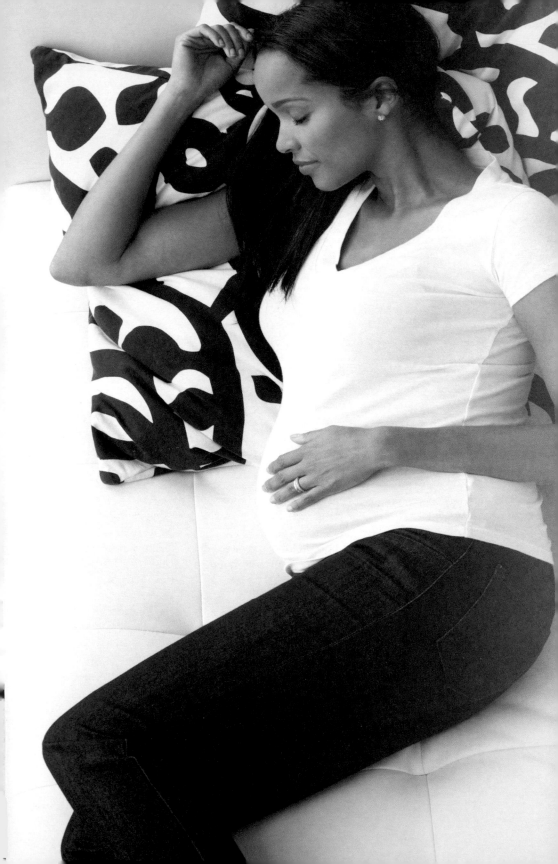

CHAPTER 13

Month 10: Weeks 37 to 40

I think nature's way of making us look forward to labor is to make the final month extremely uncomfortable. I can handle a few more weeks, but I'm definitely ready to have this child.

— *Kris*

Month 10! Pregnancy is supposed to be nine months! What's going on? In case you missed it, the introduction to Part 2 explains why this book is divided into 10 months instead of nine. Birth may happen at any time now. However, pregnancy is officially considered complete at 40 weeks.

BABY'S GROWTH

In these final weeks, your uterus finishes expanding and baby gets plump. During the final weeks, weight gain varies, depending on the child. Some babies put on more weight than do others.

Week 37 By the end of this week, your baby is considered early term. He or she isn't quite done growing yet, but the rate of weight gain is slowing a bit. As your baby's body builds more fat, it is slowly becoming rounder. A baby's sex seems to play some role in determining size at birth. If you have a boy, he'll likely weigh a bit more than a baby girl born to you at a similar length of gestation.

Week 38 In recent weeks, your baby's development has focused mainly on improving organ functioning. Your baby's brain and nervous system are working better every day. However, this developmental process continues through childhood and even into the later teen years. This month, your baby's brain has prepared to manage the complicated jobs of breathing, digesting, eating and maintaining a proper heart rate.

At 38 weeks into pregnancy, the average baby weighs in at about 7 pounds and is nearing 14 inches long from crown to rump.

Week 39 Almost there — at the end of this week, you'll have a full-term baby. Baby has now lost most of the vernix and lanugo that used to cover his or her skin, although you may see traces of them at birth. Your baby now has enough fat laid down under the skin to hold his or her body temperature as long as there's a little help from you. This fat gives baby a healthy, chubby look at birth.

The rest of the body has been catching up, but the head is still the largest part of your baby's body. That's why it's important for baby to be headfirst in a vaginal birth.

You continue to supply your baby with antibodies — protein substances that help protect against bacteria and viruses. During the first months of life, these antibodies help baby's immune system stave off infections. Some antibodies are also provided through breast milk. If you haven't gotten your tetanus, diphtheria and acellular pertussis (Tdap) booster yet (see page 159), now is the time so that baby will have those protective antibodies after birth.

By this point in pregnancy, babies vary quite a bit in size. A 39-week-old baby typically weighs 6 to 9½ pounds.

HOW BABY COMES OUT

The ideal — and most common — position for birth is shown here. In this position, the smallest dimension of the baby's head leads the way through the birth canal.

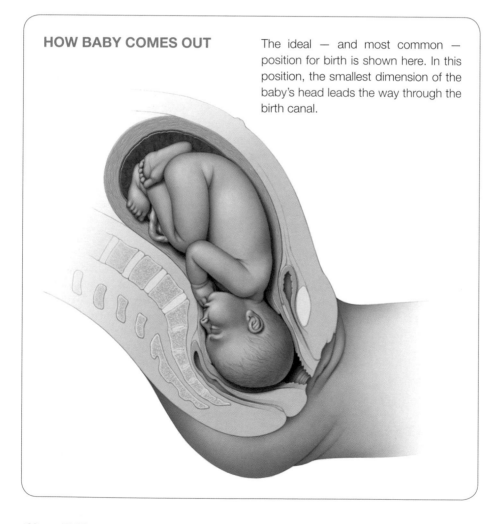

Week 40 Congratulations! Your due date arrives this week. Most women don't deliver right on their due dates — only about 4 percent do, by some estimates — but you're probably ready to meet your little one. Keep in mind that it's just as normal to have your baby a week late as it is to have him or her a week early. Try to be patient, although with all the work you've done, that may not be easy.

As labor approaches, your baby will experience many changes in order to prepare for birth, including a surge in hormones. This may help maintain blood pressure and blood sugar levels after birth. It may also have something to do with communicating to your uterus that the time has come.

With labor, the blood flow to the placenta will decrease a bit during each contraction. But by now, the baby can tolerate these interruptions so long as they aren't too frequent and don't last too long. Your little one is ready for all the amazing changes he or she will experience at birth.

At 40 weeks, the average baby weighs about 7½ to 8 pounds and measures about 20 inches long with legs fully extended. Your own baby may be smaller or larger and still be normal and healthy.

YOUR BODY CHANGES

Before you were pregnant, your uterus weighed only about 2 ounces and could hold less than a half-ounce. At term, it will have multiplied in weight by a factor of 20, to about 2½ pounds and will have stretched to hold your baby, your placenta and almost a quart of amniotic fluid.

What's happening and where Sometime around the end of this month, after roughly 40 weeks of growth and change, you'll go through labor and delivery and give birth to a new human being.

Respiratory system You may still experience shortness of breath. If your baby drops lower into your pelvis before labor begins, which is more common among first-time moms, you may feel less pressure on your diaphragm. However, many women experience shortness of breath throughout pregnancy because as baby grows, pressure is exerted under the rib cage.

Digestive system As it has for the past several months, your digestive system continues to operate at a slowed pace. You may still experience heartburn and constipation. If your baby drops this month, these symptoms may improve. With less pressure on your stomach, digestion may be easier.

Breasts Stimulated by the hormones estrogen and progesterone, your breasts are fully prepared to feed your baby. As delivery approaches, your nipples may start leaking colostrum — the yellowish protein fluid your breasts first produce.

Over the course of pregnancy, some women's nipples become inverted, dimpling back into their breasts. If this happens to you, don't worry. A lactation consultant can help prepare your nipples for breast-feeding.

Uterus This month, your uterus will complete its expansion. When you reach term, it will extend from your pubic area to the bottom of your rib cage. If this is your first baby, the baby may drop lower into your pelvis (lightening) weeks before you go into labor. If you've been through childbirth before, lightening and the onset of labor tend to happen closer together.

Urinary tract You may find it difficult to get a good night's sleep because you have to get up so often to urinate. You're probably also continuing to leak urine, especially when you laugh, cough or sneeze. Hang in there. Your pregnancy is almost over.

Bones, muscles and joints The aptly named hormone relaxin, which is produced by your placenta, continues to relax and loosen the ligaments holding your three pelvic bones together. This will allow your pelvis to open wider during childbirth — wide enough to accommodate your baby's head as it passes through. Until then, the effects of relaxin may manifest themselves in clumsiness, back and pelvic pain, and loose-feeling limbs.

If your baby drops a couple of weeks before labor begins, which is more common among first-time moms, you may also feel some pressure or aches and pains in your pelvic joints.

Vagina At some point over the next several weeks, your cervix will begin to open (dilate). It may start a couple of weeks before labor begins, or just a few hours before. Ultimately, your cervix will dilate from 0 (closed) to 10 centimeters (fully dilated) so that you can push the baby out.

In these final weeks, you may feel an occasional sharp pain inside your vagina. You may also feel pressure, aches or sharp twinges in your perineal area — the area between your vaginal opening and anus — as your baby's head presses on your pelvic floor.

As the cervix thins and relaxes, you may lose the mucous plug that's been in place at the cervical opening during your pregnancy, helping to keep bacteria from getting into your uterus. There isn't a strong relationship between the loss of the mucous plug and the beginning of labor. It can happen up to two weeks before labor begins — or it can happen right before. When it happens, you may notice a thick discharge or stringy mucus that's clear, pink or blood tinged. Don't worry if you don't notice this change. Some women don't realize when they've lost their mucous plug.

Among a few pregnant women, the amniotic sac breaks or leaks before labor begins, and the fluid that has cushioned the baby comes out as a trickle or a gush. If this happens to you, follow your care provider's instructions. He or she will probably want to evaluate you and your baby as soon as your water breaks (membranes rupture). In the meantime, don't do anything that could introduce bacteria into your vagina, such as using tampons or having sexual intercourse.

If the fluid coming from your vagina is anything other than clear and colorless, let your care provider know right away. For example, vaginal fluid that's greenish or yellowish and foul smelling could be a sign of a uterine infection or that your baby has passed a bit of stool (meconium) into the fluid.

Weight gain Your baby is actually gaining weight more slowly this month. As a result, you may notice that your own weight gain has slowed or even stopped. Some women even lose a pound or so at the very end of the pregnancy. For a reminder of where all that weight has been going over the past 10 months, see page 45.

YOUR EMOTIONS

By this point, you're likely tired of being pregnant. You may be having trouble sleeping because you can't find a comfortable position. Once you do drift off, your bladder may be waking you up every couple of hours. Time may seem to be standing still.

To deal with the anticipation and discomfort, try to keep busy. Find a project, read the latest best-seller, wrap up work before taking a break from your job, and spend time with friends and family. Make sure you're well-stocked on groceries and diapers, your hospital bag is packed, and your car seat is ready to go. Keeping your mind active will help the days move more quickly until you're finally in labor. Plus, it may be a while before you have time to yourself again!

TIME TO RELAX

It's a fact: If you're frightened and anxious during labor, you'll have a more difficult labor. Stress sets in motion a whole range of reactions in your body that can ultimately interfere with labor. Childbirth educators call it the fear-tension-pain cycle. To keep yourself from becoming too stressed, you need to find ways to relax. There are many ways you can do this. The right music can be soothing. So can a cool evening breeze or an evening with your feet up watching a funny movie.

Techniques to keep you calm There are also different relaxation techniques that you can use to help you keep calm. You may have learned about these techniques in your childbirth course, but here's a quick refresher:

- *Progressive muscle relaxation.* Beginning with your head or feet, relax one muscle group at a time, moving toward the opposite end of your body.
- *Touch relaxation.* Starting at your temples, have your partner apply firm but gentle pressure for several seconds. Then move to the base of your

skull, shoulders, back, arms, hands, legs and feet. As your partner touches each part of your body, relax the muscle group in that area.

- *Massage.* Your partner massages your back and shoulders, making sweeping motions down your arms and legs and small circular motions on your brow and temples. These movements will help relax your muscles and cause your brain to release chemicals called endorphins, which help enhance your sense of well-being. Experiment with different techniques until you find a form of massage that feels good.
- *Guided imagery.* Imagine yourself in an environment that gives you a feeling of peacefulness, relaxation and

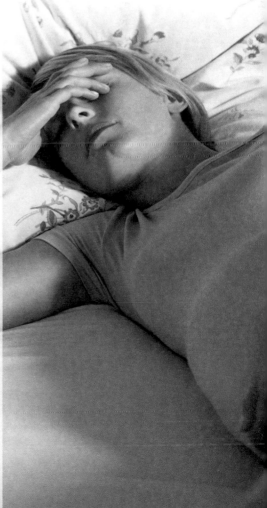

well-being. Concentrate on the details, such as the smells, colors or sensations on your skin. To enhance the imagery, play nature sounds or soft music.

▸ *Meditation.* With this mind and body technique, you focus your attention on your breathing or on repeating a word, phrase or sound. This is done to interrupt the stream of thoughts that normally occupies the conscious mind. When your thoughts are suspended, you enter a state of physical relaxation and mental calmness.

▸ *Breathing techniques.* Inhale through your nose, envisioning cool, pure air rushing into your lungs. Exhale slowly through your mouth, imagining yourself blowing all your tension away. Practice breathing both more slowly and more quickly than normal. You can use both these techniques, and others, during labor.

Practice relaxation techniques often this month. When you do, make sure the environment is peaceful and that you're comfortable. Use pillows if you want, or turn on some soft music.

PRENATAL CHECKUP

You'll likely see your care provider weekly now until baby arrives. A routine pelvic exam is not typically part of this checkup, but your care provider may check your cervix if he or she thinks you may be in the early stages of labor. This exam is reported in numbers and percentages. For example, your care provider may tell you that you're 3 centimeters (cm) dilated and 30 percent effaced. When you're ready to push your baby out, your cervix will be 10 cm dilated and 100 percent effaced.

Don't put too much stock in these numbers. You may go for weeks dilated at 3 cm, or you may go into labor without any dilation or effacement beforehand. However, measures of your cervix do help your care provider determine which medications or methods to use for induction of labor, should you need to be induced.

When to call During the last month of pregnancy, these signs and symptoms require immediate medical attention:

Vaginal bleeding If you have bright red bleeding of more than a spot or two at any time this month, call your care provider right away. It could be a sign of placental abruption, a serious problem in which your placenta separates from the wall of your uterus. This condition is a medical emergency. However, try not to confuse this kind of bleeding with the slight bleeding you may have after a pelvic exam or with the blood and mucus you may see as the cervix thins.

Constant, severe abdominal pain If you have constant, severe abdominal pain, contact your care provider immediately. Although uncommon, this can be another sign of placental abruption. If you also have a fever and vaginal discharge along with the pain, you may have an infection.

Decreased movement It's normal for the vigor of your baby's activities to decrease somewhat during the last few days before birth. It's almost as if your baby is resting and storing up energy for the big day. But the number of movements shouldn't drop a great deal. Decreased frequency of movement may be a signal that something is wrong. To check your baby's movements, lie on your left side and count how often you feel the baby move. If you notice fewer than four movements in an hour or if you're otherwise

EXERCISE OF THE MONTH

Wall pushup

This move strengthens your shoulders, arms, chest and core so that you're ready for lots of lifting and holding the baby.

1. Stand facing a wall and place your hands on the wall at the level of your shoulders. Hands and feet should be about shoulder-width apart.
2. Tighten your core. Slowly bend your elbows and lower your chest until your chin is near the wall. Hold the position briefly.
3. Return to the starting position. Repeat five to 10 times.

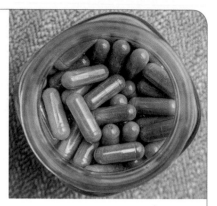

PLACENTOPHAGY

In recent years, particularly in the United States, there has been growing interest in ingesting the placenta after birth — a practice known as placentophagy. Among other perceived benefits, new moms have reported that consuming the placenta helped to increase their milk production, ward off postpartum depression, decrease postpartum bleeding, restore iron levels and improve their energy overall. As your due date draws near, you may be curious about this trend.

The placenta is a complex organ that nourishes your baby during pregnancy. Delivery of the placenta typically follows within five to 30 minutes after baby has arrived. For consumption, the placenta is then stored in an airtight container and kept cold to help prevent bacterial growth until it can be processed. Many women hire a company to cook or dehydrate the placenta and process it into capsules. Others may eat it raw, cooked, dehydrated or blended into smoothies.

However, scientific research has not yet found evidence that human placentophagy has any of the benefits reported anecdotally or in self-reported surveys. Few controlled studies have examined the effects, and those in existence have shown no benefit to maternal mood, fatigue or iron levels from taking placenta pills. In fact, data have shown that some nutrients in the placenta are likely lost during processing, and the remaining amounts are unlikely to have a clinical benefit.

There's another reason to approach this trend with caution — your baby's safety. The processing of the placenta may not destroy bacteria that can be dangerous for your newborn, such as group B streptococcus (GBS). The Centers for Disease Control and Prevention has reported one case in which a previously healthy infant experienced serious complications from GBS present in the mother's placenta pills. Bacteria in placenta pills could possibly make you ill, too.

Because eating the placenta carries significant risks with no proven benefits, experts advise against it.

---

worried about your baby's decreased movement, call your care provider.

What to do when baby's overdue
Your due date has come and gone — and you're still pregnant. What's going on? Although your due date may seem to have magical qualities, it's simply an educated guess about when your baby is most likely to arrive. It's perfectly normal to give birth one to two weeks before — or after — your due date. If your pregnancy continues one full week past your due date, it's known as late term. Once you're two full weeks past your due date, your pregnancy is officially postterm.

You may be more likely to have an overdue pregnancy if:
▶ The exact date of the start of your last menstrual period isn't known and the

gestational age wasn't confirmed with an early ultrasound, so your due date may be off by several days

▶ This is your first pregnancy
▶ You've had previous overdue pregnancies
▶ Overdue pregnancies tend to run in your family
▶ Your baby is a boy

Rarely, an overdue pregnancy may be related to problems with the placenta or the baby.

You will continue your prenatal visits if your pregnancy extends beyond your due date, and your care provider will continue to monitor your health. To encourage labor to begin, he or she may offer membrane sweeping or stripping. In this procedure, your care provider gently inserts a finger through the partially open cervix and "sweeps" it around the inner portion of the cervix or the lower uterus. This separates the membranes (amnion) at the lowest portion of the uterus and triggers a release of chemicals and hormones, such as oxytocin, associated with the onset of labor. Research has shown that membrane sweeping decreases the number of women who need to undergo late-term and postterm induction of labor.

If you're more than one week past your due date, your care provider may also track your baby's heartbeat with an electronic fetal monitor or use ultrasound to observe your baby's movements and to measure the amount of amniotic fluid.

Giving baby a nudge Sometimes it's better to deliver your baby sooner rather than later — particularly if your care provider is concerned about your health or your baby's health or if your pregnancy continues more than two weeks past your due date.

Why the concern about two weeks? At this point in your pregnancy, your ba-by's size may complicate a vaginal delivery. After 42 weeks, there is also a slightly increased chance that aging of the placenta can compromise the baby's ability to thrive in the womb. And an overdue baby is more likely to pass and inhale fecal waste (meconium), which can cause breathing problems after birth.

If you are overdue, your care provider may recommend inducing labor — taking steps to try to kick-start your labor. You may be given medication to help your cervix soften and open. If your amniotic sac is still intact, your care provider may break your water by creating an opening in the sac with a thin plastic hook. The process doesn't hurt, but you may feel a warm gush of fluid when the sac breaks.

If necessary, you may also be given medication to promote contractions. A common choice is a synthetic version of the hormone oxytocin (Pitocin), which causes the uterus to contract. The dosage may be adjusted to regulate the strength and frequency of your contractions.

For more information on inducing labor, see page 451.

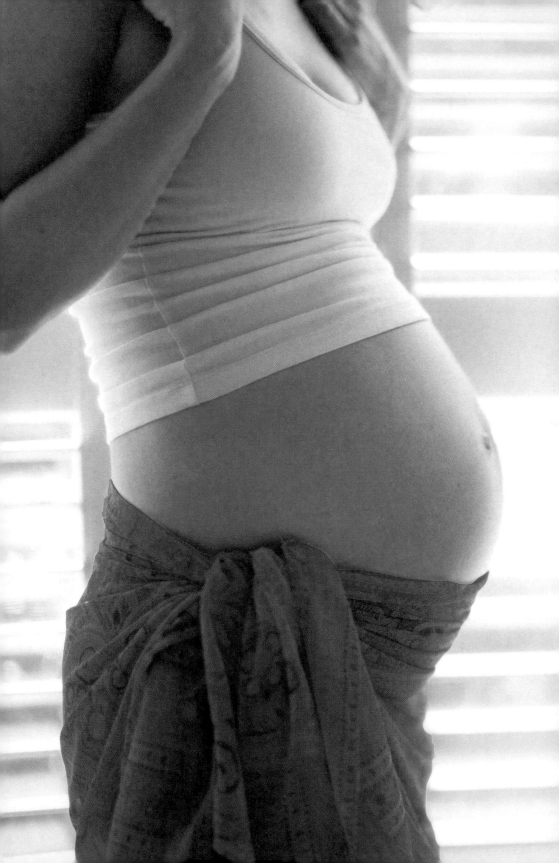

CHAPTER 14

Labor and childbirth

The last weeks of pregnancy may feel like a time of endless waiting. This is especially true if your baby is overdue. As you anticipate the start of labor, it may seem as if time is slowing down.

WHILE YOU WAIT

There's plenty to do while you wait for that little one to arrive. Here's a list of some helpful tasks to check off.

Review your birth plan Make sure you've discussed your birth preferences with your care provider and that you've also familiarized yourself with standard practices where you will be delivering. For example, when would medication be used to accelerate labor? Is your care provider comfortable with birthing positions other than the traditional one of lying on your back? Under what circumstances would a cut to enlarge the vaginal opening (episiotomy) be performed?

In addition, find out when you should notify your care provider once you're in labor. Should you go directly to the hospital, call ahead to the hospital or call the care provider's office first? Are there any other steps your care provider wants you to take?

And remember, not everything may go according to plan. If you've never given birth before, you may not know how you'll cope with the pain of labor. Even if you have given birth before, every pregnancy and labor is different. In addition, problems may occur that no one expected. Control what you can — but be ready to let go of what you can't control.

Preregister at the hospital Ask about preregistering at the hospital or birthing center where you plan to deliver. Filling out the necessary paperwork and sorting out insurance matters ahead of time can save you extra work when the big day finally arrives. Face it; it's no fun to be doing paperwork between contractions.

Pack your bag Because your due date isn't a given, it's a good idea to have your bag packed and ready for the hospital ahead of time. Here are some items you may want to have on hand:

- A watch or a phone app that counts seconds, for timing contractions
- A copy of your birth plan
- Socks or slippers — labor rooms are often kept cool
- Glasses — you may have to remove your contact lenses
- Lip balm for dry lips
- A camera or video camera and charger
- A phone charger
- Pajamas or a nightgown that opens in front to allow for easy breast-feeding
- A robe
- A nursing bra or, if you plan to bottle-feed, a supportive bra
- Several pairs of underwear large enough to fit over maternity pads
- Moisturizer, other toiletries, any cosmetics you'll want and a hair dryer

- Comfortable clothes to wear at the hospital and loose clothing for going home — probably a midpregnancy outfit
- Baby clothes, including a hat, and a seasonally appropriate going-home outfit
- A baby blanket
- Snacks and drinks for your stay after baby arrives

If you don't want to put everything into your bag yet — your cosmetics, for example — make a list so that you can gather items easily when you prepare to leave. Normally, you don't have to rush — you might even have time to shower beforehand — but it's best to be organized. Your partner will also want to be prepared to stay with you, with his or her own clothes, snacks and toiletries set aside. In addition, have a car seat installed for baby's ride home.

Try to relax Most women greet the end of their pregnancies with a mixture of anticipation and nervousness. But try not to worry. Women's bodies are made to accommodate labor and delivery. Labor, as the name implies, is work; that's true. But you can help make the experience go as smoothly as possible by trying to relax.

Many women experience a spurt of energy in the last weeks of pregnancy, a behavior often referred to as nesting. You may find yourself cleaning like mad and anxious to start any projects that you've put off. Even though the thought of coming home to a clean house may be tempting, don't wear yourself out.

Focus on savoring this time you have before your baby arrives. Treat yourself to a nice dinner or fun outing. Indulge in a favorite hobby. Read a good book. Cuddle with your partner. Staying busy but relaxed will help time move along.

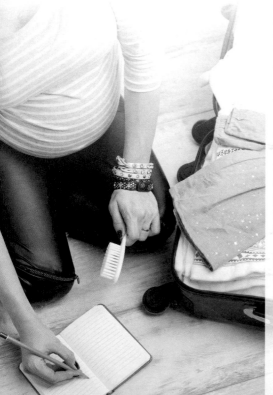

COMMON QUESTIONS

When discussing labor and childbirth with your care provider, don't be embarrassed by any question. For example, you may be wondering:

What if I have to go to the bathroom during labor? Some women will be able to get up and urinate every few hours. Your care provider will probably encourage you to do so because a full bladder may slow down the baby's descent. However, it may be difficult to sense a full bladder when you're having contractions, especially if you've had an epidural. Or you may not want to move, out of fear that doing so will worsen the contractions. Your care team may provide you with a bedpan or empty your bladder with a catheter. Occasionally, a small amount of stool is expelled during birth. This is perfectly normal and nothing to worry about.

Will my pubic hair be shaved? Not likely. Shaving a pregnant woman's pubic hair used to be standard practice, to clean the site for delivery. Now shaving is rarely, if ever, done. You don't need to shave at home beforehand.

Will I have to bare myself in front of a lot of strangers? During labor, the team caring for you will perform periodic vaginal exams to check how you're progressing. A newborn care provider also may be present to examine the baby after birth. Who else you have in the labor room or birthing room is largely up to you. Medical professionals who help deliver babies see births almost every day, so they're used to the messy but awesome experience of birth. At some university hospitals, medical or nursing students may observe a labor and delivery, if it is OK with the laboring mother. Remember that medical students are also professionals and may be able to lend a hand or extra support, so consider their presence an advantage.

What if I make loud noises during labor? Labor is a physical act that requires your participation. You may make straining or grunting noises during the workout of labor. Birth is rarely silent; it takes too much physical and emotional effort to expect quiet. It's perfectly normal to make noise during labor and delivery. Medical professionals who help deliver babies won't be shocked in the least.

Does labor hurt my baby? During the most difficult phases of labor and delivery, your baby is squeezed and pushed down the narrow vaginal canal. Your baby must also corkscrew through the bony passageway of the mother's pelvis. However, it's unlikely that this hurts the baby. During intense labor, the baby's heartbeat slows down intermittently in response to the stress of the journey. This is expected and not serious.

HOW YOUR BODY PREPARES

As labor approaches, your body undergoes certain changes that signal that your baby likely will be born soon.

Early signals Some of the changes to watch for include:

Lightening As you approach your due date, you may feel that the baby has settled deeper into your pelvis. This natural step is called lightening. The profile of your abdomen may change — your belly may seem lower and tilt more forward. (Friends and family may even note that the baby has dropped!) You may find that it's easier to breathe with less pressure on your diaphragm.

In exchange, you'll likely feel increased pressure on your bladder from the baby as it drops down into your pelvis. You may feel twinges of pain as the baby bumps against your pelvic floor. And your center of gravity may feel lower, throwing you off balance slightly.

Don't worry if you don't feel or notice baby dropping. Some women don't experience these changes. This is especially true of women who are already carrying their babies low. And after your first pregnancy, lightening generally occurs much later in subsequent pregnancies. The baby may drop into position just hours before the onset of labor or even during labor itself.

Braxton Hicks contractions Throughout your second and third trimesters of pregnancy, you may experience occasional, usually painless contractions — a sensation that your uterus is tightening and relaxing. They're especially noticeable when you place your hand on your abdomen. These false labor pains are Braxton Hicks contractions, and they're your body's way of warming up for labor. Your uterus is exercising its muscle mass to build strength for the big job ahead. As you approach your due date, these contractions typically become stronger and may even become painful at times.

Bloody show During pregnancy, the opening to your uterus (cervix) is blocked by a thick plug of mucus. This plug forms part of the barrier between your vagina and uterus, helping to prevent bacteria from entering the uterus. A few weeks, days or hours before labor begins, this plug may discharge and you may have what's called bloody show. You may notice a small amount of blood-tinged, brownish discharge from your vagina. Some women don't notice any change in discharge. Bloody show may be a sign that things could happen soon, although labor could still be a week or more away.

Signs you're in labor It's one of the most common questions care providers hear from expectant mothers: "How will I know when I'm in labor?" You may have heard other mothers say that you'll just know, but that may not be very comforting. Subtle signs often announce the start of labor, but it's the onset of painful contractions that lets you know labor is underway — you'll feel them!

Thinning and softening of the cervix One sign that labor is starting is that your cervix begins to thin (efface) and soften (ripen) in preparation for delivery. As labor progresses, the cervix eventually will go from an inch or more in thickness to paper-thin. Effacement is measured in percentages. If your care provider says, "You're about 50 percent effaced," it means that your cervix is half its original thickness. When your cervix is 100 percent effaced, it's completely thinned out.

Dilation of the cervix Your care provider may also tell you that your cervix is beginning to open (dilate). Dilation is measured in centimeters, with the cervix opening from 0 to 10 centimeters (4 inches) during the course of labor (see page 207). Thinning, softening and dilation of the cervix often precede other signs of labor. They can also occur days, even weeks, before actual contractions begin. With a first pregnancy, effacement usually begins before dilation. With subsequent pregnancies, the opposite is often true.

Breaking of water At some point during labor, the bag of water (amniotic sac) housing your baby either begins to leak or it fully breaks. Then the fluid that has cushioned your baby flows out of your vagina in a trickle or a gush.

You may fear that your water will break and your labor start while you're out in public. In reality, few women experience a dramatic breaking of water, and if they do, it usually happens at home.

Most often, a woman's water breaks while she's in active labor and already at the hospital. In fact, your care provider may even break your water for you during labor to help move things along or allow more careful monitoring of the baby.

Contractions At the beginning of labor, the uterus begins to squeeze (contract). These contractions are what move your baby down the birth canal. Labor pains (contractions) often begin with cramping

PRESENTATION, POSITION AND STATION

As the end of your pregnancy nears, your care provider may talk to you, in medical terms, about the presentation, position and station of your baby.

Presentation refers to the part of the fetus entering the pelvis, for example, the baby's head or feet. Throughout your pregnancy, your baby floats in your uterus and changes position somewhat freely. But, usually between the 32nd and 36th week of pregnancy, the baby rotates to — ideally — a headfirst position, settling into place for labor and delivery. Sometimes, though, babies may descend feet-first (breech presentation) or lie sideways (transverse lie) within the uterus.

Position refers to the relationship of the presenting part of the fetus to the mother's pelvis. In other words, is baby facing to the front or back or to the left or right?

Station refers to how far your baby's head has moved into the pelvic cavity in preparation for childbirth. Station is measured in centimeters, with each station being 1 centimeter. A baby high up in the pelvic cavity is said to be at a -5 station. A baby at 0 station is midway through the pelvis. Once actual labor begins, the baby's head continues through the pelvis to +1, +2 and +3 stations. At the +5 station, the baby's head crowns, emerging from the vagina and completing its passage through the pelvic cavity. For most women experiencing their first labor, the baby will already be at 0 station at the onset of labor. For women who are having their third or fourth babies, this may not happen until labor has progressed for several hours.

or discomfort in your lower back and abdomen that doesn't stop when you change position. Over time, the contractions become stronger and more regular. To distinguish between false and true labor, consider:

Frequency of your contractions. Using a watch, clock or phone app, time your contractions — from the beginning of one to the beginning of the next. True labor will develop into a regular pattern, with your contractions becoming closer together. In false labor, contractions remain irregular.

Length of your contractions. Measure the duration of each contraction by timing when it begins and when it stops. True contractions last about 30 to 60 seconds at the onset and get progressively longer and stronger. False labor contractions vary in length and intensity.

IT'S TIME! — OR IS IT?

Once you've started having regular contractions, the next question is: Is it time to leave for the hospital or birthing center, or call your care provider?

Your care provider probably will give you instructions about whom to call and at what point. For example, you may be told to call your care provider when it becomes difficult for you to walk or talk through the contractions. Many women are told to go to the hospital or birthing center after an hour of contractions that come five minutes apart. You may need to leave sooner if your labor seems to be progressing rapidly or your water breaks.

As your due date approaches, keep your car's gas tank full. You might even make a practice run to the hospital or birthing center if you're not familiar with the route. If you have other children,

---

CAN YOU KICK-START LABOR?

Most pregnant women have heard of at least one folk remedy for starting labor. Perhaps you've gotten advice on things you can do to help get labor going, such as:

- Frequent walking
- Having sex
- Exercising
- Using a laxative
- Stimulating your nipples
- Eating spicy foods
- Driving on a bumpy road
- Fasting
- Being frightened
- Consuming castor oil
- Drinking herbal tea

Keep in mind that most folk remedies aren't based in science and simply don't work. Some are even ill-advised. For example, fasting really isn't good for you or the baby. A few folk remedies have some basis in science. Nipple stimulation, for example, may cause uterine contractions, similar to what happens when a baby breast-feeds right after birth. It's also biologically plausible that sex might trigger contractions because semen contains substances similar to those used in labor-inducing medications. But that doesn't mean that your care provider will advise that you try either of these methods. Generally, the best advice is to be patient and let nature takes its course.

make arrangements for them while you're in the hospital, including a friend or family member to come to the house in case you have to leave in the middle of the night.

Ready; set; not yet! You might leave for the hospital or birthing center with regular contractions that are five minutes apart, and after you arrive, they may stop or decrease in intensity. You may even be sent home if your contractions aren't to the stage called active labor and your cervix isn't dilating. If this happens, don't feel embarrassed and try not to feel frustrated. Think of it instead as a good practice run.

Sometimes, telling real labor from false labor can be tricky. When in doubt, call your care provider or go to the hospital. If your water breaks, most care providers want you to come to the hospital. If there are concerns about your health,

WHAT'S THAT FOR?

If you've never been hospitalized, you may find medical surroundings slightly intimidating. But if you understand what's going on around you, you can better relax. Here's a list of equipment and supplies often found in a typical delivery room and what each item is used for during the birthing process.

Birthing bed A birthing bed (delivery bed) is usually a twin bed that's high off the ground. Delivery beds are designed to be practical. The bed can be raised or lowered, and the end of the bed can be removed to facilitate delivery. The bed may have a bar that you can hold on to while you push. Most delivery beds have stirrups that can be pulled out. Sometimes the stirrups are helpful during delivery, or you may need them if you require stitches after the birth.

Fetal monitor This piece of equipment helps your care team keep track of how baby is doing. In external fetal monitoring, one device measures and records the frequency of your contractions. Another device records the baby's heart rate. The two are connected to a monitor that displays and prints out both tracings at the same time so that their interactions can be observed. Specific patterns suggest that labor may be negatively affecting your baby and intervention may be needed.

Blood pressure monitor This device measures your blood pressure throughout your labor and delivery. A cuff goes around your arm just above the elbow and is attached to a measuring instrument.

Other items Your room may also have extra comforts, such as a rocking chair or a birthing chair, stool or ball. You can request extra pillows, blankets and towels. Some rooms have a tub or shower for your use during labor. At some point, a bassinet may be brought into the room for baby to be placed in once he or she is born.

your care provider may also instruct you to go to the hospital or birthing center sooner rather than later.

If you are sent home, it likely won't be long before true labor sets in and you're back at the hospital — this time to stay.

STAGES OF LABOR AND CHILDBIRTH

Labor is a sequence of events, or a process, that takes place over the span of an hour to as long as several days. How long your labor will last depends on many factors. As a rule, labor is usually longer with first babies. That's because the openings of the uterus (cervix) and birth canal (vagina) of first-time mothers are less flexible. For women giving birth for the first time, labor often lasts between 12 and 24 hours, although it can be longer. For women who have given birth before, labor often lasts eight to twelve hours or more.

How long labor lasts and how it progresses differs from woman to woman and from birth to birth. However, even though every labor is unique, the se-quence of events that takes place remains roughly the same. Labor is formally divided into three natural stages. Stage 1 occurs when the uterus opens the cervix to allow descent of the baby. Stage 2 is pushing and delivery — the birth of your baby. Stage 3 is delivery of the placenta (afterbirth).

Stage 1 The first stage of labor is the longest of the stages and is, itself, divided into three phases — early labor, active labor and transition.

Early labor Early labor begins with the start of contractions. During this early phase, as you're having contractions, your cervix dilates gradually to about 6 centimeters (cm). This period is usually the least intense phase of labor. The contractions of the uterus cause the cervix to thin and pull up around the baby's head. Repeated contractions will eventually stretch the cervix to a full 10 cm, an opening large enough for the baby's head to pass through.

Your contractions during early labor may last about 30 to 60 seconds. They may be irregular or regular, ranging between five and 20 minutes apart. They're

WHAT DOES LABOR FEEL LIKE?

Except for perhaps menstrual cramps, labor pain (contractions) may be unlike anything you've experienced. That's because you're not accustomed to feeling your uterine muscles contracting.

A contraction usually begins high in the uterus — close to your diaphragm — and radiates down the abdomen and into the lower back. You may feel the pain in your lower abdomen, lower back, hips or upper thighs. This sensation has been described as an aching, pressure, fullness, tightening, cramping and backache.

For some women, labor pains seem like very strong menstrual cramps. For others, they take on a whole different feeling.

usually mild to moderately strong. You may also experience a backache, upset stomach and, possibly, diarrhea. Some women report a sensation of warmth in the abdomen as labor begins.

Early labor can last for hours, so you may need to be patient. Your cervix needs to soften before it can dilate. Labor doesn't always begin when your contractions start. You may have irregular, painful contractions for hours or even several days before your cervix dilates, especially if this is your first baby.

How you may feel. With the onset of your first real contractions, you may be giddy with excitement. At the same time, though, you may be scared about the unknown. Try to remain relaxed.

What you can do. Until your contractions pick up in frequency and intensity, do household chores, watch television or a movie, or make phone calls. You may want to relax in a chair or get up and move around. Walking is a great activity because it may help relieve your discomfort. You may also find it helpful to take a shower or listen to relaxing music. It's OK to drink water or have a light snack.

If you're experiencing low backache, try ice packs or heat, or switch between hot and cold. Use a tennis ball or rolling pin to apply pressure to the lower back.

The timing and intensity of your contractions will help you know when it's time to go to the hospital or birthing center or to call your care provider.

At the hospital or birthing center. You will likely be taken to your room, often a labor room, where admission procedures are completed. After you've changed into a hospital gown or your own shirt or bra, you'll probably be examined to determine how dilated your cervix is. You may be connected to a fetal monitor to time your contractions and check your baby's heart rate. Your vital signs — your pulse, blood pressure and temperature — may be taken at regular intervals throughout your labor and delivery.

You may have an intravenous (IV) line placed into a vein, usually on the back of your hand or arm. The line may be attached to a plastic tube leading to a bag of fluid that drips into your body. The bag hangs on a movable stand, which you can wheel with you when you take a walk or go into the bathroom. The fluid

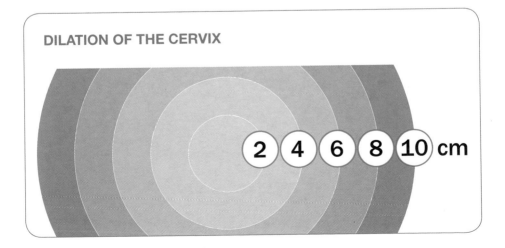

DILATION OF THE CERVIX

2 4 6 8 10 cm

LABOR POSITIONS

There's no best position for labor. Once you're in labor, experiment to find what's most comfortable for you. Listen to your body to discover what feels good. One tip: Give each new position a chance. The first few contractions may feel stronger until you get used to a new position. Contrary to what you may think, lying flat on your back generally isn't recommended for labor or childbirth. It can cause the weight of your uterus to compress major blood vessels and decrease blood flow to your uterus.

Here are examples of different labor positions you may want to try.

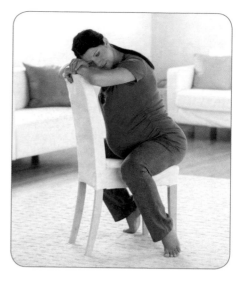

Leaning forward If your back hurts, leaning forward may feel good. Straddle a chair or lean over a table or countertop.

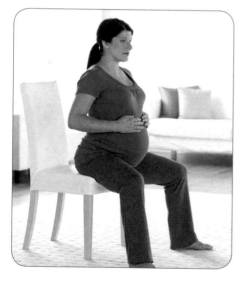

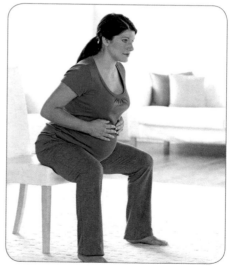

Rocking Gently rock forward and then back while sitting on a sturdy chair, the edge of a bed or a birthing ball. Rhythmic motions can be soothing.

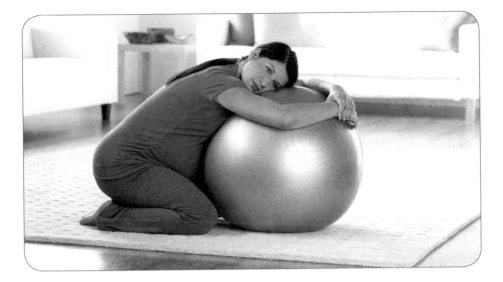

Kneeling Using a birthing ball or a pile of pillows, kneel on the floor and rest your arms and upper body on top of the ball or pillows.

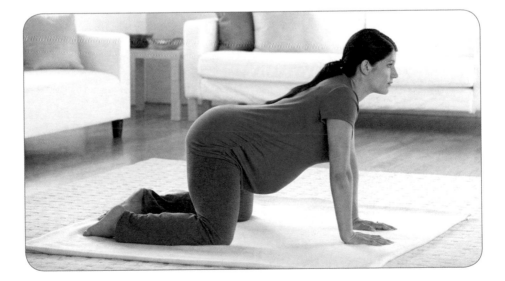

Hands and knees This position takes the pressure off your spine, which can ease back pain. It may boost baby's oxygen supply as well.

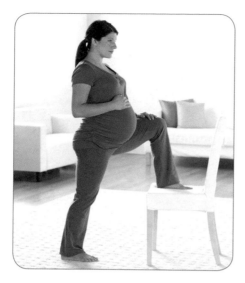

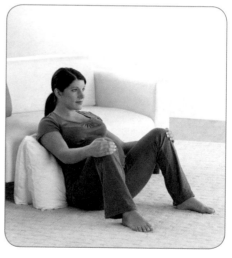

Lunging Raise one foot on a sturdy chair. During the next contraction, gently lean toward the raised foot. If a chair is too high, use a footstool.

Sitting Sit in a sturdy chair and prop one foot up on a stool. During each contraction you may want to lean toward the foot that's raised.

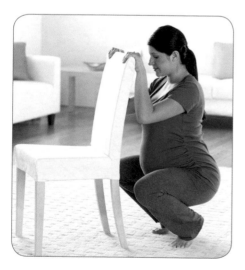

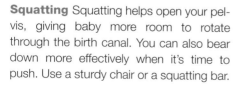

Squatting Squatting helps open your pelvis, giving baby more room to rotate through the birth canal. You can also bear down more effectively when it's time to push. Use a sturdy chair or a squatting bar.

Semisitting Prop yourself up with pillows, or ask your partner to sit behind you for support. During each contraction, lean forward and use your hands to draw your knees toward your body.

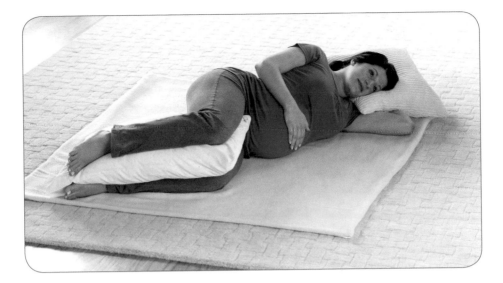

Lying on side Lie on your left side and place one or more pillows or a peanut ball between your knees. This maximizes blood flow to your uterus and may ease back pain.

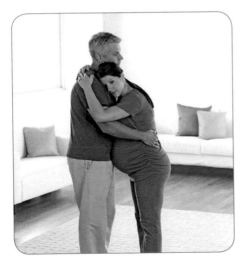

Swaying Lean on your partner for support during contractions, or wrap your arms around your partner's neck and start swaying, as though you were slow dancing.

FACTORS THAT CAN SPEED OR SLOW LABOR

Many factors can affect how your labor will progress. They include:

Size of your baby's head Because the bones of the skull aren't yet fused together, your baby's head molds itself to the shape and size of your pelvis as it moves through the birth canal (vagina). If the head moves through at an awkward angle, it can affect the length of your labor.

Position of your baby Babies' heads may not be in the most ideal position, and sometimes they're breech with their buttocks or feet coming first. They may even be sideways in the uterus. See Chapter 28 for more information.

Ability of your cervix to thin and open In most labors, the cervix opens as expected, but the speed of that dilation may vary considerably.

Medication Certain medications for pain relief can both help and hinder labor. Some care providers believe that if medications relieve pain early on, they can leave you rested and better equipped for the work of getting baby out. Some medications may interfere with your ability to push, slowing the pushing stage of labor.

Shape and roominess of your pelvis Your pelvis must be roomy enough for your baby's head to pass through. Fortunately, babies are generally well-matched to the size of their mothers. Women who have smaller frames, for example, tend to have smaller babies. In rare instances, the size of the pelvis can be a problem and slow labor.

Your ability to push Because you use your abdominal muscles to help push the baby out, the better shape you're in physically, the more you can assist. If you've had a long labor and you're tired, your pushing may be less effective.

Your physical state If you go into labor healthy and well-rested, you'll have more strength to work through your contractions. If you're ill or tired, or the early phase of your labor is particularly long, you may already be exhausted when it's time to push.

Your outlook If you have a positive outlook and you're actively involved in your labor and delivery, you'll cope better and the process may progress more quickly.

Support from staff and your labor coach An atmosphere of caring support helps you remain calm and can enhance your coping skills. A doula, someone who is specifically trained as a labor coach, may be particularly helpful. Some studies have shown that continuous support during childbirth, such as from a doula, may be associated with shorter labors. For more information about doulas, see page 349.

you receive through the IV helps to keep you hydrated. Medications also can be administered through your IV, if needed.

Contractions may start and stop regularly, but then stop for an extended period. If this happens, your care provider may suggest that you take a nap or go for a walk. If labor doesn't start again, your care provider may break your water, if the membranes haven't already ruptured, or start medication to try to get things moving again.

Active labor During this phase, your cervix dilates more quickly than during early labor, typically after about 6 cm dilation. Your contractions will become stronger and progressively longer. They may last 45 seconds to a minute or longer. They may be three to four minutes apart, or perhaps even two to three minutes apart. There's less rest between contractions.

The good news is that your contractions are accomplishing more in less time. Your baby is on the move down through your pelvis as your cervix continues to open. The average woman in her first labor generally dilates at least 1 cm an hour once she reaches 5 to 6 cm. If you've had a baby before, progression is typically faster. Active labor may last four to eight hours or more.

Throughout active labor, you'll have occasional pelvic exams to see how your cervix is changing. Your vital signs will likely be checked on a regular basis. If your amniotic sac hasn't broken already, it may break as your cervix dilates further. Or your care provider may break the water for you.

How you may feel. During active labor, your contractions become more painful, and you may feel increasing pressure in

---

BACK LABOR

Some women experience back labor — intense back pain, especially during active labor and transition. Often, back labor occurs when the baby is not in the most common position, occiput anterior, as it enters the birth canal. The baby's head may be pressing against the mother's tailbone (sacrum). But that isn't always the cause. Some women simply feel more tension in their backs than do others.

To relieve back labor:

▶ Have your labor coach apply counterpressure to your lower back. Have him or her massage the area or use hands or knuckles to apply direct pressure.

▶ Apply counterpressure by placing a tennis ball or rolling pin — if you brought either with you — under your tailbone.

▶ Have your labor coach apply heat or cold, whichever feels better to you, to your lower back.

▶ Change to a more comfortable position.

▶ If possible, take a shower and direct the warm water spray on your lower back.

▶ Ask for pain medication if you wish to try to relieve the pain.

your back. You may be unable to talk through your contractions now. Between contractions you may still be able to talk, watch television or listen to music, at least during the early part of active labor. You may feel excited and encouraged that things are starting to happen.

As your labor advances, your excitement may give way to concentrating on coping as your labor progresses and the pain intensifies. Your smile may fade as you become inwardly focused. You may feel tired and restless. Some women report feeling sensitive and irritable. You may reach a point that you no longer want to talk much. You may even need to have the room quiet and the lights dimmed so that you're completely free to concentrate on the job at hand.

During active labor, you may need greater help from your labor coach, seeking encouragement as your contractions peak and wane. Or you may react in the opposite manner. You may resist being touched or coached, in an attempt to stay focused and in control.

What you can do. Use your breathing and relaxation techniques. If you haven't practiced or learned natural childbirth techniques, your health care team will provide you with coaching. Give the suggested tricks a try. However, no single strategy works for everyone, so if what is recommended doesn't work for you, ask for another idea.

Some women find that as the pain intensifies, rocking in a rocking chair, rolling on a birthing ball, or taking a warm shower or bath helps them relax between contractions. Changing your position may also help your baby descend. Some women find walking helpful. If walking feels comfortable, continue with it, stopping to breathe through contractions. Vary your activities because no single ap-

proach is likely to work throughout labor. If these measures aren't effective, don't be afraid to request pain medication.

Try to concentrate on relaxing between your contractions. Doing so will help you stay energized through each stage of labor and delivery. Your labor won't last forever, and the only way through labor and delivery, really, is to go through it with as much determination and concentration as possible.

You may feel slightly nauseated during active labor. Try sucking on ice chips or hard candy to manage any nausea. This will also help to keep your mouth and throat from becoming dry as you're breathing harder during labor. Apply lip balm to your lips to keep them moist.

Transition The later part of the active phase of labor is called transition. It may be the shortest but most difficult phase. During transitional labor, your cervix opens the remaining few centimeters (cm), dilating all the way to 10 cm.

During transition, your contractions increase in strength and frequency with little break between. It may seem like there is time for only a hurried breath before the next one arrives. Your contractions reach peak intensity almost immediately, and they now last 60 to 90 seconds. In fact, it may feel as if your contractions never completely disappear.

Transition is a demanding time, and you'll likely feel a lot of pressure in your lower back and rectum. In addition, you may feel nauseated and vomit. One minute you may feel hot and sweaty, the next, cold. Your legs may begin to shake or cramp, which is fairly common.

As you get closer to your baby's birth, your pain medication options become more limited, but you still have choices. Trust your care provider to help you make decisions about pain medication.

How you may feel. Transition can go quickly. You may suddenly be past it and ready to push. During this phase of labor, don't worry if you feel exhausted and somewhat overwhelmed. That's normal. Try to stay focused as best you can. Until it's safe to push, relax those muscles that you have control over, and save your energy.

What you can do. During transition, concentrate on getting through each contraction. If it helps, focus on getting through just the first half of each contraction. After a contraction peaks, the second half gets easier. If your contractions are being monitored, your partner can watch their progress, letting you know when they've peaked so that you know when the hardest part is over.

During transition, you may not want things like a radio or television distracting you. Don't think about the next contraction. Just take each one as it arrives.

If you feel the urge to push, try to hold back until you've been told you're fully dilated. This will help prevent your cervix from tearing or swelling, which can delay delivery. Instead of pushing, try to pant (blow air out in short breaths) through the contraction.

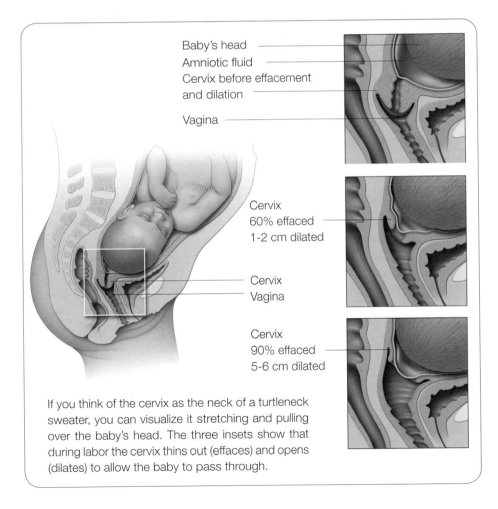

Baby's head
Amniotic fluid
Cervix before effacement and dilation
Vagina

Cervix
60% effaced
1-2 cm dilated

Cervix
Vagina

Cervix
90% effaced
5-6 cm dilated

If you think of the cervix as the neck of a turtleneck sweater, you can visualize it stretching and pulling over the baby's head. The three insets show that during labor the cervix thins out (effaces) and opens (dilates) to allow the baby to pass through.

HOW BABY COMES OUT

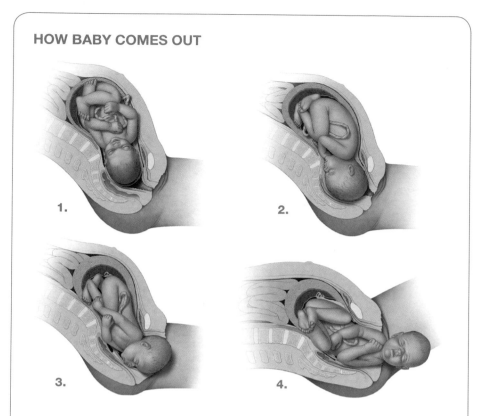

1.

2.

3.

4.

The human pelvis has a complex shape, making your baby negotiate several maneuvers during labor and delivery. Your pelvis is widest from side to side at the top (inlet) and from front to back at the bottom (outlet). The baby's head is widest from front to back, and the shoulders are widest from side to side. As a result, your baby must twist and turn on the way through the birth canal.

Because almost every mother's pelvis is widest side to side at the entrance, most babies enter the pelvis looking left or right (illustration 1). The exit from the pelvis is widest from front to back, so babies almost always turn faceup or facedown (illustration 2). These maneuvers occur as a result of forces of labor and the resistance provided by the birth canal.

In addition to making these turning maneuvers, the baby is simultaneously descending farther down the vagina. Finally, the top of your baby's head appears (crowns), stretching your vaginal opening (illustration 3). When the vulva has stretched enough, the baby's head will emerge — usually by extending the head, lifting its chin off the chest and thus emerging from under your pubic bone. The baby usually emerges facedown but will turn to one side very quickly as the shoulders turn to take the same route (illustration 4).

Next, the shoulders are born one at a time, and with a great slippery rush, the rest of the body is delivered — and now you can hold your new baby.

WHAT EXACTLY TRIGGERS LABOR?

Actually, the answer to that question is still somewhat of a medical mystery. Somehow your body knows — accurately, most of the time — when your baby has matured enough to live outside the uterus.

Our current understanding of how labor begins involves certain chemical signals produced by your body, called prostaglandins. These signals thin, soften and dilate your cervix, and at the right time, your body begins to produce prostaglandins in large amounts. It's the high levels of prostaglandins that cause uterine contractions to become more frequent and stronger. The contractions, in turn, trigger the production of even more prostaglandins, and the cycle accelerates into labor.

It's very likely that these steps evolve from a complex interplay — a cross-talk between the baby's glandular system, the placenta and the mother's uterus — that sets into motion increased prostaglandin production.

Stage 2: The birth of your baby
Once your cervix is fully dilated and you are instructed to, you can push. It isn't unusual, especially with your first birth, to have to push for one to two hours or more before the top of your baby's head appears (crowns) at the opening of your vagina. It may still take another few minutes and a few pushes to deliver the baby.

After you push the baby's head out, you'll probably be instructed to stop pushing for a moment while your care provider makes sure that the baby's umbilical cord is free.

You may find it difficult to stop pushing when told to, but try. It may help to pant instead of pushing. Slowing down gives your vaginal area time to stretch rather than tear. To stay motivated, you may be able to put your hand down and feel the baby's head or see it in a mirror. You're very close now! When you're told to, push again and your baby will be born!

Immediately after birth At birth, your baby is still connected to the placenta by the umbilical cord. Often the parents can assist with the clamping and cutting of the cord. If you'd like to assist, make your wishes known, and you'll be shown what to do. For a healthy baby without complications, a delay of 30 to 60 seconds before cord clamping is recommended to allow more cord blood to flow into the baby. Then two clamps are placed on the cord, and a scissors is used to snip painlessly between the clamps. If the umbilical cord has looped snugly around the baby's neck, the cord may be clamped and cut before the shoulders are delivered.

Immediately after birth, your baby may be placed in your arms or on your abdomen. Placing the baby directly on your skin helps to keep baby warm and facilitates early bonding with you. Occasionally, the baby may be passed to a nurse or pediatrician for evaluation and attention.

Eventually, your baby is weighed and examined. He or she is dried off and then wrapped in blankets to keep him or her warm. Apgar scores (see page 242) are taken and recorded at one- and five-minute intervals. An identification band is placed on your baby so that there's no mix-up in the hospital. This is just the first of many safeguards to ensure no mistake in identification is made.

In most cases, you'll be able to hold and breast-feed your baby right after birth. But if your baby shows any signs that help is needed, such as trouble breathing, he or she may need to be evaluated more thoroughly in the nursery.

Stage 3: Delivery of the placenta
After your baby is born, a lot is happening. You and your partner are celebrating the excitement of the birth. You're likely both decompressing, relieved that labor and childbirth are finally over. Meanwhile, a care provider in the background is examining your baby as he or she takes the first breaths and you hear those wonderful first cries.

The third, and final, stage of labor and childbirth is delivery of the placenta. The placenta is the organ inside the uterus attached to the baby by the umbilical cord. It's the organ that has nourished your baby throughout your pregnancy.

For most parents, the placenta — also called the afterbirth — is of little significance. For the medical personnel attending the birth, though, delivering the placenta and ensuring that the mother doesn't bleed excessively are important.

What's happening. After your baby is born, you'll continue to have contractions, but they're mild. These contractions are necessary for several reasons — one of which is to help you deliver the placenta.

Usually about five to 10 minutes after the birth, the placenta separates from the wall of the uterus. Your final contractions push the placenta out from the uterus and down into the vagina. You may be asked to push one more time to deliver the placenta, which usually comes out with a small gush of blood. Sometimes it may take up to 30 minutes for the placenta to detach and be expelled.

Your care provider may massage your lower abdomen after you have delivered your baby. This is to encourage your uterus to contract, to help expel the placenta.

After delivery of your placenta, you may be given a medication such as oxytocin by injection or by intravenous (IV) drip to encourage uterine contractions. Uterine contractions after birth are important. Sometimes additional medications are needed to help firm your uterus to decrease blood loss.

During birth, it's not uncommon to experience a small tear in your perineal tissue. After your placenta has been delivered, your care provider will evaluate the need for any stitches. If they're needed, your care provider will make sure you have adequate pain control. The stitches will eventually dissolve on their own.

How you may feel. You shouldn't feel much pain while your uterus contracts to push out the placenta. The hardest part may be simply being patient as you wait for the delivery of the placenta. The deep massages of your abdomen by your care provider may hurt.

What you can do. You can help expel the placenta by pushing when directed. As you push, your care provider may pull gently on the remaining umbilical cord attached to the placenta. In most instances, delivery of the placenta is a routine part of childbirth, but complications can arise if your placenta doesn't spontaneously detach from the uterine wall (retained placenta). In this situation, the care provider must reach inside the uterus and remove the placenta by hand.

Once the placenta is out, your care provider examines it to make sure it's normal and intact. If it's not intact, he or she must remove any remaining fragments inside the uterus. Rarely, surgery is needed to remove placental fragments. Remnants that aren't removed could cause bleeding and infection.

After delivery and a brief inspection, the placenta is then typically sent to a pathology lab for evaluation and possibly for preservation and storage. Most women never see the placenta, but if you're interested you can ask to. It's usually round and red, about 6 to 8 inches in diameter and about 20 ounces in weight. If you're interested in taking your placenta home (see page 196), talk to your care provider. You may have to complete a consent or release form.

In multiple pregnancies, the babies' cords may be attached to one single placenta or to separate placentas, so there may be more than one placenta to deliver.

At last. For most parents, all of the preparation, pain and effort that went into bringing a newborn into the world are quickly forgotten as they hold their newborn child. This is one of the most significant moments in your life. You are now a parent, and a new human being has taken his or her place in your family. It truly is an absolute miracle. Savor this moment, cherish it and embrace the joy that nothing else in life can quite match.

IF YOU'RE THE LABOR COACH

You may be a partner, parent, sibling or friend. Whatever your other roles, your job as labor coach is to support the mother-to-be both physically and emotionally during her labor and delivery. Here are some ways that you can help.

During early labor Through the first phase of childbirth:

Time her contractions Measure the time from the beginning of one contraction to the next. Keep a record. When contractions are coming five minutes apart and have been that way for an hour, it's usually time to call your care provider or go to the hospital.

Keep her calm Once contractions begin, you both may feel some initial butterflies. After all, it's the big moment you've been anticipating for the past 10 months. But during labor and delivery, your goal is to keep the expectant mother relaxed. That means staying as calm as possible yourself. Take some deep breaths together. Between contractions, practice the relaxation techniques you learned in childbirth class. For example, suggest that she let her muscles go limp or that she concentrate on relaxing her jaw and hands. Try massaging her back, feet or shoulders.

Help distract her Suggest activities — such as watching television or taking a walk — that will help keep her mind off labor. When appropriate, humor can be a great distraction, too. Enjoying some laughs together may be good for both of you.

Ask her what she needs If you're unsure what to do for your partner, ask her what would make her more comfortable. If she isn't sure what she needs, do your best to suggest something that you think might make her feel better. But don't take it personally if she doesn't take you up on your suggestions or focuses inward during contractions.

Give encouragement Offer her encouragement and praise through each contraction. Remind her that with each contraction, and with each passing hour of labor, she's getting closer to meeting the baby. What you don't want to do is criticize her or pretend that the pain doesn't exist. She needs your empathy and support, even if she's not complaining.

Take care of yourself, too To keep up your strength, have some refreshments periodically. But respect that your partner may not want you to eat in front of her or to leave her for an extended period to eat. If you feel faint at any time during labor and delivery, sit down, and then tell someone on the health care team.

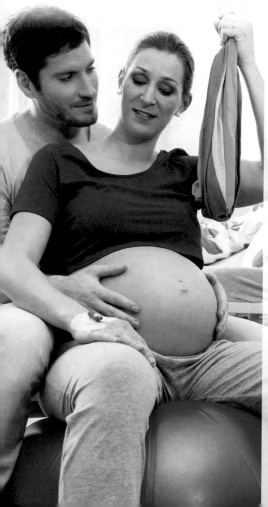

During active labor As labor progresses to the next stage:

Quiet the room If it's possible, keep the labor room or birthing room as calm as possible by keeping the doors closed and the lights dimmed. Some women find it relaxing to listen to soft music during labor.

Help her through contractions Learn to recognize the start of your partner's contractions. If she's on a fetal monitor, ask someone how to read it. Or place your hand on your partner's abdomen and feel for the telltale tightening of the uterus. You can then alert your partner when a contraction is beginning. You can also offer encouragement as each contraction peaks and wanes. If it helps her, breathe with her through difficult contractions. Try to make her more comfortable by massaging her abdomen or lower back or by using counterpressure or any other techniques you've learned.

Some women prefer not to be touched during labor, so take your cues from your partner. If she's uncomfortable, suggest a change of position or a walk — if possible — to help labor progress. Offer her water or ice chips if she's allowed to have them. Place a cool, damp cloth on her forehead or on the back of her neck if that sounds appealing to her.

Be an advocate As much as possible, serve as your partner's go-between with the health care team. Don't be afraid to ask questions about how her labor is progressing or to ask for explanations about any procedures or the need for medications. If your partner requests pain medication, ask her care providers to discuss pain relief options. Remember: Childbirth isn't a test of pain endurance. A woman doesn't fail at labor if she chooses pain relief medication.

Continue to give encouragement By the time a woman is in active labor, she's likely feeling quite tired and uncomfortable, and perhaps edgy. As in early labor, be supportive and encouraging by saying things such as: "You did a great job getting through that last contraction," or "You're doing great! I'm really proud of you."

Don't take things personally Things may be said in labor that aren't meant. Don't take it personally if your partner seems irritated with your thoughtful attempts to comfort her or if she doesn't respond to your questions. Your presence alone is comforting and sometimes is all that's needed.

During transition During this particularly difficult stage of labor:

Continue to help her through contractions Transition, as the baby progresses down the birth canal, is usually the hardest time for the mother. Now is the time to give her even more encouragement and praise. Remind her to take it one contraction at a time. If it helps her, talk her through each contraction or breathe with her. Some women find they don't want to have someone coaching them as contractions intensify. Give space, if needed. In fact, holding her hand, making eye contact or simply saying, "I love you," may be the support that means the most to her.

Put her needs first Throughout labor and delivery, stay conscious of her needs. Offer her water or ice chips, if allowed. Massage her body. Suggest position changes periodically. Keep her informed of how labor is progressing and how well she's doing. It's more important for you to take care of her than to record everything on camera or call friends and family.

During pushing and delivery When you get to this last phase:

Help guide her pushing and breathing Using cues from the health care team or from what you learned in childbirth classes, guide her breathing while she pushes. You might also support her back or hold one of her legs while she's pushing.

Stay close by A lot may happen quickly when it's time for her to push. Or she may have to keep pushing on and off for several hours. Once she gets ready to push, don't feel that you're in the way as your partner's care provider takes charge. Your presence is important, particularly as labor nears completion.

Point out her progress As the baby's head crowns, if allowed, hold up a mirror so that she can see for herself how she's progressing. Or tell her how close the baby is to being born!

Cut the cord, if desired If offered the opportunity to cut the cord, don't panic. You'll get clear directions from medical staff about what to do. Don't feel pressured to do this if you're uncomfortable with the idea.

Celebrate! Once the baby has arrived, enjoy bonding with the new baby. But don't forget to give your partner some well-earned words of praise, and congratulate yourself, too, for a job well-done!

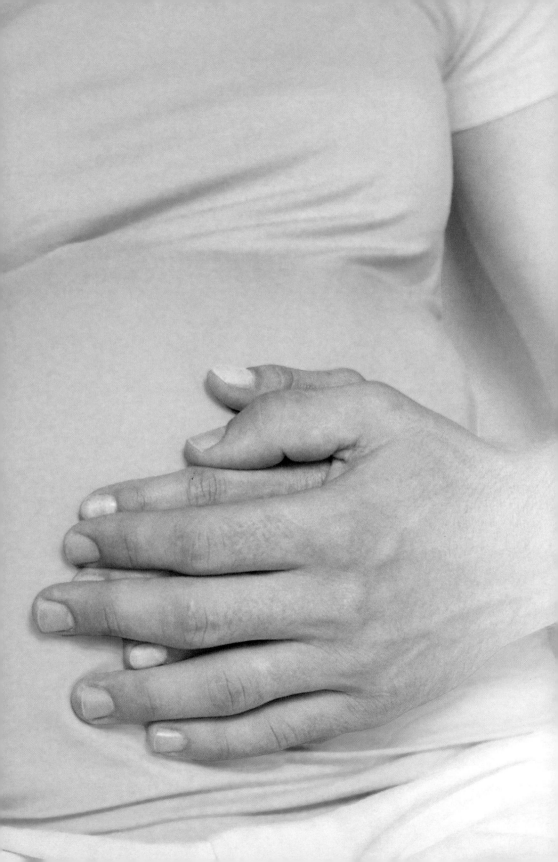

CHAPTER 15

Cesarean birth

There are times when giving birth the natural way isn't the best option. Cesarean delivery — commonly known as a C-section — is a surgical procedure used to deliver your baby through an incision in your abdomen, rather than vaginally. Cesarean deliveries now represent nearly one-third of all births in the United States. Some C-sections are planned due to pregnancy complications or because you've had a previous C-section. Some women choose to have a cesarean birth instead of a vaginal delivery (see Chapter 24). However, in many cases, the need for a C-section doesn't become obvious until labor has already started.

Knowing what to expect can help you prepare if a C-section is necessary.

WHEN IS A C-SECTION DONE?

There are many different reasons why cesarean births are performed. The decision to have a C-section may have to do with your health, while other times it's related to concerns about your baby.

Labor isn't progressing normally One of the most common reasons that doctors deliver babies by C-section is because active labor isn't progressing as it should — it's moving along too slowly or stops altogether. The causes of slow or stalled labor are varied. Your uterus may not be contracting vigorously enough to dilate your cervix completely. Or your baby's head may simply be too big to fit through your pelvis.

Baby has an abnormal heart rate pattern Certain fetal heart rate patterns are very reassuring in labor. Other patterns can indicate a problem with the baby's oxygen supply. If heart rate patterns cause concern, your care provider may recommend a C-section. Abnormal fetal heart rate patterns can arise when the baby isn't getting enough oxygen, the umbilical cord is compressed or the placenta isn't functioning optimally.

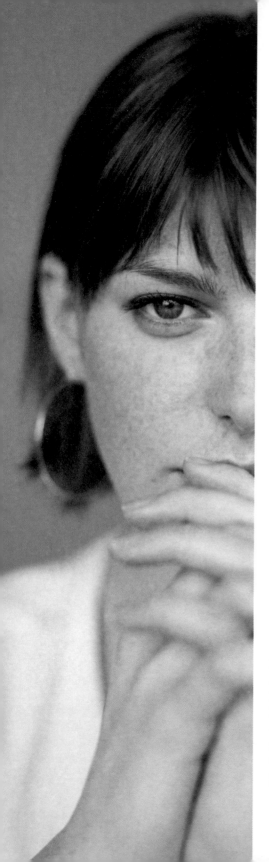

Sometimes, abnormal fetal heart rate patterns occur but aren't a signal of any real risk to your baby. At other times, the findings can indicate a serious problem. One of the most difficult decisions in obstetrics is determining when the risk is genuine. To help make that decision, your care provider may try certain maneuvers, such as massaging the baby's head during a vaginal exam, to see if this triggers an improvement in the heart rate.

Deciding when a C-section is necessary depends on many variables, such as how long labor is likely to continue before delivery and what other problems may add to the significance of the abnormal patterns.

Baby is in a difficult position Babies whose feet or buttocks enter the birth canal before the head are in what's known as the breech position. Most of these babies are born by C-section, because of an increased risk of complications with a vaginal breech delivery. Sometimes, a care provider is able to turn the baby to a head-down (cephalic or vertex) position by pushing firmly on the mother's abdomen. This procedure, an external cephalic version (ECV), is done before labor starts. If your baby is lying horizontally across your uterus, the position is called a transverse lie. This position, too, calls for a C-section unless ECV is able to turn the baby.

For more information on breech and transverse positions, see Chapter 28.

Baby's head isn't ideally positioned Ideally, your baby's chin should be tucked down to the chest so that the back of the head, which has the smallest diameter, is leading the way. If your baby's chin is up or head is turned so that the smallest dimensions aren't leading the way, a larger diameter of the head has to fit through your pelvis. For some women, having baby faceup instead of facedown doesn't pose a problem, but for others, complications can develop.

Before a C-section is done, your care provider might have you get on your hands and knees with your buttocks in the air, a position that causes the uterus to drop forward and seems to help babies turn. Sometimes a care provider may try to turn the baby's head by way of a vaginal exam, or with forceps.

You have a serious health problem A C-section may be performed if you have diabetes, heart disease, lung disease or high blood pressure. With these conditions, situations may arise where it becomes preferable to deliver the baby earlier in the pregnancy. If starting (inducing) labor isn't successful, a C-section may be necessary. If you have a serious health problem, discuss your options with your care provider early in your pregnancy.

Another unusual cause for a C-section is to protect a baby from acquiring herpes simplex infections. If a mother has herpes in the genital tract, it can be passed to a birthing baby, giving rise to serious disease. A cesarean birth can prevent that complication.

You're carrying multiples Cesarean birth is more likely for women delivering twins or other multiples. In recent years in the United States, approximately 75 percent of women carrying twins have had C-sections, either planned or during labor. Twins can be born vaginally, depending on their position, estimated weight and gestational age. Triplets and other multiples are often a different story. Studies show the vast majority of triplet births are done by C-section.

Each multiple pregnancy is unique. If you're carrying multiples, discuss your birth options with your care provider and decide together what's best for you. Remember to stay flexible. Sometimes the second baby changes position or has heart rate problems after the first baby is born.

There's a placental problem Two problems with the placenta may warrant C-section: placental abruption and placenta previa.

Placental abruption occurs when your placenta detaches from the inner wall of your uterus before or during labor. It can cause life-threatening problems for you and your baby. If electronic fetal monitoring shows that your baby is not in

WHAT ABOUT ELECTIVE C-SECTIONS?

Some healthy women choose to have cesarean deliveries — typically to avoid labor or the possible complications of vaginal birth. Sometimes doctors even suggest a C-section so that baby can be born at a more convenient time for mom or doctor or both.

These are called elective C-sections and they aren't performed for health reasons. Instead, they're done for other reasons, such as fear of vaginal delivery or wanting to make specific plans for delivery.

As elective C-sections have become more common, they've also become more controversial. For more information, see Chapter 24.

immediate trouble, you may be hospitalized and monitored closely. If your baby is in jeopardy, immediate cesarean delivery will likely be necessary.

With placenta previa the placenta lies low in your uterus and partially or completely covers the opening of your cervix. The placenta can't be delivered first because the baby would no longer have access to oxygen. Therefore, a C-section is almost always done.

There's an umbilical cord problem Once your water has broken, it's possible that a loop of umbilical cord can slip out through your cervix, before your baby is born. This is called umbilical cord prolapse, and it poses significant danger to your baby. As your baby presses against your cervix, the pressure on the protruding cord can block your baby's oxygen supply. If the cord slips out after your cervix is completely dilated and if birth is imminent, you might still be able to deliver vaginally. Otherwise, a C-section is the only option.

Similarly, if the cord is wrapped around your baby's neck or is positioned between your baby's head and your pelvic bones, or if you have decreased amniotic fluid, each uterine contraction can squeeze the cord, slowing blood flow and the delivery of oxygen to your baby. In these cases, a C-section may be the best option, especially if cord compression is prolonged or severe. This is a common cause of abnormal heart rate patterns, but it usually isn't possible to know for sure where the umbilical cord is until after birth.

Baby is very large Some babies are too large to deliver safely vaginally. Baby's size may be of particular concern if you have an abnormally small pelvis, which may prevent his or her head from passing through. This is rare unless you've had a pelvic fracture or another deformation of the pelvis.

If you've developed gestational diabetes during pregnancy, your baby may have gained a lot of weight. A cesarean birth is more likely for an overly large baby.

Baby has a health problem If your baby has been diagnosed in the womb with a health condition, such as spina bifida, your care provider may recommend a C-section. Discuss the factors that apply in your situation and your options with your care provider.

You've had a previous C-section If you've had a C-section before, you may need to have one again. But this isn't always the case. Sometimes a vaginal birth is possible after a cesarean delivery (see Chapter 25).

THE RISKS

It's important to remember that any childbirth carries risks for both the mother and the baby. Complications can arise even during or after labor and vaginal delivery in a low-risk pregnancy.

Cesarean birth is generally considered a very safe procedure. Still, it's major surgery, which carries certain risks. Keep in mind that C-sections are often performed to resolve serious problems. Therefore, it's to be expected that more complications would arise in women who have cesarean deliveries, compared with vaginal births.

Risks for you The risks of complications for women who have C-sections include:
▶ *Increased bleeding.* On average, blood loss during a C-section is about twice that of a vaginal birth. However, blood transfusions are rarely needed.

- *Reactions to anesthesia.* The medications used during surgery, including those used for anesthesia, can sometimes cause unexpected responses, including breathing problems. In rare cases, general anesthesia can lead to pneumonia if a woman aspirates stomach contents into her lungs. But general anesthesia is not often used in C-sections, and precautions are taken to avoid these complications.
- *Injury to your bladder or bowel.* These surgical injuries are rare, but can occur.
- *Endometritis.* This condition, which causes an inflammation and infection of the membrane lining your uterus, is the most frequent complication associated with cesarean birth. It occurs when bacteria that normally inhabit your vagina make their way into your uterus.
- *Urinary tract infection.* Urinary tract infections, such as bladder infections and kidney infections, rank second to endometritis as a cause of complications after a C-section.
- *Decreased bowel function.* Sometimes the drugs used for anesthesia and pain relief may cause the bowel to slow down after surgery, resulting in temporary distention of the abdomen, bloating and discomfort.
- *Blood clots in your legs, lungs or pelvic organs.* The risk of developing a blood clot inside a vein is about three to five times greater after a C-section than a vaginal delivery. Left untreated, a blood clot in the leg can travel to your heart and lungs where it can obstruct blood flow, causing chest pain, shortness of breath and even death. Clotting can also occur in the pelvic veins.
- *Wound infection.* Wound infection rates following cesarean birth vary. Your chances of developing a wound infection after a C-section are higher if you misuse alcohol, have type 2 diabetes or are obese.
- *Wound opening (disruption).* When a wound is infected or healing poorly, it's more likely to split open along the surgical suture lines.
- *Placenta accreta and hysterectomy.* With placenta accreta, the placenta is attached too deeply and firmly to the wall of the uterus to separate normally

IS THERE A LIMIT?

Most women can safely have up to three C-sections. Each repeat C-section is generally more complicated than the last, however.

For some women, the risk of surgical complications — such as infection or heavy bleeding — increases only slightly from one C-section to the next. If you had a long and difficult labor before your first C-section, a repeat C-section may be less physically taxing, although the healing process will be similar in length. For other women — such as those who have significant internal scarring — the risk of each repeat C-section increases substantially.

Repeat C-sections appeal to many women. But after you've had three or more C-sections, it's important to carefully weigh the surgical risks of another C-section against your desire for more children.

after birth. If you've had a C-section, your risk of developing placenta accreta in a subsequent pregnancy is increased. Placenta accreta is currently the most common reason why removal of the uterus (hysterectomy) is done after a cesarean birth.

▶ *Rehospitalization.* Compared with women who deliver vaginally, women who deliver by C-section may be more likely to be hospitalized again in the first few months after giving birth.

Risks for your baby Cesarean birth also can pose potential risks for your baby.

▶ *Premature birth.* With an elective C-section, it's important the gestational age is accurate so that the baby is not born before an optimal age. Delivering a baby prematurely may lead to difficulty breathing and low birth weight.

▶ *Breathing problems.* Babies born by C-section are more likely to develop a minor breathing problem called transient tachypnea. This condition is marked by abnormally fast breathing during the first few days after birth.

▶ *Fetal injury.* Rarely, accidental nicks to the baby can occur during surgery.

WHAT YOU CAN EXPECT

Whether your C-section is planned or unexpected, it will likely go as follows:

Preparation A series of discussions and procedures will take place to prepare you for the surgery. In an emergency, some of these steps might need to be cut short or left out entirely.

Anesthesia options An anesthesiologist or a nurse anesthetist may come to your hospital room to discuss your anesthesia options. Spinal, epidural and general anesthesia may all be used for C-sections.

DEALING WITH THE UNEXPECTED

Getting the unexpected news that you need a C-section can be stressful, both for you and your partner. In an instant, your expectations about giving birth may abruptly change. To make things worse, this news often comes when you're tired and discouraged after many hours of labor. In addition, there may not be much time for your care provider to explain the procedure and answer your questions.

It's normal to have some worries about how you and your baby will fare during a cesarean birth, but don't let these worries get the better of you. Almost all mothers and babies recover well after a C-section, with few problems. Although you would probably have preferred a vaginal birth, remind yourself that your health and the health of your baby are much more important than is the method of delivery.

If you're feeling anxious about a scheduled repeat cesarean birth, discuss your fears with your care provider, childbirth educator or partner. Some hospitals may be able to offer measures to help you feel comfortable and engaged in the birth. Also, tell yourself that you made it through once before — and you can do it again. Recovery may seem easier this time around because you know what to expect.

Spinal and epidural anesthesia numb your body from the chest down, and you remain awake for the procedure. You feel little or no pain, and little or no medication reaches your baby.

The differences between spinal and epidural anesthesia are fairly small. With a spinal block, pain-relieving medication is injected into the fluid surrounding your spinal nerves. With an epidural, a thin tube (catheter) is inserted just outside the fluid-filled space surrounding your spinal cord. Medication can then be given through the catheter. An epidural takes about 20 minutes to administer, and relief can last until after the catheter is removed. A spinal block can be performed more quickly but usually lasts only about two hours.

General anesthesia, in which you're completely unconscious, may be used in emergency C-sections, when your baby needs to be delivered quickly. Some of the medication does reach your baby, but this generally doesn't cause any problems. Most babies show no effect of general anesthesia since the mother's brain absorbs the medication promptly. If necessary, your baby can be given medications to counteract any effects of the anesthesia.

Other preparations Once you, your doctor and the anesthesiologist have decided which type of anesthesia you'll have, preparations begin in earnest. These typically include:

▶ *An IV.* An intravenous (IV) needle is inserted into your hand or arm. This will allow you to receive fluids and medications during and after surgery.
▶ *Blood samples.* Sometimes, blood samples are taken and sent to the hospital lab for analysis. These tests give your doctor a more complete picture of your presurgery condition.
▶ *Antacid.* You may be given an antacid to neutralize your stomach acids. This

greatly diminishes the possibility of damage to your lungs if you were to vomit during anesthesia and stomach contents were to enter your lungs.
▶ *Monitors.* Your blood pressure will be monitored during surgery. You will also be hooked up to a cardiac monitor through electrodes stuck to your chest, to monitor your heart rate and rhythm during surgery. A saturation monitor will be attached to your finger to monitor the oxygen level in your blood.
▶ *Urinary catheter.* A thin tube is inserted into your bladder to drain urine so that your bladder will stay empty during surgery.

The operating room Most C-sections are performed in operating rooms designed specifically for that purpose. The atmosphere may be a lot different from what you might have experienced in the birthing room. Because surgery is a team effort, many more people will be there. If you or your baby has a complex medical problem, members from several medical teams may be present.

For planned or nonurgent cesarean births, some hospitals now offer measures in the operating room to improve the experience. These measures aim to engage parents in the birth in certain ways and encourage successful breastfeeding and bonding. For example, your IV and monitors may be placed so that at least one arm can move and hold the baby immediately after birth, if possible.

Getting ready If you're going to have an epidural or spinal block, you may be asked to sit up with your back rounded or lie curled up on your side. The anesthesiologist will likely scrub your back with antiseptic solution and inject a medication to numb the site. Then he or she can administer the medication by inserting a needle between two vertebrae and through the tissue next to your spinal column.

You may receive just one dose of medication through the needle, which will then be removed. Or your anesthesiologist may thread a narrow catheter through the needle, slide the needle out and tape the catheter to your back to keep it in place. This allows you to receive repeat doses of anesthetic as needed.

If you need general anesthesia, all preparations for surgery will be done before you receive the anesthetic. Your anesthesiologist will likely administer the medication through your IV. Once you're anesthetized, you'll be placed on your back with your legs positioned securely in place. A wedge may be placed under the right side of your back so that you're turned to the left. This shifts the uterine weight left, which can help ensure good uterine blood flow.

To prepare the surgical site, a nurse may clip a portion of your pubic hair, if it will interfere with surgery. Your abdomen will be scrubbed with an antiseptic solution and draped with sterile cloths. Typically, a curtain will also hang above your chin to help keep the surgical field clean.

Abdominal incision Once you're ready, the surgeon makes the first incision. This is the abdominal incision, made in your abdominal wall. The incision will probably be about 6 inches long, going through your skin, fat and muscle to reach the lining of your abdominal cavity (peritoneum). Bleeding blood vessels can be sealed with heat (cauterized) or tied off.

The location of your abdominal incision will depend on several factors, such as whether your C-section is an emergency and whether you have any previous abdominal scars. Your baby's size or the position of placenta also is considered.

The most common incisions are:

- *Low transverse incision.* Also known as a bikini incision, this type of incision curves across your lower abdomen along the line of an imaginary bikini bottom and is the preferred abdominal incision. It heals well and causes the least pain after surgery. It's also preferred for cosmetic reasons and gives your surgeon a good view of the lower pregnant uterus.

- *Vertical incision.* Sometimes, this type of incision is the best option. A vertical incision allows faster access to the lower portion of your uterus, allowing your surgeon to remove your baby more quickly. Occasionally, time is of the essence.

Uterine incision Once your abdominal incision is complete, a surgeon moves your bladder off the lower part of the uterus and makes an incision in the wall of your uterus. Your uterine incision may or may not be the same type as on your abdomen. The uterine incision is usually smaller than the abdominal incision.

As with the abdominal incision, the location of the uterine incision will depend on several factors, such as whether your delivery is an emergency, how big your baby is, and how your baby or the placenta is positioned inside the uterus.

The low transverse incision, made horizontally across the lower portion of the uterus, is the most common, used in the majority of cesarean births. It provides ease of entry, bleeds less than incisions higher on the uterus and poses less risk of bladder injury. It also forms a strong scar, presenting little danger of rupture during future labors.

In some cesarean births, a vertical uterine incision is more appropriate. A low vertical incision — made in your lower uterus where the tissue is thinner —

may be used if a baby is positioned feet-first, rump-first or sideways in your uterus (breech or transverse lie). It may also be used if your surgeon thinks your incision may need to be extended to a high vertical incision — what doctors sometimes call a classical incision.

A classical incision may be called for to provide access to an extremely pre-term baby, before the lower uterus is well-developed. A classical incision may also be needed if there are known placental complications, such as placenta previa, or, occasionally, to avoid bladder injury.

Birth With your uterus open, the next step is to open the amniotic sac so that your baby can make his or her grand appearance. If you're awake, you'll probably feel some tugging or pressure as your baby is pulled out. You shouldn't feel any pain.

After your baby is born and the umbilical cord has been clamped, your baby will likely be handed to another member of your health care team. This person makes sure your baby's nose and mouth are free of fluids and that he or she is breathing well. In just a matter of minutes, you'll have your first look at your baby.

After birth Once your baby is delivered, the next step is generally to detach and remove the placenta from the uterus, followed by closure of your incisions, layer by layer.

The stitches on your internal organs and tissues usually can dissolve on their own and won't need to be removed. For the incision on your skin, your surgeon may use stitches or a type of staples to close it. Throughout this repair, you may feel some movement or pressure but no pain. Some types of staples are absorbable and do not need to be removed, but other types will be removed by your doctor or nurse several days after delivery.

Seeing your baby While a cesarean birth typically takes about 45 minutes to an hour to perform, your baby will likely be born in the first five to 10 minutes of the procedure. If you're feeling up to it and are awake, you may be able to hold your baby as your surgeon closes the incisions in your uterus and abdomen. At the very least, you'll probably be able to see your baby snuggled into your partner's arms. Before giving your baby to you or your partner, your health

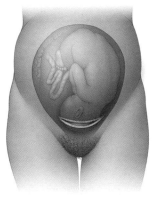

Low transverse incision

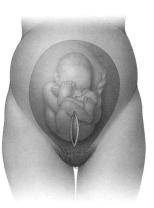

Low vertical incision

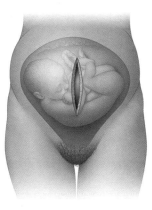

Classical incision

care team may suction your baby's nose and mouth and do the first Apgar test, which is a quick assessment of a baby's appearance, pulse, reflexes, activity and respiration taken at one minute after birth.

The recovery room After surgery, you'll be taken to another room — it may be a birthing room or a postoperative room — for recovery. There, your vital signs are monitored until the anesthesia has worn off and your condition is stable. This generally takes an hour or two. During your time in recovery, you and your partner may have a few minutes alone with your baby so that you can get acquainted.

If you've chosen to breast-feed your baby, you may be able to do it for the first time in the recovery room, if you're feeling up to it. When it comes to breast-feeding, the sooner you start, the better. However, if you've had general anesthesia, you may be groggy and uncomfortable for a few hours after surgery. You may want to wait until you're more awake and have received pain medication before beginning breast-feeding.

AFTER SURGERY

After a couple of hours in recovery, you'll likely be moved to a room in the maternity unit of the hospital. Over the next 24 hours, your care provider and nurses will monitor your vital signs, the condition of your abdominal dressing, the amount of urine you're producing and the amount of post-pregnancy bleeding you're experiencing. Your health care team will con-

VAGINAL SEEDING

The vaginal microbiome is a rich ecosystem of bacteria and other microorganisms that may affect women's health in various ways. Recent research has suggested that exposure to these organisms (microbiota) in the birth canal may play a role in infant health as well, contributing to lower risks of allergies, asthma and autoimmune disease among babies born vaginally.

A new practice called vaginal seeding aims to give the same possible health benefits to babies born via C-section. It involves taking a swab from the mother's vagina and applying it to the skin, eyes and mouth of a cesarean-born baby. The theory is that exposing newborns to these bacteria may boost their own microbiomes in protective ways.

However, vaginal seeding carries serious risk — among other bacteria, it may transfer infectious organisms such as group B streptococci to the baby. Until further research shows the safety and benefit of the practice, experts advise against it.

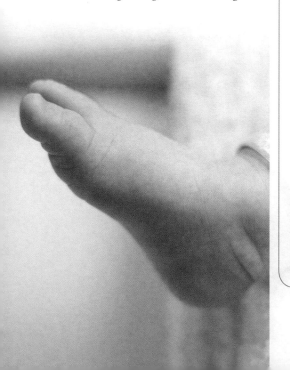

tinue to carefully monitor your condition for the remainder of your stay in the hospital.

Recovery The typical hospital stay after a cesarean birth is two to four days. During your hospital stay and when you return home, it's important that you take good care of yourself to speed your recovery. Most women recover from a C-section with few, if any, problems.

Pain As the anesthesia wears off after surgery, other types of pain medication can help you stay comfortable in the hospital. It's important to have pain relief so that you can rest effectively. This is especially crucial during the first several days of recovery, when your incision is beginning to heal. If you're breast-feeding and you have questions or concerns about taking pain medication, talk with your care provider about your options.

If you're still experiencing pain when it's time for you to be discharged, your care provider may prescribe a small supply of pain medication for you to take at home.

Eating and drinking You may be allowed only ice chips or sips of water for the first few hours after your surgery. Once your digestive system starts to function more normally again, you'll be able to drink more fluids and eat some food.

Walking You'll probably be encouraged to take a brief walk a few hours after surgery, if it's not too late in the day. Walking may be the last thing you feel like doing, but it's good for your body and an important part of your recovery. It helps clear your lungs, improve circulation, promote healing, and get your urinary and digestive systems back to normal. If you're having gas pains, walking can help relieve

A C-SECTION: YOUR PARTNER'S INVOLVEMENT

If your C-section isn't an emergency requiring general anesthesia, your partner may be able to come into the operating room with you. Many hospitals allow this. Your partner may be thrilled by the idea, or he or she may be squeamish or downright scared. It can be difficult to be so close to surgery when it involves someone you know and love.

If your partner chooses to be present for your C-section, he or she will have to wear surgical scrubs, a hair covering, shoe covers and a face mask. He or she may watch the procedure or sit near your head and hold your hand, behind the anesthesia screen. Having your partner close by will probably make you feel more relaxed. There is, however, a potential disadvantage: Partners have been known to faint in the delivery room, giving rise to a second patient who can't be given too much immediate attention.

Most hospitals encourage taking photos of your baby, and the surgical team may even take some shots for you. Many hospitals, though, don't allow direct filming of the operation. Before your partner starts snapping photos or taking a video, make sure he or she asks permission.

them. Walking also helps prevent blood clots, a possible complication of surgery.

After your first little stroll, you'll probably be encouraged to take brief walks a couple of times a day until it's time for you to go home.

Vaginal discharge After your baby's birth you'll experience what's called lochia — a red, brown or clear discharge that lasts for several weeks. Some women who have C-sections are surprised by the amount of vaginal discharge they experience. Even though the placenta is removed during the operation, the uterus still needs to heal and this discharge is part of the process.

Incision care The bandage on your incision will likely be removed the day after surgery, when your incision has had enough time to seal shut. During your hospital stay, your care team will probably check the incision frequently. As your incision begins to heal, it may itch, but don't scratch it. Applying lotion is a better and safer alternative.

If you have surgical staples that need to be removed, that will likely happen before you go home. Once you're home, shower or bathe as usual. Afterward, dry the incision thoroughly with a towel or a hair dryer at a low setting.

Your scar will be sore and sensitive for a few weeks. You'll probably want to wear comfortable, loose clothing that doesn't rub. If clothing does tend to irritate the scar, placing a light gauze dressing over the wound may help. Occasional pulling or twitching sensations around the incision site are normal. As the scar heals, you can expect it to itch and even burn.

Breast-feeding Certain techniques may be helpful when you start breast-feeding after a C-section. For example, you may

want to try the football hold (see page 332), in which you hold your baby much the way a running back tucks a football under his arm. This breast-feeding position is popular among moms who've had C-sections because it keeps your baby from putting pressure on your still-sore abdomen. The first few days after your C-section, you may also want to try nursing while lying down (see page 333).

Restrictions During the first week at home after a cesarean section it's important to restrict your activities and concentrate on taking care of yourself and your newborn.

▶ *Avoid heavy lifting or other activities that could put a strain on your healing incision.* Also make sure to support your abdomen. Use good posture when you stand and walk. Hold your abdomen near the incision during sudden movements, such as when coughing, sneezing or laughing. Use pillows or rolled up towels for extra support while breast-feeding.

▶ *Take medication as needed.* Your care provider may recommend acetaminophen (Tylenol, others) or ibuprofen (Advil, Motrin IB, others) to relieve pain. If you're constipated or bowel movements are painful, an over-the-counter stool softener or a mild laxative, such as milk of magnesia, may be helpful.

▶ *Ask your care provider for recommendations about what activities you can and can't do.* You might feel very tired when you first try to exert yourself. Give yourself a chance to heal. After all, you just had surgery. For many women, once they begin to feel better, they find it difficult to adhere to activity restrictions.

▶ *Until you can make quick movements with your legs or torso without pain, don't drive.* Although some women recover from a C-section more quickly than do others, the typical period of time to avoid driving is one to two weeks.

- *Avoid sex.* Don't have sex until your care provider gives you the green light — often four to six weeks after surgery. You don't have to give up on intimacy in the meantime, though. Spend time with your partner, even if it's just a few minutes in the morning or after the baby goes to sleep at night.

- *Once your care provider gives you the OK, begin exercising.* But take it easy. Swimming and walking are good choices. By the third or fourth week after leaving the hospital, you'll likely feel like resuming your normal activities at home.

Possible complications In general, report these signs and symptoms to your care provider if they occur once you're home from the hospital:

- Fever of 100.4 F or higher
- Painful urination
- Vaginal discharge (lochia) that's heavier than a normal period
- A tear in your incision
- Redness or oozing at the incision site
- Severe abdominal pain

WELCOME, LITTLE ONE

No matter how your baby is born, meeting the newest member of your family and bringing him or her home is a thrilling experience. Enjoy moments of bonding while you and baby get to know each other. As you juggle your recovery and life with a newborn, don't be afraid to ask for or accept help from friends and family in providing nutritious meals, running errands, or taking care of other tasks around your home. Usually, they'll be more than glad to help in exchange for a peek at the baby! Or if what you need is a break from visitors or quiet time with the baby to rest and settle in, trust that friends and family will understand. Remind yourself that you've grown another human — you've earned a break, whatever that means for you.

PART 3

Baby is finally here

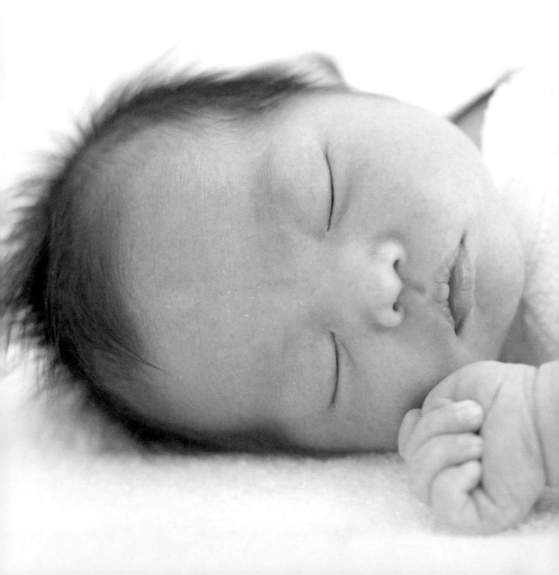

CHAPTER 16

Your newborn

The wait is over. For the last 10 months, you've spent endless hours in preparation and anticipation of the day you'd look into your baby's face. And now that day is here.

Your labor and delivery — whether it was a marathon session or shockingly short — is behind you. Now is the time to snuggle, enjoy and get to know that precious little person you've been waiting for so long to meet.

Even though you're probably eager to go home and start your new life, take advantage of your time in the hospital or birthing center. Many mothers are surprised by how much private time they want after birth. Although your family and friends will want to see you and hear about how you and the baby are doing, you might want to limit calls and visits. It's OK to turn off the phone and set limited visiting hours. The nurses can help restrict visitors to ensure your privacy. Friends and family — especially if they're parents themselves — will understand if you need time for yourself and your baby.

Think about it — your body has been through a significant workout. So sit back and let the hospital staff wait on you and help take care of you and baby. It's a luxury you probably won't have for long.

Your time in the hospital is also an opportunity to ask questions — you'll likely have many! Answers are usually just down the hall. Part of the job of hospital staff is to help you make the transition to parenthood, whether this is your first baby or your fourth. Take advantage of their expertise.

In addition, many hospitals provide literature and videos about the care of newborns, ranging from feeding your baby to car seat safety. Your nurse can suggest which materials might be most helpful to you. If you have the opportunity, take some time to review this information. Once you get home, spare moments may be few and far between.

Many hospitals allow your baby to room in with you. This is a wonderful opportunity to get to know and spend time with your newborn. However, talk with your care team if you feel you aren't getting the quiet time you need for your body to rest and recover from giving birth. Once you go home, you won't have much time to rest.

In this chapter, you'll learn about your newborn's first days of life — what he or she may look like, and what exams and immunizations your baby may undergo. The chapter also discusses common conditions often seen in newborns and, if your son or daughter is born prematurely, possible complications.

YOUR BABY'S APPEARANCE

Considering what they've just been through during labor and childbirth, it's no wonder that newborns don't look like the sweet, clean babies seen in the media. Instead, your newborn will first appear somewhat messy looking. If your baby is like most, his or her head will be a bit misshapen and larger than you expected. The eyelids may be puffy, and his or her arms and legs may be drawn up as they were in the uterus. He or she may be somewhat bloody, wet and slippery from amniotic fluid.

In addition, most babies will be born with some of the lotion-like covering (vernix) that protected them in the uterus. It'll be most noticeable under your baby's arms, behind the ears and in the groin. Most of this vernix will be washed off during your baby's first bath.

Head At first, your baby's head may appear flat, elongated or crooked. This peculiar elongation is one of the common features of a newly born baby.

A baby's skull consists of several sections of bone that are flexibly joined so that the head shape can change to correspond to the shape of your pelvis as your baby moves through the birth canal. A long labor usually results in an elongated or tall skull shape at birth. The head of a breech baby may have a shorter, broader appearance. If a vacuum extractor was used to assist in the birth, your baby's head may look particularly elongated. Sometimes you can feel ridges where the sections of bone have overlapped. As baby's head shape normalizes over the first few days, these ridges will go away.

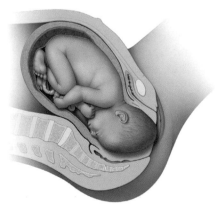

Head elongation

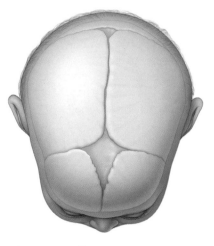

Fontanels

Fontanels When you feel the top of your baby's head, you'll notice two soft areas. These soft spots, called fontanels, are where your baby's skull bones haven't grown together yet.

The fontanel toward the front of the scalp is a diamond-shaped spot roughly the size of a quarter. Though it's usually flat, it may bulge when your baby cries or strains. In nine to 18 months, this fontanel will typically be filled in with hard bone. The smaller, less noticeable fontanel at the back of the head is about the size of a dime and it closes much quicker — by six to eight weeks after birth.

Skin Most babies are born with some bruising, and skin blotches and blemishes are common.

A rounded swelling of the scalp is usually seen on the top and back of the baby's head when a baby is born the usual way — headfirst. This puffiness of the skin disappears within a day or so.

JENNIFER'S STORY

When I was pregnant, I couldn't wait to get my baby home — to dress him in his new clothes, put him to sleep in his beautiful new crib, and nurse him in the brand-new rocking chair we'd spent hours trying out and had placed in the sunniest spot in the living room. But, actually, arriving home was different from what I expected. I had a red-faced, screaming baby who spit up on all of those new outfits. My breasts were engorged from my milk coming in. And there was a sudden, overwhelming feeling that my husband and I were on our own to survive as parents.

The first couple of weeks home were not the wonderful, hazy days I dreamed they would be. To be honest, they were overwhelming, and at times I felt like I was barely conscious. When my milk came in, I was so shocked I called my pediatrician's office to ask if it was normal and how could I possibly get my son to latch on? When my son cried and was inconsolable each day from 5 to 6 p.m., I called again to ask if this was normal and what we could do to try to help him. During nighttime feedings, I was so tired that I fell asleep with the baby at my breast and woke up with a stiff, kinked neck.

It took us a couple of weeks to settle into our routine. Thankfully, my husband was very supportive. I was in charge of "input" and my husband was in charge of "output" — I nursed the baby and he changed the diapers. Within two days, my breast engorgement had resolved and my baby was happily nursing. I tried to nurse as much as I could on my side, so at least I was off my feet and resting. Once we got past the immediate rush of visitors, when people asked me what they could do to help, I happily replied, "Why don't you bring us dinner." It was great not to cook and to have some social interaction with other adults.

By my six-week postpartum visit, I was happy to report that my baby was starting to smile and coo. That made all the difference in the world. I had gone from being just a milk supplier and diaper changer to someone he actually recognized — his mom.

Pressure from your pelvis during labor can cause a bruise on your baby's head. The bruise may be noticeable for several weeks, and you might feel a small bump that persists for several months. You may also see scrapes or bruises on your baby's face and head if forceps were used during delivery. These bruises and blemishes should go away within a couple of weeks.

Other skin conditions common in newborns include:

▸ *Milia.* These are tiny white pimples on the nose and chin. Although they appear to be raised, they are nearly flat and smooth to the touch. Milia disappear in time, and they don't require treatment.

▸ *Cradle cap.* Also called seborrheic dermatitis, this greasy, flaky plaque often occurs on the scalp. It occurs during baby's first month of life and usually resolves on its own after a couple of months. For more information, see page 268.

▸ *Salmon patches.* These red patches may be found over the nape of the neck, between the eyebrows or on the eyelids. They can become especially red when baby cries or is upset. Also called stork bites or angel kisses, they usually disappear over the first few months.

▸ *Erythema toxicum.* It sounds scary, but erythema toxicum is the medical term for a skin condition that's typically present at birth or appears within the first few days after birth. It's characterized by small white or yellowish bumps surrounded by pink or reddish skin. The condition causes no discomfort and is not infectious. Erythema toxicum disappears in a few days.

▸ *Newborn acne.* Newborn (neonatal) acne refers to the red bumps and blotches similar to acne that are seen on the face, neck, upper chest and back. It's most noticeable at 1 or 2 months and typically disappears without treatment within another month or two.

- *Dermal melanosis.* Also known as the blue-gray macule of infancy, these are large, flat gray or blue areas that contain extra pigment and often appear on the lower back or buttocks. They're especially common in black, American Indian and Asian infants and in babies with dark complexions. Dermal melanosis doesn't change color or fade like a bruise would, but it generally goes away in later childhood.

- *Pustular melanosis.* These spots look like small white sesame seeds that quickly dry and peel off. They may look similar to skin infections (pustules), but pustular melanosis isn't an infection and disappears without treatment. The spots are most commonly seen in the folds of the neck and on the shoulders and chest. They're more common in babies with darker skin.

- *Strawberry hemangiomas.* Caused by overgrowth of blood vessels in the top layers of skin, strawberry hemangiomas are red, raised spots that may resemble a strawberry. Usually not present at birth, a hemangioma begins as a small, pale spot that becomes red in the center. A strawberry hemangioma enlarges during the baby's first few months and eventually disappears without treatment.

Hair Your baby may be born bald, with a full head of thick hair, or almost anything in between! Don't fall in love with your baby's locks too quickly. The hair color your baby is born with isn't necessarily what he or she will have six months down the road. Blond newborns, for example, may become darker blond as they get older, and their hair may develop a reddish tinge that isn't apparent at birth.

You may be surprised to see that your newborn's head isn't the only place he or she has hair. Downy, fine hair called lanugo covers a baby's body before birth and may temporarily remain on your newborn's back, shoulders, forehead and temples. Lanugo is especially common on premature babies. It disappears in the weeks after birth.

Eyes It's perfectly normal for your newborn's eyes to be puffy. In fact, some infants have such puffy eyes that they aren't able to open their eyes wide right away. But don't worry, within a day or two, your baby will be able to look into your eyes.

You may also notice that your new baby sometimes looks cross-eyed. This, too, is normal and will be outgrown within several months.

Sometimes babies are born with red spots on the whites of their eyes. These spots are caused by the breakage of tiny blood vessels during birth. The spots are harmless and won't interfere with your baby's sight. They generally disappear in a week to two.

As with hair, a newborn's eyes give no guarantee of future color. Although most newborns have dark bluish-brown, blue-black, grayish-blue or slate-colored eyes, permanent eye color may take six months or even longer to establish itself.

NEWBORN CARE

From the moment your little one is born, he or she is the focus of much activity. Your care provider or a nurse will clean your baby's face. To make sure your baby can breathe properly, his or her nose and mouth are cleared of fluid immediately after birth.

While baby's airway is being cleared, his or her heart rate and circulation can be checked with a stethoscope or by feeling the pulse in the umbilical cord. All newborns look somewhat bluish-gray for the first several minutes, especially on their lips and tongue. By five to 10 minutes after birth, they become pink.

Your baby's umbilical cord is clamped with a plastic clamp, and you or your partner may be given the option to cut it. Research has shown that allowing baby to remain attached to the umbilical cord for 30 to 60 seconds after delivery may improve baby's development by preventing low iron levels. In premature infants, delayed cord clamping may help prevent

complications such as anemia, bleeding and bowel problems. However, this practice can also increase the risk of jaundice. Talk to your care provider during your prenatal visits if you would prefer delayed cord clamping. Keep in mind that it may not be possible at the time of delivery if baby needs emergency care. And if you're considering cord blood banking, be aware that delayed clamping reduces the amount of cord blood, so the cord may not meet donation criteria.

The next day or two after birth will be busy for baby. The medical team will conduct newborn examinations, administer screening tests and give preventive treatments. Here's what to expect.

Examinations One of the first examinations of your baby will be determining his or her Apgar scores.

Apgar scores A quick evaluation of a newborn's health — an Apgar score — is given at one minute and five minutes after birth. Developed in 1952 by anesthesiologist Virginia Apgar, this brief examination rates newborns on five criteria: color, heart rate, reflexes, muscle tone and respiration.

Each of these criteria is given an individual score of 0, 1 or 2. Then all scores are totaled for a maximum possible score of 10. Higher scores indicate healthier infants, while scores below 5 mean an infant needs help at birth.

While Apgar scores assess a baby immediately after delivery, they don't predict long-term health. Most babies with low Apgar scores are ultimately perfectly healthy.

Other checks and measurements Soon after birth, your newborn's weight, length and head circumference are measured. Your baby's temperature may be taken, and breathing and heart rate measured.

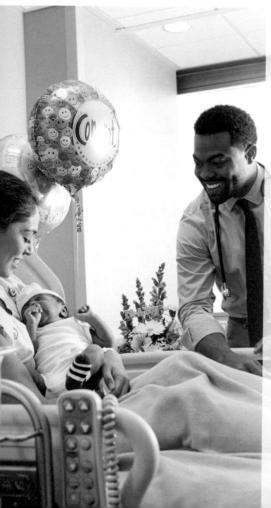

Then, usually within 12 hours after your baby's birth, a physical exam is conducted to detect any problems or abnormalities.

Treatments and vaccinations To prevent disease, the following protections are generally taken:

Eye protection To avert the possibility of gonorrhea or certain other infections being passed from mother to baby, all states require that infants receive a protective eye treatment immediately after birth. Gonorrheal eye infections were a leading cause of blindness until early in the 20th century, when treatment of newborns' eyes became mandatory. Typically, an antibiotic ointment containing erythromycin is placed onto baby's eyes. These preparations are gentle to the eyes and cause no pain.

Vitamin K injection In the United States, vitamin K is routinely given to infants shortly after they're born. Vitamin K is necessary for normal blood coagulation, the body's process for stopping bleeding after a cut or bruise. Newborns have low levels of vitamin K in their first few weeks. An injection of vitamin K can help prevent the rare possibility that a newborn would become so deficient in vitamin K that serious bleeding might develop. This problem is not related to hemophilia.

Hepatitis B vaccination Hepatitis B is a viral infection that affects the liver. It can cause such illnesses as cirrhosis and liver failure, or it can result in the development of liver tumors. Adults contract hepatitis through sexual contact, shared needles or exposure to the blood of an infected person. Babies, however, can contract hepatitis B from their mothers during pregnancy and birth.

The hepatitis B vaccine can protect infants if they are exposed to the virus.

Therefore, your baby will be given the vaccine in the hospital or birthing center shortly after birth.

Newborn screening (NBS) Before your baby leaves the hospital, newborn screening will be completed. Testing involves a heel stick to obtain a small sample of baby's blood, a hearing test and screening for congenital heart problems.

The blood sample is sent to the state health department or a private laboratory working in collaboration with the state. The blood sample is analyzed to detect the presence of rare but important genetic diseases. Results of the NBS are typically completed within a couple of days.

Occasionally, test results are out of the normal range and additional testing is recommended for your baby. Don't be alarmed if this happens to your newborn. To ensure that every newborn with any of these conditions is identified, even borderline results are evaluated. Retesting is especially common for premature babies.

Each state independently operates its NBS program, resulting in slight differences in tests offered. The Advisory Committee on Heritable Disorders in Newborns and Children, which works with the U.S. Department of Health and Human Services, has recommended NBS for about 60 disorders and conditions. Some of the more common diseases that can be detected by the NBS panel include:

▸ *Phenylketonuria (PKU).* Babies with PKU retain excessive amounts of phenylalanine, an amino acid found in the protein of almost all foods. Without treatment, PKU can cause intellectual and physical disability, poor growth rate, and seizures. With early detection and treatment, growth and development should be normal.

▸ *Congenital hypothyroidism.* About 1 in 2,000 to 4,000 babies have a thyroid hormone deficiency that slows growth and brain development. Left untreated, it can result in intellectual disability and stunted growth. With early detection and treatment, though, normal development is possible.

- *Congenital adrenal hyperplasia (CAH).* This group of disorders is caused by a deficiency of certain hormones. Signs and symptoms may include lethargy, vomiting, muscle weakness and dehydration. Infants with mild forms are at risk of reproductive and growth difficulties. Severe CAH can cause kidney dysfunction and even death. However, lifelong hormone treatment can suppress the disease.
- *Galactosemia.* Babies born with galactosemia can't metabolize galactose, a sugar found in milk. Although newborns with this condition typically appear normal, they may develop vomiting, diarrhea, jaundice and liver damage within a few days of their first milk feedings. Untreated, the disorder may result in intellectual disability, blindness, growth failure and, rarely, death. Treatment includes eliminating milk and all other dairy (galactose) products from the diet.
- *Sickle cell disease.* This inherited disease prevents blood cells from circulating easily throughout the body. Affected infants will have an increased susceptibility to infection and slow growth rates. The disease can cause bouts of pain and damage to vital organs such as the lungs, kidneys and brain. With early medical treatment, the complications of sickle cell disease can be minimized.
- *Medium-chain acyl-CoA dehydrogenase (MCAD) deficiency.* This rare hereditary disease results from the lack of an enzyme required to convert fat to energy. Serious life-threatening signs and symptoms and even death can occur. But with early detection and monitoring, most children diagnosed with MCAD can lead normal lives.
- *Cystic fibrosis.* Cystic fibrosis is a genetic disease that causes the body to produce abnormally thickened mucous secretions in the lungs and digestive system. Signs and symptoms generally include salty-tasting skin, persistent coughing, shortness of breath and poor weight gain. Affected newborns can develop life-threatening lung infections and intestinal obstructions. With early detection and treatment, infants diagnosed with cystic fibrosis can live longer and in better health than they did in the past.

Hearing screening Most hospitals will also test your baby's hearing as part of the NBS. This screening can detect possible hearing loss in the first days of a baby's life. If possible hearing loss is found, further tests may be done to confirm the results. Hearing loss is relatively common, and detecting it early is important for your baby's development.

These two tests are used to screen a newborn's hearing. Both are quick (about 10 minutes), painless and can be done while your baby sleeps.

- *Automated auditory brainstem response.* This test measures how the brain responds to sound. Clicks or tones are played through soft earphones into the baby's ears while electrodes taped on the baby's head measure the brain's response.
- *Otoacoustic emissions.* This test measures responses to sound waves presented to the ear. A probe placed inside the baby's ear canal measures the response when clicks or tones are played into the baby's ear.

Critical congenital heart defect (CCHD) screening Before leaving the hospital, your baby will likely also be screened for any heart defects. Ultrasounds can identify many heart defects during a pregnancy. However, some issues may be missed or cannot be detected until after a baby is born.

For this test, an oxygen sensor (pulse oximeter) is placed on your baby's hands or feet. The test is quick and does not cause discomfort to your baby. If the oxygen levels are low or different on the right and left sides, your baby's care provider will most likely recommend additional testing.

CIRCUMCISION

If you have a baby boy, one of the decisions you'll face soon after birth is whether to have him circumcised. Circumcision is a surgical procedure performed to remove the skin covering the tip of the penis. Knowing about the procedure's potential benefits and risks can help you make an informed decision.

Issues to consider Although circumcision is fairly common in the United States, it's still somewhat controversial. According to the American Academy of Pediatrics, current evidence of the medical benefits of circumcision outweigh the risks. However, the benefits may still be low for most baby boys, so it is an elective procedure.

Consider your own cultural, religious and social values in making this decision. For some people, such as those of the Jewish or Islamic faith, circumcision is a religious ritual. For others, it's a matter of personal hygiene or preventive health. Some parents choose circumci-

sion because they don't want their son to look different from his peers. Others feel that circumcision is unnecessary. Some people feel strongly that circumcision is disfiguring to the baby's normal appearance.

As you decide what's best for you and your son, consider these potential health benefits and risks.

Potential benefits of circumcision Some research suggests that circumcision provides certain benefits. These include:

▶ *Decreased risk of urinary tract infections.* Although the risk of urinary tract infections in the first year is low, studies suggest that such infections may be up to 10 times more common in uncircumcised baby boys than in those who are circumcised. Uncircumcised boys are also more likely to be admitted to the hospital for a severe urinary tract infection during the first three months of life than are those who are circumcised.

▶ *Decreased risk of cancer of the penis.* While this type of cancer is very rare, circumcised men show a lower incidence of cancer of the penis than do uncircumcised men.

▶ *Decreased risk of some sexually transmitted infections.* Studies have shown a lower risk of human immunodeficiency virus (HIV), human papillomavirus (HPV) and herpes simplex virus infections in circumcised men. However, safe sexual practices are much more important in the prevention of sexually transmitted infections than is circumcision.

▶ *Prevention of penile problems.* Occasionally, the foreskin on an uncircumcised penis may narrow to the point where it's difficult or impossible to retract, a condition called phimosis. A narrowed foreskin can also lead to inflammation of the head of the penis (balanitis). While circumcision can help prevent these issues, they can still occur from the remaining foreskin in some circumcised boys.

▶ *Ease of hygiene.* Circumcision makes it easy to wash the penis. But even if the foreskin is intact, it's still quite simple to keep the penis clean. Normally the foreskin adheres to the end of the penis in a newborn, then gradually stretches back during early childhood. Wash your baby's genital area gently with soap and water. Lat-

er, when the foreskin easily retracts, your son can learn to wash this area by gently pulling the foreskin back and cleansing the tip of the penis.

Potential risks of circumcision Circumcision is considered a safe procedure. However, circumcision does have some potential drawbacks, including:

▶ *Risks of minor surgery.* All surgical procedures, including circumcision, carry certain risks, such as excessive bleeding and infection. There's also the possibility that the foreskin may

HOW IT'S DONE

If you decide to have your son circumcised, his care provider can answer questions about the procedure and help you make arrangements at your hospital or clinic. Usually, circumcision is performed before you and your son leave the hospital. At times, circumcision is done in an outpatient setting. The procedure itself takes about 10 minutes.

Typically, the baby lies with his arms and legs restrained. After the penis and surrounding area are cleansed, a local anesthetic is injected into the base of the penis. A special clamp or plastic ring is attached to the penis, and the foreskin is trimmed away. An ointment, such as petroleum jelly, is applied. This protects the penis from adhering to the diaper.

If your newborn is fussy as the anesthetic wears off, hold him gently — being careful to avoid putting pressure on the penis. It usually takes about seven to 10 days for the penis to heal.

Before circumcision (left), the foreskin of the penis extends over the end of the penis (glans). After the brief operation, the glans is exposed (right).

be cut too short or too long, or that it doesn't heal properly. If the remaining foreskin reattaches on the end of the penis, a minor surgery may be needed to correct it. However, these occurrences are uncommon.

▶ *Pain during the procedure.* Circumcision does cause pain. Typically a local anesthetic is used to block the nerve sensations. Talk to your care provider about the type of anesthesia used and what your baby may experience.

▶ *Difficult to reverse.* It's difficult to recreate the appearance of an uncircumcised penis.

▶ *Cost.* Some insurance companies don't cover the cost of circumcision. If you're considering circumcision, check whether your insurance company will cover it.

▶ *Complicating factors.* Sometimes, circumcision may need to be postponed, such as if your baby is born prematurely, has severe jaundice or is feeding poorly. It also may not be feasible in certain situations, such as in the rare instance when baby's urethral opening is in an abnormal position on the side or base of the penis (hypospadias). Other conditions that may prevent circumcision include ambiguous genitalia or a family history of bleeding disorders.

Circumcision doesn't affect fertility. There is also no evidence to suggest that sexual function or satisfaction is affected by circumcision. Whatever your choice in considering circumcision for your baby, negative outcomes are rare and mostly minor.

CIRCUMCISION CARE

If your newborn boy was circumcised, the tip of his penis may seem raw for the first week after the procedure. Or a yellowish mucus or crust may form around the area. This is a normal part of healing. A small amount of bleeding is also common the first day or two.

Clean the diaper area gently and apply a dab of petroleum jelly to the end of the penis with each diaper change. This will keep the diaper from sticking while the penis heals. If there's a bandage, change it with each diapering. At some hospitals, a plastic ring is used instead of a bandage. The ring will remain on the end of the penis until the edge of the circumcision has healed, usually within a week. The ring will drop off on its own. It's OK to gently wash the penis or bathe your baby as the penis heals.

Problems after a circumcision are rare. But call your baby's care provider in the following situations:

▶ Your baby doesn't urinate normally six to eight hours after the circumcision.
▶ Bleeding or redness around the tip of the penis is persistent.
▶ The penis tip is swollen.
▶ A foul-smelling drainage comes from the penis tip, or there are crusted sores that contain fluid.
▶ The ring is still in place two weeks after the circumcision.

NEWBORN ISSUES

Some babies have a bit of trouble adjusting to their new world. Fortunately, most of the problems they experience are minor and soon resolve.

Jaundice More than half of all newborn babies develop jaundice, a yellow tinge to the skin and eyes. Signs generally develop a few days after birth, and the condition may last several weeks.

A baby develops jaundice when bilirubin, which is produced by the breakdown of red blood cells, accumulates faster than the liver can break it down and pass it from the body. All babies have their bilirubin level checked before leaving the hospital, either with a blood draw or by measuring the yellowing of the skin.

Jaundice usually disappears on its own, and it doesn't cause any discomfort to your baby. Your baby may develop jaundice for a few reasons:

- Bilirubin is being produced more quickly than the liver can react.
- The baby's developing liver isn't able to remove bilirubin from the blood.
- Too much of the bilirubin is reabsorbed from the intestines before the baby gets rid of it in a bowel movement.

Although mild levels of jaundice don't require treatment, babies with more-severe cases can require a newborn to stay longer in the hospital. Jaundice may be treated in several ways:

- You may be asked to feed the baby more frequently, which increases the amount of bilirubin passed with bowel movements.
- A doctor may place your baby under a bilirubin light. This treatment, called phototherapy, is quite common. A special lamp helps rid the body of excess bilirubin.

- Your baby may be given intravenous immune globulin to decrease the severity of the jaundice if the bilirubin level becomes extremely high.
- Rarely, an exchange blood transfusion is done to reduce the bilirubin level.

Infection A newborn's immune system isn't adequately developed to fight infection. Therefore, any type of infection can be more dangerous for newborns than for older children or adults.

Serious bacterial infections, which are uncommon, can invade any organ or the blood, urine or spinal fluid. Prompt treatment with antibiotics is necessary, but even with early diagnosis and treatment, a newborn infection can be life-threatening.

For this reason, doctors are cautious when treating a possible or suspected infection. Antibiotics often are given early, and their use is stopped only when an infection doesn't seem likely. Although the majority of the test results come back showing no evidence of infection, it's better to err on the side of safety by quickly treating a baby than to risk not treating a baby with an infection soon enough. If you tested positive for group B streptococcus (GBS) near the end of your pregnancy, or you were diagnosed with an infection in labor, this may influence the decision to start your baby on antibiotics in the hospital. (For more on GBS, see page 444.)

Viruses can cause infections in newborns, although viral infections are less common than are bacterial infections. Certain newborn viral infections such as herpes, varicella, HIV and cytomegalovirus may be treated with antiviral medication.

Learning to eat Whether you choose to breast-feed or bottle-feed, you may find it difficult to interest your newborn in eating during the first few days. This is fairly common. Some babies seem to adopt a slow-and-sleepy approach to eating. If you're concerned that your baby isn't getting enough nourishment, talk to your baby's nurse or doctor. Occasionally, slow eaters require tube feedings to help them along for a few days. But soon they catch on and breast-feed or bottle-feed with enthusiasm.

Over the first week, a newborn will lose about 10 percent of his or her birth weight before gradually gaining that weight back, and more!

THE PREMATURE NEWBORN

Every parent dreams of having a healthy, full-term baby. Unfortunately, that dream isn't always the reality. Although most infants are born full term and free of medical problems, some are born too early. Prematurity — defined as being born before 37 weeks of gestation — is often, though not always, accompanied by medical complications.

The outlook for these newborns is much more hopeful than it was years ago. In fact, more than two-thirds of babies born at 24 to 25 weeks can survive with the proper medical care. Still, many of these very premature babies have long-term health problems. This section explains some of the types of problems and treatments that can arise with prematurity.

The setting Your first close-up look at your premature baby will likely be in the neonatal intensive care unit (NICU). You'll probably be amazed, overwhelmed — and perhaps a little shocked — by this first look.

You may first notice the array of tubes, catheters and electrical leads taped to your tiny baby. This equipment may seem scary or intimidating. It's important to remember that it helps keep your baby healthy and the medical staff informed about your baby's condition.

THE NEONATAL INTENSIVE CARE UNIT TEAM

In the neonatal intensive care unit (NICU), your baby is cared for by many specialists and other health care professionals. The team attending to your baby may include:

- Neonatal nurses — registered nurses with special training in caring for premature and high-risk newborns
- Neonatal respiratory therapists — staff trained to assess respiratory problems in newborns and adjust ventilators and other respiratory equipment
- Neonatologists — pediatricians who specialize in the diagnosis and treatment of problems of the newborn
- Pediatric surgeons — surgeons trained in the diagnosis and treatment of newborn conditions that may require surgery
- Pediatricians — doctors who specialize in treating children
- Pediatric resident physicians — doctors receiving specialized training in treating children

Because premature babies have less body fat than do full-term babies, they need help staying warm. They're often placed in an infant incubator, an enclosed and warmed plastic box called an isolette, to help them maintain a normal body temperature.

In the NICU, your baby will receive specialized care, including a feeding plan tailored to your baby's needs. For the first few days after delivery, premature babies are usually fed intravenously because their gastrointestinal and respiratory systems may be too immature for formula feedings. When your baby is ready, the intravenous feeding will end and a new form of feeding, called tube feeding, will likely be the next step. With tube feedings, your baby receives breast milk or formula through a tube that delivers the food directly to the stomach or upper intestine.

What baby may look like You'll definitely notice your baby's tiny size. He or she may be considerably smaller than a full-term infant.

Your baby's features will appear sharper and less rounded than a full-term baby's. A premature baby's skin also has a number of notable characteristics. The skin and cartilage that form baby's outer ears will be very soft and pliable. The skin may be covered with more fine body hair (lanugo) than is common in full-term babies, and it may look thin, fragile and somewhat transparent, allowing you to see baby's blood vessels.

These characteristics will be easy to see because most premature babies aren't dressed or wrapped in blankets. This is so the nursery staff can closely observe their breathing and general appearance.

Getting involved Become physically involved with your baby as early as possible. Loving care is important to your baby's growth and development.

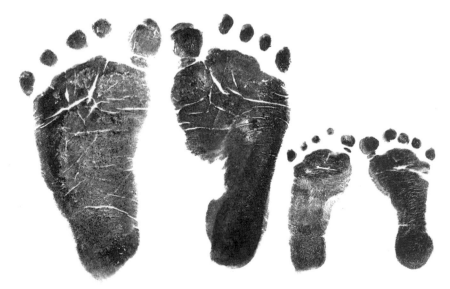

Footprints of a full-term baby girl whose birth weight was 8 pounds, 4 ounces.

Footprints of a premature baby boy whose birth weight was 1 pound, 8 ounces.

When you were pregnant, you probably daydreamed about holding, bathing and feeding your new baby. As the parent of a premature baby, you may not be able to spend these first weeks with your baby in the way you had envisioned. Still, you can be involved with your baby in important ways.

You can reach through the openings in the isolette to hold your baby's hand or gently stroke him or her. Gentle contact with your premature baby can help him or her thrive. Help your newborn get to know you by humming a lullaby or talking softly to him or her.

As your baby's condition improves, you'll be able to hold and rock your baby. Skin-to-skin contact, sometimes called kangaroo care, can be a powerful way to bond with your baby. In kangaroo care, a nurse can help place your baby on your bare chest, then loosely cover him or her with a blanket. Studies have shown that premature babies respond positively to this skin-to-skin contact with their parents and that kangaroo care can improve babies' recovery times.

Another way you can be involved in your baby's health is by providing breast milk, which contains proteins that help fight infection and promote growth. In the NICU, your baby will likely be fed every one to three hours through a tube that goes from the nose or mouth to the stomach. A nurse can show you how to pump breast milk, which can be refrigerated and used as your baby needs it.

Complications of prematurity Not all premature babies develop complications, but the earlier a child is born, the greater the chances a problem may occur.

WHEN YOUR BABY IS HOSPITALIZED

- Spend time touching and talking to your newborn. Premature babies respond positively to skin-to-skin contact.
- Learn as much as you can about your baby's medical condition, especially what parents should watch for and how you as parents can help care for the condition.
- Take an active role in your baby's care, especially as your baby becomes close to leaving the hospital.
- Don't be afraid to ask questions. Medical terminology can be confusing and intimidating. Have your baby's doctor or nurse write down any key diagnoses. Ask for printed patient information sheets or recommendations of websites you can visit for further information.
- Lean on someone. Talk the situation over with your partner or other family members. Invite family members and friends to join you at the hospital. Ask to meet with the hospital social worker.
- Inquire if public health nurses or visiting nurses can assist with your baby's care after you're home.
- Ask if your baby should be enrolled in special infant follow-up or infant development programs.

Some complications are apparent at birth, while others may not develop for weeks or months. Some of these conditions may include:

Respiratory distress syndrome Respiratory distress syndrome (RDS) is the most common breathing problem among newborns, occurring almost exclusively in premature infants. With RDS, a baby's immature lungs lack an important liquid substance called surfactant, which gives normal, fully developed lungs the elastic qualities required for easy breathing.

RDS is usually diagnosed within the first minutes to hours after birth. The diagnosis is based on the extent of breathing difficulty and on abnormalities seen on the baby's chest X-ray.

Treatment. Babies with RDS require various degrees of help with their breathing. Supplemental oxygen is usually required until the lungs improve.

A ventilator, also called a respirator, can give the baby carefully controlled breaths. These can range from a few extra breaths per minute to entirely taking over the work of breathing.

Some babies benefit from breathing assistance called continuous positive airway pressure (CPAP). A plastic tube that fits in the nostrils provides additional pressure in the air passages to keep the tiny air sacs in the lungs properly inflated.

Babies with severe RDS are often given doses of surfactant preparation directly into the lungs. Other medications that increase urine output, rid the body of extra water, reduce inflammation in the lungs, reduce wheezing and minimize pauses in breathing (apnea) also may be used.

Bronchopulmonary dysplasia A premature baby's lung problems generally improve within several days to several weeks. Babies who still require help with ventilation or supplemental oxygen a month after birth are often described as having bronchopulmonary dysplasia (BPD). This condition is also called chronic lung disease.

Treatment. Babies with BPD continue to need supplemental oxygen for an extended period. If they develop a bad cold or pneumonia, they may need breathing assistance, such as that provided by a ventilator. Some of these babies may need to continue using supplemental oxygen, even after they go home from the hospital. As these babies grow, their need for supplemental oxygen lessens and their breathing becomes easier. However, they're more likely than are other children to have episodes of wheezing or asthma.

Apnea and bradycardia Premature babies typically have immature breathing rhythms that cause them to breathe in spurts: 10 to 15 seconds of deep breathing followed by five- to 10-second pauses. This condition is called periodic breathing. Sometimes, a pause in baby's breathing (apnea) can result in a slowed heartbeat (bradycardia).

Treatment. The reduced breathing, heart rate and oxygen saturation in a premature baby with apnea and bradycardia typically return to normal on their own. If they don't, a nurse may gently stimulate the baby by rubbing or wiggling him or her awake. In more-severe spells, the baby may need brief assistance with breathing.

Patent ductus arteriosus Before birth, babies receive oxygen from the placenta rather than through the lungs, so the lungs require minimal blood flow. Because of this, a short blood vessel called the ductus arteriosus diverts blood away from the lungs and eventually back to the placenta.

Before birth, a chemical compound called prostaglandin E (PGE) circulates in the baby's blood, keeping the ductus arteriosus open. Once a full-term infant is born, levels of PGE fall sharply, causing the ductus arteriosus to close. This allows for the change from pre-birth circulation to after-birth (postpartum) circulation.

Occasionally, especially in premature babies, PGE circulates at higher than normal levels. This causes the ductus arteriosus to remain open and can result in respiratory or circulation difficulties.

Treatment. Patent ductus arteriosus is often treated with a medication that stops or slows the production of prostaglandin E. If this medication isn't effective, an operation might be needed.

Intracranial hemorrhage Premature babies who are born at less than 34 weeks are at risk of bleeding in their brains. The earlier a baby is born, the higher the risk of this complication. Therefore, if premature birth seems inevitable, the mother may be given certain medications to help lessen the likelihood of a severe intracranial hemorrhage in the newborn.

Treatment. Babies with minor degrees of intracranial hemorrhage require only observation. Those with serious degrees of bleeding may undergo various treatments. Babies with severe intracranial hemorrhage are at risk of developmental problems such as cerebral palsy, spasticity and intellectual disability.

Necrotizing enterocolitis For reasons that aren't entirely clear, some premature babies — usually those born at less than 28 weeks of gestation — develop a problem called necrotizing enterocolitis. In this condition, a portion of the baby's intestine develops poor blood flow. This can lead to infection in the bowel wall. Signs include a bloated abdomen, feeding intolerance, breathing difficulty and bloody stools.

Treatment. Babies with this condition may be treated with intravenous feedings and antibiotics. In severe cases, an operation may be required to remove the affected portion of the intestine.

Retinopathy of prematurity Retinopathy of prematurity (ROP) is abnormal growth of the blood vessels in an infant's eyes. It's most common in very premature babies. Most babies born at 23 to 26 weeks of gestation, for example, will experience at least some ROP, and babies beyond about 30 weeks of gestation rarely develop ROP.

During fetal life, the retina develops from the back of the eye forward, and the process is complete just about the time a baby is full term. When a baby is born prematurely, the retinal development isn't finished, which may allow a number of factors to disturb it.

Treatment. If your baby is at risk of ROP, an eye specialist (ophthalmologist) can examine the eyes after 6 weeks of age. Fortunately, most cases of ROP are mild and will resolve without additional treatment. More-severe degrees of retinopathy are often successfully treated with procedures such as laser treatment or cryotherapy. Fortunately, today, blindness is uncommon and affects only the smallest and most unstable premature babies.

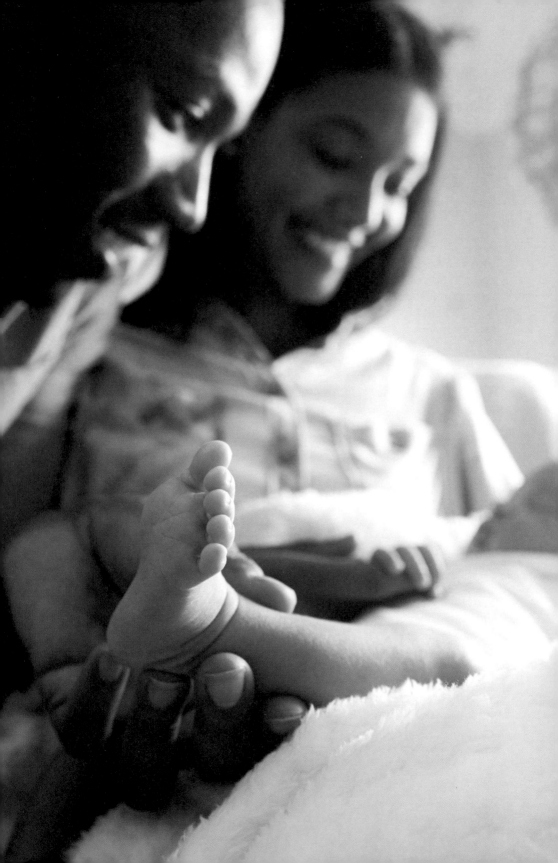

CHAPTER 17

Taking baby home

Finally, the moment you've been anticipating is here — you're bringing home the newest member of your family! You've set up the crib and nursery, bought and borrowed cute baby outfits, and stocked up on diapers, wipes, blankets and other supplies. You've been thinking about all of the changes this new person will bring to your life, and you're likely feeling both excited and scared.

Now you wonder: Am I ready? Are we ready? Probably not — and that's perfectly normal.

No matter how many pregnancy and baby care books you've read or how meticulous you've been in getting everything in place, nothing can fully prepare you for the first few weeks after your baby's birth — a time that's often exciting and overwhelming.

During the first weeks after your baby is born (postpartum), you're dealing with many different physical, emotional and practical issues all at once. You're getting used to this new being and trying to understand his or her needs and habits. At the same time, your body is recovering from pregnancy and childbirth.

Given all of these changes, the several weeks after you bring your baby home are likely to be one of the most challenging times of your life. It may take weeks or months to feel back to normal. Be patient with yourself and your baby. You'll get there in your own way and in your own time.

Having a new baby in your life is a special experience. This chapter gives you a glimpse into your newborn's world and offers some advice on taking care of your baby and keeping him or her safe.

YOUR BABY'S WORLD

During the first few weeks of a newborn's life, it may seem like all he or she does is eat, sleep, cry and keep you busy changing diapers. But your baby is also taking in the sights, sounds and smells of his or her new world, learning to use his or her muscles and expressing a number of innate reflexes.

As soon as babies are born, they begin to communicate with you. Infants can't use words to communicate their needs, moods or preferences, but they have other ways of expressing themselves, especially by crying.

You may not always know how your newborn is feeling, and sometimes it may seem as though he or she is communicating in a foreign language. But you can learn about how your baby experiences the world and relates to you and others. In turn, your baby will learn your language of touching, holding, and making sounds and facial gestures.

Reflexes Newborns are just learning to enjoy the freedom of movement outside the cramped quarters of the uterus. In their first few days, they may seem a bit reluctant to experiment with their new mobility, preferring to be wrapped and held snugly. Over time, however, your baby will begin to explore a range of movements.

Babies are born with a number of reflexes — automatic, involuntary movements. Some of these movements, such as turning the head to avoid suffocating, seem to be protective responses. Some may be preparing babies for voluntary movements. Most reflexes diminish after a few weeks or months and then disappear completely as they're replaced with new, learned skills.

In the meantime, watch for some of these reflexes:

- *Rooting.* This reflex prompts babies to turn in the direction of the food source, whether it's a breast or bottle. If you gently stroke a newborn's cheek, he or she will turn in that direction, with his or her mouth open, ready to suck.

- *Sucking.* When a breast, bottle nipple or pacifier is placed in a baby's mouth, he or she will automatically suck. This reflex not only helps the newborn eat but also can calm him or her.

- *Stepping.* When you hold infants under their arms and let the soles of their feet touch the ground, they may place one foot in front of the other as if they're walking. This stepping reflex is most apparent after about the fourth day and disappears at about two months. Most babies won't actually learn to walk until they're almost 1 year old.

- *Startle (Moro reflex).* When startled by a noise or sudden movement, babies may throw both arms outward and cry. You may notice this if you put your baby in the bassinet or crib too quickly.

- *Fencing (tonic neck reflex).* If you turn your baby's head to one side while he or she is lying on his or her back, you may see this classic baby pose, in which one arm is crooked and raised behind the head and the other is straightened and extended away from the body in the direction the head is turned. Your baby may also clench the fist of the extended arm.

▸ *Smiling.* In the first few weeks of life, most of a newborn's smiles are involuntary, but it won't be long before the baby begins smiling in response to a person or situation.

If you're observant, you may notice some of these reflexes, but don't worry if you don't notice them. Your baby's care provider may check for them during physical examinations.

You can encourage your baby's movement by gently cycling the arms and legs as he or she lies on his or her back. Or you might let the baby kick at your hands or a squeaky toy.

Senses It's a new world for your baby, and all of his or her senses are coming alive to explore and make sense of it. You'll notice when an object, light, sound, smell or touch engages your baby. Watch for him or her to settle down or become quiet when something new is introduced.

Sight Your newborn is nearsighted and sees objects best at 8 to 12 inches away. That's the perfect distance for seeing the most important things to babies — their parents' faces as they hold or feed them. Your baby will love to fixate on your face, and it will be the favorite entertainment for a while. Give your newborn plenty of face-to-face time to get to know you.

In addition to being interested in human faces, newborns are also engaged by brightness, movement and simple, high-contrast objects. Many toy stores sell black-and-white and brightly colored toys, mobiles, and nursery decorations.

Because newborns can't fully control their eye movements, they may appear to be cross-eyed at times. This is normal. Your baby's eye muscles will strengthen and mature during the next few months.

When your baby is quiet and alert, provide simple objects for him or her to look at. Try slowly moving an object to the right or left in front of him or her. Most babies will briefly follow moving objects with their eyes and sometimes with their heads. Don't overload your child — one item at a time is plenty. If your baby is tired, hungry or overstimulated, he or she won't want to play this game.

Hearing Once baby is born, new sounds will capture his or her attention. In response to noises, babies may pause in sucking, widen their eyes or stop fussing. They may startle at a loud noise such as a dog barking, and they may be soothed by the hum of the vacuum cleaner or the whirring of the clothes dryer. Babies can easily adapt and tune out noises, so they may react to a particular sound only once or twice.

Newborns can tell the difference between human voices and other sounds. Babies are most curious about their parents' voices. Your baby will learn quickly to associate your voice with food, warmth and touch. He or she will listen carefully when you talk to him or her — even infants enjoy being read to. Talk to your baby whenever you can. Even though he or she won't understand what you're saying, the sound of your voice is reassuring and calming.

Most hospitals now routinely test every baby's hearing as part of newborn screenings. Early screening is an important tool to identify hearing loss before it affects language and social development.

Touch Infants are sensitive to touch and can detect differences in texture, pressure and moisture. They respond quickly to changes in temperature. They may startle when cold air blows across their skin and become quiet again when they're wrapped warmly. Your touch provides comfort and reassurance to your baby and can rouse a sleepy baby for feeding.

Smell and taste Infants have a good sense of smell. A baby can recognize his or her mother by scent at a very young age. Babies may show interest in a new smell by a change in movement or activity. But they easily become familiar with a new smell and no longer react to it.

The sense of taste is closely related to the sense of smell. Although newborns aren't exposed to many tastes beyond breast milk or formula, research shows that from birth, babies prefer sweet tastes over others.

Crying Crying is the first and primary form of communication that newborns use. And they do plenty of it — young babies typically cry on average from one to four hours a day. It's a normal part of adjusting to life outside the womb.

Common reasons for crying include:
- *Hunger.* Most babies eat six to 10 times in a 24-hour period. For at least the first three months, babies usually wake for night feedings.
- *Discomfort.* Your baby may cry because of wet or soiled diapers, gas or indigestion, and uncomfortable temperatures or positions. When babies are uncomfortable, they may look for something to suck on. But feeding won't stop the discomfort, and a pacifier may help only briefly. When the discomfort passes, your baby will probably settle down.
- *Boredom, fear and loneliness.* Sometimes, a baby will cry because he or she is bored, frightened or lonely and wants to be held and cuddled. A baby

seeking comfort may calm down with the reassurance of seeing you, hearing your voice, feeling your touch, being with you, being cuddled or being offered something to suck on.
- *Overtiredness or overstimulation.* Crying helps an overtired or overstimulated baby to shut out sights, sounds and other sensations. It also helps relieve tension. You may notice that your baby's fussy periods occur at predictable times during the day, often between early evening and midnight. It seems that nothing you do at these times can console him or her, but afterward baby may be more alert than before and then may sleep more deeply. This kind of fussy crying seems to help babies get rid of excess energy.

As your baby matures, you'll be able to distinguish the different messages in your baby's cries.

Calming a crying baby In general, during the first few months of life, it's best to respond promptly to your infant when he or she cries. You won't spoil your baby by doing so. Studies show newborns who are quickly and warmly responded to cry less overall.

When your baby's crying seems prolonged, run down a simple list to determine what might be needed:
- Is baby hungry?
- Does baby need a clean diaper?
- Does baby need to be burped?
- Is baby too warm or too cold?
- Does baby need to suck on something for comfort?
- Does baby need some tender care — walking, rocking, cuddling, stroking, gentle talking, singing or humming?
- Does baby need to be moved to a more comfortable position? Is something pinching, sticking or binding him or her?

SWADDLING BABY

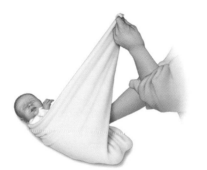

Step 1. Bring one corner of the blanket up and pull it taut. Bring the blanket across your baby's body with one arm tucked inside. Tuck the corner under your baby's bottom snugly.

Step 2. Fold the bottom point up, leaving some room for your baby's hips and legs to move freely.

Step 3. Bring up the other corner of the blanket, pull it taut, and tuck it around your baby's other arm and under his or her body.

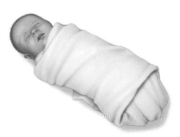

Step 4. A cozy bundle.

▶ Has there been too much excitement or stimulation? Does baby just need to cry for a while?

Try to meet your baby's most pressing needs first. If hunger seems to be the problem, feed him or her. If the crying is shrieking or panicky, check to make sure nothing is poking or pinching your baby. If your baby is warm, dry, well-fed and well-rested but still wailing, these suggestions may help:

▶ Try swaddling baby snugly in a blanket.

▶ Gently talk to or sing to your baby face-to-face.

▶ Gently stroke baby's head or rub or pat his or her chest or back.

▶ Offer your baby your finger or a pacifier to suck on as you rock him or her.

- Use a gentle motion, such as rocking your baby in your arms, walking with him or her against your shoulder, or carrying him or her in a front carrier.
- Play soft music.
- Hold baby tummy down on your lap.
- Hold baby in an upright position on your shoulder or against your chest.
- Put baby in his or her car seat and go for a drive.
- Give baby a warm bath or put a warm — not hot — water bottle on his or her stomach.
- Go outside. Take your baby for a walk in a stroller or carriage.
- Reduce the noise, movement and lights in the area where your baby is. Or try introducing white noise, such as the continuous, monotonous sound of a vacuum cleaner or a recording of ocean waves. This can relax and lull babies by blocking out other sounds.

If your baby is dry, full, comfortable and wrapped snugly but is still crying, he or she may just need a 10- to 15-minute period alone. Stay within earshot, and check on the baby every few minutes from a distance. Although many parents find it difficult to let their babies cry, it may give the infants an opportunity to wind down and let off steam.

Remember that you won't always be able to calm your baby, especially when the fussing is simply a way to release tension. Babies do cry; it's a normal part of being a baby. Rest assured that the crying won't last forever — the amount of time your baby spends crying usually peaks at about six weeks after birth and then gradually decreases. By 3 to 4 months of age, there is often a marked improvement.

It's also a normal part of parenting to find excessive crying frustrating. Make arrangements with family, friends or a baby sitter for needed breaks. Even an hourlong break can renew your coping strength.

If your baby's crying is making you feel out of control, put your baby in a safe place, such as a crib. Then contact your care provider, your hospital emergency room or a local crisis intervention service. No matter how impatient or angry you get, never shake a baby. And never let anyone else shake a baby. Shaking an infant can cause blindness, brain damage or even death.

Eating and sleeping Two important items on a newborn's agenda are eating and sleeping. Because most of a baby's energy goes into growing, many non-sleeping hours are spent eating.

Eating patterns During the first several weeks, most babies will want to eat six to 10 times a day. Their stomachs don't hold enough breast milk or formula to satisfy them for long. That means you could be feeding your baby every two or three hours, including during the night. However, there's tremendous variation among infants in how often and how much they eat.

Your baby probably won't have a feeding routine at first. Although you can roughly estimate the amount of time between feedings, the baby's schedule will be erratic. During growth spurts, feedings will be more frequent for a day or two.

You'll soon learn to read the signals that your baby is hungry, such as crying, opening its mouth, sucking, putting a fist in its mouth, fidgeting and turning toward your breast. Babies will also let you know when they've had enough by pushing the nipple or bottle out of their mouths or turning their heads away.

Sleep patterns and cycles As with eating, it takes awhile for newborns to

COPING WITH COLIC

Every baby is fussy at times, but some babies cry much more than do others. If your baby is healthy but has frequent fussy episodes, especially during the evening, or has prolonged, inconsolable crying for three or more hours a day, chances are your baby has colic. It's not a physical disorder or disease — colic is just the term for recurring bouts of crying that are difficult to relieve.

A colicky baby's crying is not simply due to hunger, a wet diaper or any other apparent cause, and the baby can't be calmed down. Experts aren't sure what causes the condition. Colic typically peaks at about six weeks after birth and usually goes away by 3 months of age.

For parents of a baby with colic, it may seem that the baby will never outgrow this phase. It's common to feel frustrated, angry, tense, irritable, worried and fatigued.

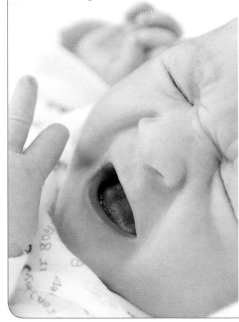

What to do No treatment consistently provides relief to infants with colic. Experiment with various methods to calm your baby, and try not to get discouraged if many of your efforts seem futile. Remember that your baby will eventually outgrow colic. And having a fussy newborn doesn't necessarily mean anything about your child's temperament later in life. Many colicky babies turn out to be happy, smiling, easygoing toddlers and children.

During your baby's crying spells, the more relaxed you are, the easier it'll be to console your child. Listening to a newborn wailing can be agonizing, but your own anxiety, frustration or panic may only add to the infant's distress.

Take a break and allow others to watch your baby so that you can relax. Sometimes a new face can calm the baby when you've used up all your usual tricks.

When it may not be colic Sometimes it can be difficult to determine if your baby has colic or if his or her crying is related to something else. Call your baby's care provider if:

- Your baby seems to cry for an unusual length of time
- The cries sound odd to you
- The crying is associated with decreased activity, poor feeding, or unusual breathing or movements
- The crying is accompanied by other signs of illness, such as vomiting, fever and diarrhea

Also call your care provider if you or someone else in your household is having trouble staying calm around the baby.

develop a schedule for sleeping. During the first month, they usually sleep and wake round-the-clock, with relatively equal periods of sleep between feedings.

In addition, newborns don't know the difference between night and day. It takes time for them to develop circadian rhythms — the sleep-wake cycles and other patterns that revolve on a 24-hour cycle. As a baby's nervous system gradually matures, so do his or her phases of sleep and wakefulness.

Although newborns don't usually sleep for more than about $4^1/2$ hours at a stretch, altogether they sleep 12 or more hours a day. They generally stay awake long enough to feed, or for up to about two hours, before falling asleep again. By the time your baby is 2 weeks old, you'll likely notice that the periods of sleeping and wakefulness are lengthening. By 3 months, many babies shift more of their sleep to nighttime, much to the relief of their parents.

You can help adjust your baby's body clock toward sleeping at night by:

▶ Avoiding stimulation during nighttime feedings and diaper changes. Keep the lights low, use a soft voice, and don't play or talk with your baby. This reinforces the message that nighttime is for sleeping.

▶ Establishing some kind of bedtime routine. This might be singing, having a quiet time or reading for an hour before putting your baby to bed.

DEVELOPING GOOD SLEEPING HABITS

Drooping eyelids, rubbing the eyes and fussiness are the usual signs that a baby is tired. Many babies cry when they're put down for sleep, but if left alone for a few minutes, most will eventually quiet themselves.

If your baby is not wet, hungry or ill, try to be patient with the crying and encourage self-soothing. If you leave the room for a while, your baby will probably stop crying after a short time. If not, try comforting him or her and allow the baby to settle again.

In the first few months, it's common for a pattern to evolve in which a baby is fed and falls asleep in a parent's arms. Many parents enjoy this closeness and snuggling. But eventually this may be the only way the baby is able to fall asleep. When the baby wakes up in the middle of the night, he or she can't fall asleep again without being fed and held. To avoid these associations, put your baby in bed while he or she is drowsy but still awake. When babies fall asleep in bed without assistance when they're first laid down, they're more likely to learn to fall asleep on their own after waking in the middle of the night.

Keep in mind that young babies who stir during the night aren't necessarily distressed. Infants typically cry and move about when entering different sleep cycles. Parents sometimes mistake a baby's stirrings as a sign of waking up, and begin unnecessary feeding. Instead, wait a few minutes to see if your baby falls back to sleep.

SAFE SLEEP

Always place your baby on his or her back to sleep, even for naps. This is the safest sleep position for reducing the risk of sudden infant death syndrome (SIDS). Sometimes called crib death, SIDS is the sudden and unexplained death of a baby under 1 year of age.

Research shows that babies who are put to sleep on their stomachs are much more likely to die of SIDS than are babies placed on their backs. Infants who sleep on their sides also are at increased risk, probably because babies in this position can roll onto their stomachs. Since 1992, when the American Academy of Pediatrics began recommending the back-sleeping position for infants, the incidence of SIDS in the United States has declined significantly.

The only exceptions to the back-sleeping rule are babies who have health problems that require them to sleep on their stomachs. If your baby was born with a birth defect, spits up often after eating, or has a breathing, lung or heart problem, talk to your baby's care provider about the best sleeping position for your child.

Make sure that everyone who takes care of your baby knows to place the infant on his or her back for sleeping. That may include grandparents, child care providers, baby sitters, friends and others.

Some babies don't like sleeping on their backs at first, but they get used to it quickly. Many parents worry that their baby will choke if he or she spits up or vomits while sleeping on his or her back, but doctors have found no increase in choking or similar problems.

Some babies who sleep on their backs may get a flat spot on the backs of their heads. For the most part, this will go away after the baby learns to sit up. You can help keep your baby's head a normal shape by alternating the direction your baby lies in the crib — head toward one end of the crib for a few nights and then toward the other. This way, the baby may not always sleep on the same side of his or her head.

Other tips that may help reduce the risk of SIDS include:

▶ *Breast-feed your baby.* Although it's not entirely clear why, breast-feeding may protect babies against SIDS.

▶ *Dress your baby in a sleep sack.* By doing this you don't need to use a blanket and worry about the blanket interfering with breathing.

▶ *Select bedding carefully.* Use a firm mattress. Avoid placing baby on thick, fluffy padding, which may interfere with breathing if baby's face presses against it. For the same reason, don't leave pillows, fluffy toys or stuffed animals in your infant's crib.

▶ *Don't smoke or expose baby to household smoke.* Infants whose mothers smoke during and after pregnancy are three times as likely to die of SIDS as infants of nonsmoking mothers.

▶ *Keep the temperature at a comfortable level.* If your baby is sweating around the neck or face, it probably means he or she is too warm.

Feeding a sleepy baby You'll no doubt have times when your baby signals that he or she is hungry, only to doze off when you begin feeding. Try these tips to feed a sleepy baby:

- Watch for and take advantage of your baby's alert stages. Feed at these times.
- A sleeping baby may squirm and root around or fuss when hungry. If your baby naps for more than three hours, watch for these subtle signs. If your baby is partially awake, gently wake him or her and encourage eating.
- Give your baby a massage by walking your fingers up his or her spine.
- Partially undress your baby. Because your baby's skin is sensitive to temperature changes, the coolness may wake him or her long enough to eat.
- Stroke a circle around your baby's lips with a fingertip a few times.
- Rock your baby into a sitting position. The baby's eyes often open when he or she is positioned upright.

Peeing and pooping New parents often wonder what's normal when it comes to their baby's urination and bowel movements. By 3 or 4 days old, a baby should typically have about six to eight wet diapers a day if he or she is getting enough to eat. As your baby gets older, he or she may have wet diapers with every feeding.

In a healthy infant, urine is light to dark yellow in color. Sometimes, highly concentrated urine dries on the diaper to a pinkish color, which may be mistaken for blood. Actual blood in the urine or a bloody spot on the diaper is cause for concern, however.

As for stools, the range of normal is quite broad and varies from one baby to another. Babies may have a bowel movement as frequently as after every feeding, as infrequently as once a week, or in no consistent pattern.

If you're breast-feeding, your baby's stools will resemble light mustard with seed-like particles. They'll be soft and even slightly runny. The stools of a formula-fed infant are usually tan or yellow and firmer than those of a breast-fed baby, but no firmer than peanut butter. Occasional variations in color and consistency are normal. Different colors may indicate how fast the stools moved through the digestive tract or what the baby ate. The stool may be green, yellow, orange or brown.

Mild diarrhea is common in newborns. The stools may be watery, frequent and mixed with mucus. Constipation is not usually a problem for infants. Babies may strain, grunt and turn red during a bowel movement, but this doesn't mean they're constipated. A baby is constipated when bowel movements are formed and hard.

FIRST BOWEL MOVEMENTS

Your baby's first soiled diaper — which should occur within 48 hours of birth — may surprise you. During these first few days, your newborn's stools will be thick and sticky — a tarlike, greenish-black substance called meconium. After the meconium is passed, the color, frequency and consistency of your baby's stools will vary depending on how your baby is fed — by breast or bottle.

BABY CARE BASICS

Once your son or daughter is home, you may wonder about even the little things. Am I holding him or her right? Is this outfit too tight or too hot? Is the bath water too cold? It's normal to feel a little nervous or anxious.

But it won't take long until you're more confident in caring for your baby's needs. You'll soon become a pro at everything from changing diapers to giving your little one a bath.

Holding your baby At first you may feel a little awkward or nervous about holding and carrying your baby. Over time you'll feel more comfortable. And you'll soon learn what positions your baby likes — all babies have their own preferences. Newborns generally love being held close, soothed by the warmth of your body. They also feel secure and calm when they're cradled in the crook of an elbow, with their head, legs and arms firmly supported.

During the first few months of life, babies differ in their abilities to control their neck muscles and heads. Until you're sure your baby can hold up his or her head quite well, lift baby gently and slowly so that his or her body is supported and the head doesn't flop back. When putting your baby down, gently support the head and neck with one hand and the bottom with the other.

With experience you'll discover the best position for calming and comforting a fussy baby. You might try holding him or her along the length of your arm, face down, with the baby's head at the bend of your elbow and his or her crotch at your hand. Or you can hold the baby face down across your lap, with his or her tummy lying against your thigh. Another comforting position is to lie on your back

and put baby face down on your chest while gently rubbing his or her back.

Your baby will probably also develop a preference for how he or she wants to be carried. Some infants enjoy facing outward, looking at the world, and others prefer the security of snuggling close to your body. Your baby may like being carried with arms and legs tucked in, or he or she may prefer a more relaxed position with just the body and head supported.

Changing diapers To parents of young babies, life often seems to be an endless round of changing diapers. Indeed, the average child goes through at least 2,500 diapers in their first year alone. That statistic is daunting, but it may help to think of those frequent changes as opportunities

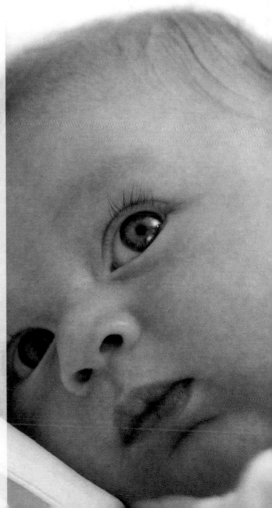

for closeness and communication with your baby. Your warm words, gentle touches and encouraging smiles help make your baby feel loved and secure, and soon your infant will be responding with gurgles and coos.

Because newborns urinate frequently, it's important to change your baby's diapers every two or three hours for the first few months. But you can wait until your baby wakes up to change a wet diaper. Urine alone doesn't usually irritate a ba-

by's skin. However, the acid content in a bowel movement can, so change a messy diaper soon after your baby awakens.

Get equipped To make diaper changing more comfortable for you and your baby, make sure you have on hand:

▶ *Diapers.* Stock an adequate supply of diapers. You can buy cloth or disposable diapers, including compostable options, or you can use a diaper service. Most diaper services use cloth

DIAPER RASH

All babies get red or sore bottoms from time to time, even with frequent diaper changes and careful cleaning. Diaper rash may be caused by many things, including irritation from stools or from a new product, such as disposable wipes, diapers or laundry detergent. Sensitive skin, a bacterial or yeast infection, and chafing or rubbing from tightfitting diapers or clothing also can cause a rash.

Diaper rash usually is easily treated and improves within a few days. The most important factor in treating diaper rash is to keep your baby's skin as clean and dry as possible. Thoroughly wash the area with water during each diaper change. While your baby has a diaper rash, avoid washing the affected area with soaps and disposable, scented wipes. Alcohol and perfumes in these products can irritate your baby's skin and aggravate or provoke the rash.

It's also important to allow baby's bottom to air-dry before putting on a new diaper. If possible, let your child go without a diaper for short periods of time. Also avoid using plastic pants or tightfitting diaper covers when baby has a diaper rash.

In addition, use a soothing ointment that contains zinc oxide anytime pinkness appears in the diaper area. These products typically are applied in a thin layer to the irritated region several times throughout the day to soothe and protect the baby's skin. If the rash doesn't improve within a few days, check with your baby's care provider.

Don't use talcum powder or cornstarch on a baby's skin. An infant may inhale talcum powder, which can be very irritating to a baby's lungs. Cornstarch can contribute to a bacterial infection.

To help prevent diaper rash, avoid using superabsorbent disposable diapers because they tend to be changed less frequently. If you're using cloth diapers, be sure to wash and rinse them thoroughly. To improve circulation, select plastic pants or waterproof covers that snap on, instead of those with elastic bindings. In addition, try using moisture-wicking liners with cloth diapers.

diapers, and their fees typically cover rental of the diapers, delivery and pickup, and laundering. If you use disposable diapers, be sure to get the size corresponding to your baby's weight. You'll likely need about 80 disposable diapers a week.

If you plan to buy cloth diapers, you'll want to scope out the many options that are now available. You could still fold flat cloth diapers like your grandma might have done — but there's certainly no need to. Some kinds of cloth diapers will need plastic pants over the top, while others use absorbent cloth inserts with a cover made of waterproof material. Some can even be used with biodegradable, disposable inserts, which are convenient when you're on the go. If you know other parents who have used cloth diapers recently, ask them about their preferences and experiences. Doing research will help you to make an informed decision about what might work best for you.

The number of cloth diapers you'll need depends partly on how often you plan to wash them. For example, if you have three dozen flat diapers, you'll probably need to wash them every other day. Even if you use disposable diapers, you'll likely find it helpful to have a dozen cloth diapers on hand in case you run out of disposables. (The reverse is also true!) Older styles of cloth diapers are handy to drape over your shoulder or to put on your lap while burping your baby, too.

- *Pre-moistened baby wipes.* Although a moistened cloth also works, it's hard to beat the convenience of pre-moistened baby wipes. Choose wipes for sensitive skin to prevent irritation.
- *A diaper pail.* Various types of diaper pails are available. Look for a pail that's convenient, sanitary and holds in odors.
- *Baby lotion.* It's not necessary to use lotion at every diaper change, but it may come in handy if your baby develops diaper rash. Unscented lotions are preferable.
- *A changing table.* Choose a table with a wide, sturdy base that has compartments for storing diaper-changing supplies.

Diaper-changing basics When changing a diaper, use a flat surface — a changing table, a changing pad on the floor or a crib. If you're using a changing table, be sure to use the safety belt or keep one hand on your baby at all times.

Your baby may urinate when you're changing the diaper. If your baby is a boy, you can avoid being sprayed with urine by covering his penis loosely with a diaper or cloth while cleaning the rest of the diaper area.

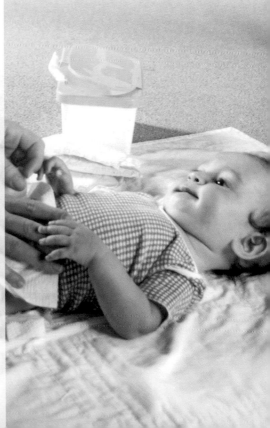

After you've removed the soiled diaper, take time to thoroughly clean your baby's bottom:

- During the cleaning, carefully grasp and hold baby's legs at the ankles with one hand.
- Use either a cotton cloth dampened with warm water or a pre-moistened baby wipe to wipe your baby's diaper area. Use alcohol-free and fragrance-free wipes to avoid drying or irritating the baby's skin.
- In case of a bowel movement, use the unsoiled front of the diaper to remove the bulk of the stool. Wipe down and away from the genitals, folding the waste inside the diaper.
- Gently finish cleaning with a cloth or wipe, using a mild soap as needed. You needn't apply lotion, unless your baby tends to develop rashes.
- Lift your baby's lower body by the ankles and slide the new diaper underneath. Fit the diaper snugly around your baby's waist and fasten the tabs on either side. For newborns, fold the top of the diaper down until the umbilical cord stump falls off.

If you're using flat or prefold cloth diapers, you can fold them several ways. Experiment with different techniques for best absorbency and fit. Folding the front narrower than the back may bring the diaper around the legs more tightly. You may also want to create extra padding in the front if you have a boy. With newer kinds of cloth diapers, you can add extra absorbency through additional layers or inserts.

Different styles of cloth diapers may use snaps, hook and loop fasteners, or a separate fastener, such as pins or a Snappi, to secure a tight fit. If you're using diaper pins, you can avoid poking the baby by keeping the fingers of one hand between the pin and your baby's body while securing the pin. Flat and prefold diapers should fit snugly because they tend to loosen as your baby moves around.

CRADLE CAP

Your baby may develop scaliness and redness on his or her scalp. This condition is called cradle cap (seborrheic dermatitis), which results when oil-producing sebaceous glands produce too much oil. Cradle cap is common in infants, usually beginning in the first weeks of life and clearing up over a period of weeks or months. It may be mild, with flaky, dry skin that looks like dandruff, or more severe, with thick, oily, yellowish scaling or crusty patches.

Shampooing with a mild baby shampoo can help with cradle cap. Don't be afraid to wash your baby's hair more frequently than before. This, along with soft brushing, will help remove the scales. If the scales don't loosen easily, rub petroleum jelly or a few drops of mineral oil onto your baby's scalp. Let it soak into the scales for a few minutes, and then brush and shampoo your baby's hair. If you leave the oil in your baby's hair, the scales may accumulate and worsen cradle cap.

If cradle cap persists or spreads to your baby's face, neck or other parts of the body, especially in the creases at the elbow or behind the ears, contact your baby's care provider, who may suggest a medicated shampoo or lotion.

Bathing Your infant doesn't need much bathing. During the first week or two, until the stump of the umbilical cord falls off, give your newborn sponge baths. After that, a complete bath is necessary only one to three times a week for the first year. More frequent baths can dry out baby's skin.

Once the umbilical area is healed, try placing your baby directly in the water. The first baths should be as gentle and brief as possible. If your infant resists baths, give sponge baths, cleaning the parts that really need attention, especially the hands, neck, head, face, behind the ears, under the arms and the diaper area. Sponge baths are a good alternative to a full bath for the first six weeks.

Bathing basics Find a time for bathing your baby that's convenient for both of you. Many people give their baby a bath before bedtime, as a relaxing, sleep-promoting ritual. Others prefer a time when their baby is fully awake. You'll enjoy this time more if you're not in a hurry and not likely to be interrupted.

Most parents find it easiest to bathe a newborn in a bathinette, sink or plastic tub lined with a clean towel. Have all of your bathing supplies ready and try to have the room warm — about 75 F — before you undress your baby. In addition to the basin of water, you'll need a washcloth, cotton balls, a towel, diaper-changing supplies and clothing to put on after the bath. Plain water baths are fine most of the time. If needed, you can use mild baby soap and shampoo that are free of fragrances and deodorants, which can irritate baby's delicate skin. Use these at the end of the bath.

Before filling the tub or basin, test the water temperature with your elbow or

---

UMBILICAL CORD CARE

After your newborn's umbilical cord is cut, all that remains is a small stump. Usually it will dry up and fall off one to three weeks after birth. Until then, keep the area as clean and dry as possible. It's a good idea to give sponge baths rather than full baths until the cord falls off and the navel area heals.

Traditionally, parents have been instructed to swab the cord stump with rubbing alcohol. Some research indicates that leaving the stump alone may help the cord heal faster, so many hospitals now recommend against this practice. If you're unsure about what to do, talk to your baby's care provider.

Exposing the cord to air and allowing it to dry at its base will hasten its separation. To prevent irritation and keep the navel area dry, fold the baby's diaper below the stump. In warm weather, dress a newborn in just a diaper and T-shirt to let air circulate and help the drying process.

It's normal to see a bit of crusted straw-colored discharge or dried blood until the cord falls off. But if your baby's navel looks red or has a foul-smelling discharge, call your baby's care provider. When the stump falls off, you may see a little blood, which is normal. But if the navel continues to bleed, have it examined by your baby's care provider.

wrist. The water should feel warm, not hot. Fill the tub with a couple of inches of warm water. Undress your baby, removing the diaper last. If the diaper is dirty, clean your baby's bottom before setting him or her in the bath. Use one hand to support your baby's head and the other to guide him or her in, feet first, then gently lower the rest of the body in. It's important to support the head and torso, to provide safety and a sense of security.

It's not necessary to shampoo your baby's hair with every bath — once or twice a week is plenty. Massage the entire scalp gently. When you rinse soap or shampoo from the baby's head, cup your hand across his or her forehead so that the suds run toward the sides, not the eyes. Or tip your baby's head back a bit.

Use a soft cloth to wash your baby's face and hair with clear water. Use a damp cotton ball to wipe each eye from the inside to the outside corner. Gently

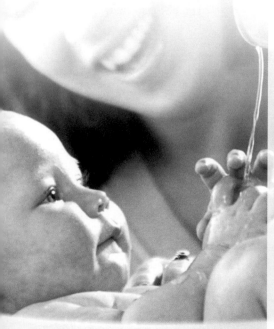

pat the face dry. Wash the rest of the body from the top down, including the inside folds of skin and the genital area. For a girl, gently spread the labia to clean. For a boy, lift the scrotum to clean underneath. If he's uncircumcised, don't try to retract the foreskin of the penis. Let your baby lean forward on your arm while you clean his or her back and bottom, separating the buttocks to clean the anal area.

Be careful handling your infant when he or she is wet and slippery. As soon as you're done bathing, wrap the baby in a towel or a baby towel with a built-in hood and gently pat him or her dry.

Skin care Many parents expect their newborns' skin to be flawless. More commonly, you'll see some blotchiness, bruising from birth and skin blemishes that are unique to newborns, such as baby acne (milia). Most young infants have dry, peeling skin, especially on their hands and feet, for the first few weeks. Some blueness of the hands and feet is normal and may continue for a few weeks. Rashes also are common.

Most rashes and skin conditions are treated easily or clear up on their own. If your baby has pimples, place a soft, clean receiving blanket under his or her head and wash the face gently once a day with a mild baby soap. If the baby has dry or peeling skin, try using an over-the-counter, unscented lotion.

Nail care Your baby's nails are soft, but they're sharp. A newborn can easily scratch his or her own face — or yours. To prevent your baby from accidentally scratching his or her face, you may need to trim the fingernails shortly after birth and then as often as a few times a week after that.

Sometimes you may be able to carefully peel off the ends with your fingers because baby nails are so soft. Don't worry — you won't rip the whole nail off. You can also use a baby nail clipper or a small scissors. Here are some tips to make nail trimming easier for you and your baby:

▶ Trim the nails after a bath. They'll be softer, making them easier to cut.
▶ Wait until your baby is asleep.
▶ Have another person hold your baby while you trim his or her nails.
▶ Trim the nails straight across and keep them short.

Clothing When you're buying clothes for your newborn, you may want to choose a 3-month size or larger so that the baby doesn't immediately outgrow the clothes. In general, look for soft, comfortable clothing that's washable. Avoid buttons, which are easily swallowed, and ribbons or strings, which can cause choking. Don't buy garments with drawstrings, which can catch on objects and strangle a child.

Because you'll likely be changing your baby's clothing several times a day, or at least changing diapers, make sure the outfits are uncomplicated and open easily. Look for garments that snap or zip down the front, have loosefitting sleeves, and are made of stretchy fabric.

During the first few weeks, babies are often wrapped in receiving blankets. This keeps them warm, and the slight pressure around the body seems to give most newborns a sense of security.

Dress for the weather New parents sometimes overdress their infants. A good rule of thumb is to dress your baby in the same number of layers that you would feel comfortable wearing. Unless it's hot outside, you might put the baby in an undershirt and diaper, covered by pajamas or a dressing gown, and wrapped in a receiving blanket. In hot weather — over 75 F — a single layer of clothing is appropriate, but a cover is needed when the baby is in air conditioning or near drafts.

Remember that your baby's skin will sunburn easily. If you're going to be outside for any length of time, protect your baby's skin with clothing and a cap. Keep the baby in the shade to avoid overexposure to the sun. You can use sunblock after your baby is 6 months old, but don't rely on it as the baby's only sun protection. Babies don't sweat easily and can become overheated.

TWINS, TRIPLETS OR MORE

Every year, thousands of moms bring home more than one newborn — twins, triplets or even more. Life changes for any new parent, but for parents of multiples the changes are, well, multiplied!

Having more than one new baby at once can be exciting. It's also extremely demanding. Sometimes just getting through the day can seem impossible. And multiples often are born early, which increases the risk of complications. This means you need to spend more of your time at doctor appointments than you would with a single baby.

What are some of the changes that you can expect with multiples? You'll often be tired because you'll be getting a lot less sleep, and your household standards will probably have to relax for a few years. If you have other children, the arrival of multiples can trigger more than the usual sibling rivalry. Multiple babies require an enormous amount of your time and energy, and they attract extra attention from friends, relatives and strangers on the street.

You may have some negative or difficult feelings from time to time. Having less time for each baby can make you feel guilty or sad, and those feelings may become even more pronounced if you already have another child or children. However, the joy and excitement your multiples bring will soon cancel out all of those negative moments.

Getting through the first weeks
Here are some tips for dealing with the challenges of caring for multiples:

▶ *Recruit help and accept all offers of help.* Even though this may be difficult to do, it can make a big difference. Some families hire help, some rely on extended family, and some get help from friends, neighbors, their church or organizations for parents of multiples.

▶ *Establish a list of priorities.* The list generally focuses on babies' needs, such as feeding, bathing, sleeping and cuddling. Rest and breaks for you also should be on the list.

▶ *Recognize your babies as individuals from the beginning.* Select different-colored clothing for your babies, which helps you identify each one at a glance. Avoid referring to the babies as "the twins" or "the triplets." Use their names. Be sure to take pictures of each child separately.

▶ *Use charts or checklists.* This is helpful for documenting feedings and keeping track of who has been cared for and when.

▶ *If you have older children, encourage them to be an active, helpful part of the experience.* Ask them to help with the baby chores, and tell them how special it will be to be a big sister or big brother. It's also important to regularly set aside time to spend alone with your other children. Older children also may enjoy time alone with grandparents, aunts, uncles, or other family members or friends.

▶ *Use disposable diapers or a diaper service unless you have extra household help.* If you use disposable diapers, keep at least a dozen cloth diapers on hand for emergencies.

▶ *Gather practical advice, information and support.* Feeding, bathing and dressing multiples may require some special strategies. Consider attending a local support group for parents of twins or other multiples. You'll likely get many invaluable ideas from other parents. Read books and magazines, visit websites, and get involved in social media dedicated to advice on parenting multiples.

▶ *Don't neglect your relationship with your partner.* Talk to each other about your feelings and problems. Try to give each other breaks when you can, and do what you can to have some time alone as a couple.

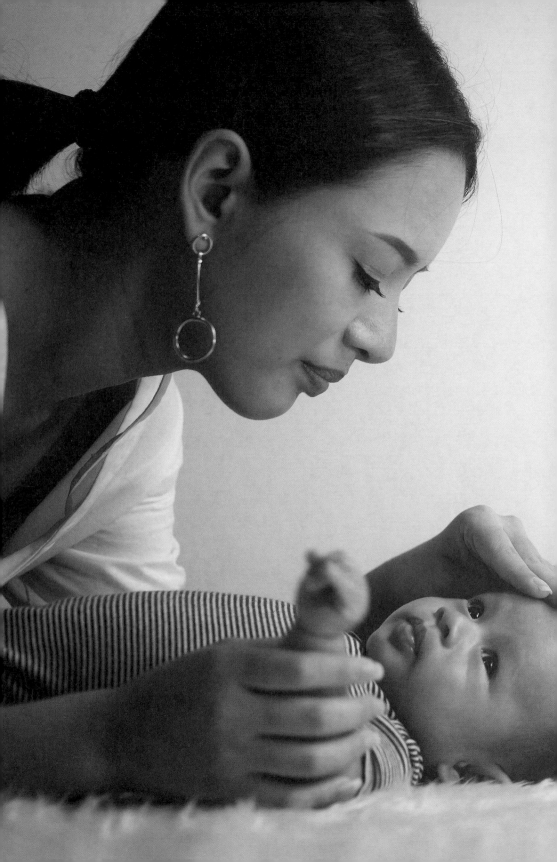

CHAPTER 18

Postpartum issues for mom

After having your baby, you may wonder if your body will ever return to normal. With a healthy lifestyle, it will! But it does take time to recover from the changes that occurred over the previous 10 months. It's not realistic to expect to bounce back quickly after giving birth, but over time you will start to feel better physically and get back in shape. This chapter discusses some of the issues you may deal with in the coming weeks as your body goes through a variety of changes.

If you had a cesarean birth, you can expect a few additional discomforts and precautions during the postpartum period. See Chapter 15 for information about recovering from a cesarean delivery.

BREAST CARE

With breast-feeding, your breasts will remain enlarged for most of the time you're nursing. This is especially evident in the first four to six weeks. To keep comfortable, wear a good-quality, well-fitting bra. Avoid using soap on your breasts in the shower, as this can aggravate cracked nipples. Water is really all you need.

If you don't breast-feed, the enlargement you noticed during pregnancy will gradually disappear during your baby's first month of life.

Engorgement For the first few days after you have given birth, your breasts contain colostrum. Within a few days, this colostrum will change to more mature milk and your breasts will feel full. They may become larger and heavier, flushed, swollen and tender, whether or not you breast-feed. If you're not nursing your baby, your breasts may be engorged and hard until you're no longer producing milk. Engorgement usually lasts less than three days, but it can be uncomfortable. Even if you're breast-feeding, your breasts may at times overfill and become engorged. To ease engorgement:

▶ Express a little milk, either manually or by feeding your baby.

- Apply cold compresses between feedings to help with discomfort.
- Wear a supportive bra.

Leaking milk If you're breast-feeding, don't be surprised if you leak milk during and between feedings. Milk may drip from your breasts anytime, anywhere and without warning. As many new mothers can attest, you might find yourself leaking when you think or talk about your baby, hear a baby cry, or go for a long stretch between feedings. Milk may leak from one breast while you nurse from the other. This is common, particularly in the early weeks. To deal with leaky breasts:

- Stock up on nursing pads, but avoid those that are lined or backed with plastic because they can irritate your nipples. Change pads after each feeding and whenever they become wet.
- Place a large towel under yourself at night when you sleep.

Sore or cracked nipples When you begin breast-feeding, your nipples may feel sore or tender. This is a common problem in the early weeks and can happen even if your baby is positioned perfectly and you're doing everything right.

Some women are surprised at how vigorously their babies suck — and how uncomfortable it can be. It takes some time to get used to the sensation of baby feeding. However, the tenderness usually disappears after a few days. If you develop a sore nipple that becomes cracked, this can be very painful.

Follow these suggestions to prevent and treat sore or cracked nipples:

- Make sure your baby is latched on to your breast correctly (see page 329). A persistent, poor latch is the main reason for cracked nipples. To help your baby get the nipple fully into his or her mouth, position your baby with the nose near the nipple, lift the breast with your fingers, and compress the areola with your thumb and fingers to help baby get the right grasp on the nipple.
- When removing your baby from the breast, slip your finger into the side of the baby's mouth to break the suction. Do this before taking the baby off the breast.
- With clean hands, express breast milk and rub it into your nipples. Breast milk has excellent healing properties. Lanolin ointment also can be used.
- Let your nipples air dry after feedings and remember to change nursing pads frequently.
- If these measures aren't helping, contact a lactation specialist or your care provider. They'll work with you to find other interventions or treatments that may be more helpful.

BREAST SELF-AWARENESS

Breast self-examination can be more difficult during pregnancy and breast-feeding, but being observant of your breast appearance and consistency is still important. Your breasts will feel very different while nursing. If you're concerned about a lump, check your breasts right after you've fed your baby, when your breasts are emptier and any abnormalities may be more obvious.

Blocked ducts In the early weeks of breast-feeding, a milk duct may become blocked as a result of engorgement, a too-tight bra or a blocked nipple opening. If you experience a blockage, you will feel a soft to somewhat dense lump that is quite tender to the touch. To clear a blocked duct, start feedings with the affected breast and gently massage it while feeding. Try positioning baby so that his or her chin is near the block, and apply a warm compress before feeding. You may also try massaging the breast toward the nipple while you take a shower.

Call your care provider if you have body aches and a fever in addition to the painful clogged duct. This may signal an infection of the breast called mastitis (see page 475).

BOWEL AND URINATION PROBLEMS

For the first few days to weeks after birth, going to the bathroom can be an uncomfortable experience. It takes a while for tissues to heal and urination and bowel movements to return to how they were before you gave birth.

Bowel movements You may not have a bowel movement for a few days after delivery. That's because of a lack of food during labor and how empty your bowels may have become during that time, and because the muscle tone in your intestines may be temporarily decreased. A delayed bowel movement is not unusual, but it increases your risk of constipation.

In addition, you may find yourself holding back from passing stool out of fear of hurting your perineum or aggravating the pain of hemorrhoids, or from fear of pain in your incision following a C-section. Straining will not disrupt the incision.

If you still haven't had a bowel movement four days after your child was born, contact your care provider.

Another potential problem for new moms is fecal incontinence — the inability to control bowel movements. This may be caused by the stretching and weakening of pelvic floor muscles, tearing of the perineum or nerve injury to the muscles around the anus. You're more likely to experience fecal incontinence if you had an unusually long labor or a difficult vaginal delivery.

Kegel exercises (see page 183) can help return tone to your anal muscles. But ask your care provider when to begin Kegels, especially if you had extensive surgical repair after delivery.

To prevent constipation and help promote regular bowel movements:

‣ Drink plenty of fluids.
‣ Eat more fiber-rich foods, including fresh fruits and vegetables and whole grains.
‣ Keep as physically active as possible.
‣ Try using stool softeners (Colace, Surfak, others) or fiber laxatives (Citrucel, FiberCon, others).

Hemorrhoids During your pregnancy you may have developed hemorrhoids. Some women may not notice hemorrhoids until after delivery. If you experience pain during a bowel movement and feel a swollen mass near your anus, you may have a hemorrhoid. Hemorrhoids are worsened by constipation and the need to strain. To help avoid these problems, try the following:

‣ Eat a fiber-rich diet, including fresh fruits and vegetables and whole grains.
‣ Drink plenty of liquids. Water is best.
‣ If your stools are still too firm, try using stool softeners or fiber laxatives.

For additional suggestions on how to relieve the discomfort of hemorrhoids, see page 406. If you continue to have problems, talk to your care provider, who might suggest a prescription medicine.

Urine leakage After pregnancy, it's not uncommon to experience a brief period of time when you leak a small amount of urine each time you laugh, cough or strain. This results from the stretching of the muscles and connective tissues of the pelvic floor that support the base of the bladder.

For most women, this is a temporary problem that improves within a few months after baby is born. In the meantime, you may need to wear sanitary pads, especially if you're physically active. Doing Kegel exercises (see page 183) can also lead to quicker recovery of your bladder control.

Difficulty urinating After giving birth, you may sometimes experience a hesitancy or a decreased urge to urinate. This may be the result of swelling or bruising of the muscles and nerves of the perineum and the tissues surrounding the bladder and urethra, perineal pain, or the fear of the sting that occurs when urine touches your tender perineal area.

To encourage urine flow:
- Squirt water over your perineum with a squirt bottle while sitting on the toilet.
- Watch the clock! Urinate every two hours whether you feel the urge or not.
- Try urinating in the shower or bathtub.
- Drink more fluids to stay hydrated.

The problem usually develops immediately after delivery. If it develops once you are home, let your care provider know. If you experience burning during urination or an intense, painful and unusually frequent urge to urinate, you may have a urinary tract infection. Contact your care provider if you have these signs and symptoms, or you suspect that you aren't completely emptying your bladder.

HEALING

You may experience some aches and pains after delivery, but generally they're mild and go away within a few days to weeks.

Uterine cramping After your baby's birth, your uterus begins shrinking immediately, decreasing to its normal size over about six weeks. Contractions of your uterine muscles (afterpains) cause this shrinking. The contractions, which may feel somewhat similar to severe menstrual cramps, are also important to prevent bleeding at the site where the placenta was attached. This cramping is often mild after the birth of your first baby. Typically, many women find that these pains intensify with subsequent births.

Uterine cramping also tends to be more intense when you're breast-feeding, because the baby's sucking triggers the release of the hormone oxytocin, which also causes your uterus to contract.

Uterine cramping after birth will subside. In the meantime, empty your bladder frequently, use heat packs on your lower abdomen, and consider taking over-the-counter medications such as acetaminophen or ibuprofen. See your care provider if you have worsening pain, fever or foul-smelling discharge, as these signs and symptoms could indicate a uterine infection.

Episiotomies and tears If you received stitches after delivery due to an incision to widen the vaginal canal (episiotomy) or due to a tear, the stitches will gradually dissolve. You may feel discomfort for up to two weeks, but it should gradually improve during this time. As with any wound, the tissue around an episiotomy or a tear takes about six weeks to regain its natural strength. Very rarely with an extensive tear, the tenderness may continue for a month or more. Those weeks can be a bit tough because it can be painful to sit while the episiotomy or tear heals, but you should experience steady improvement.

To ease your discomfort:

▶ Squirt water over your perineum after using the restroom. Gently pat dry, front to back, with tissue.

▶ Soak in a tub of comfortably hot water two to three times per day for at least 20 minutes. This keeps the area clean and is also very soothing.

▶ Ice packs to the perineum can help with swelling and pain. This is most beneficial in the first few days after giving birth.

▶ Place witch hazel pads on your sanitary pad so they are next to your stitches.

▶ Keep the wound clean. Warm baths and showers may be soothing.

▶ Unless you have been told otherwise, begin strengthening your pelvic floor muscles by doing Kegel exercises within days after birth.

▶ Use over-the-counter medications such as acetaminophen (Tylenol, others) or ibuprofen (Advil, Motrin IB, others).

▶ Keep your stools looser with adequate water intake, fiber and over-the-counter stool softeners as needed. But rest assured that your bowel movements after birth should not cause issues with your stitches.

▶ If your tear or episiotomy suddenly has increased pain or a pus-like discharge, or you develop a fever, you may have an infection. Call your care provider.

Vaginal discharge As your uterus sheds its lining and returns to its normal size after birth, you'll have a vaginal discharge known as lochia. It varies widely in amount, appearance and duration, but it typically starts off as a bright red, heavy flow of blood. After about four days, it gradually diminishes and becomes paler, changing to pink or brown, and then to yellow or white after about 10 days. The vaginal discharge can last from two to eight weeks.

To reduce the risk of infection, use sanitary napkins rather than tampons. Don't be alarmed if you occasionally pass blood clots — even if they're as large as a golf ball.

Call your care provider if:

▶ You're soaking a large sanitary pad every hour for two hours in a row or you feel dizzy due to blood loss

▶ The discharge has a foul odor

▶ Your bleeding increases and you're passing numerous clots

▶ You pass clots larger than a golf ball

▶ You have a temperature of 100.4 F or higher

▶ You have new or increased pain in your abdomen

GETTING BACK INTO SHAPE

It's one thing to look five months pregnant when you are five months pregnant, but it's no fun to look that way after you've given birth. However, that's the way it is for most women. Don't be surprised if you need to wear some of your maternity clothes the first few weeks after delivery. That's because it takes a while for your body to lose fat and regain muscle tone. It also takes time for other parts of your body, such as your skin and hair, to return to their pre-pregnancy appearance. Give yourself at least a month or more to shed that exhausted look!

Fatigue During the first weeks of caring for a newborn baby, many mothers feel a fatigue that never seems to let up and a definite lack of energy. After the tiring work of labor, you're hit with the round-the-clock rigors of taking care of the baby. Night after night of interrupted sleep and the energy required for breast-feeding and carrying around a baby can add to your exhaustion. Fatigue may be even more pronounced if you have other children, if your baby was premature or has health problems, if you had multiple babies, or if you're a single parent.

Over time, your fatigue will likely lessen as your body adjusts to the demands of motherhood, you gain experience in dealing with your baby and the baby sleeps through the night.

You most likely won't be able to completely avoid being tired, but these tips may keep fatigue from depleting you:

- Try to rest whenever you can. Take advantage of your baby's daytime naps to get some sleep yourself.
- Enlist your partner to share the work of baby care and household chores. Accept offers of help from other people, too.
- Try not to do too much. Cut back on less important tasks, such as housework.
- Limit the number of guests you have and, at first, don't try to entertain.
- Exercise regularly to increase your energy level and help you fight fatigue. Eating well also is important, but don't eat too much late at night because digestion can interfere with your sleep.
- Go to bed early and unwind by listening to music or reading.
- If your fatigue doesn't improve over time, check with your care provider.

Hair and skin You'll likely notice some changes in your hair and skin after the birth of your baby.

Hair loss For some women, one of the most noticeable changes after delivery is hair loss. During pregnancy, elevated hormone levels keep you from losing hair at the usual rate — which probably gave you an extra-lush head of hair. After the birth, your body sheds all that excess hair. Don't worry — the loss is temporary, and by the time your baby is 6 months old, your hair will probably be back to normal.

To keep your hair healthy, eat well and continue taking a vitamin supplement.

Red spots Small red spots on your face after the birth are caused by small blood vessels breaking during the pushing stage of labor. The spots usually disappear in about a week.

Stretch marks Stretch marks won't disappear after delivery, but over time they fade from reddish purple to silver or white (see page 420).

Skin darkening Skin that darkened during pregnancy, such as the line down your abdomen (linea nigra) and the mask of pregnancy (skin darkening on the face), fade slowly over several months. They rarely go away completely.

Weight loss After you give birth, you may feel very flabby and out of shape. In fact, you may look in the mirror and feel like you're still pregnant! This is perfectly normal. Very few women can slip back into a tight pair of jeans a week after having a baby. Realistically, it will probably take three to six months or longer to get back to your pre-pregnancy shape and fitness level.

You'll probably lose more than 10 pounds during birth, including the weight of the baby, the placenta and amniotic fluid. During the first week after delivery, you'll lose additional fluid weight. After that, the amount of weight you lose will depend on your diet and how much exercise you get. Look for a gradual reduction in your weight — about a pound a week — if you follow a healthy eating plan and you exercise on a regular basis.

To lose your pregnancy weight, it's important to eat well and exercise. Instead of cutting back significantly on how much you eat, skipping meals or going on a fad diet, focus on eating healthy foods, including vegetables, fruits, whole grains and low-fat sources of protein. You basically want to follow the same healthy-eating plan you did while you were pregnant, with perhaps a reduction in calories. For more on healthy eating see page 36.

Exercise Regular daily exercise is very good for you. It can help you recover from labor and delivery, restore your strength, and get your body back to its pre-pregnancy shape. In addition, exercise can increase your energy level and help you fight fatigue, and it can improve your circulation and help prevent backaches. Physical activity also brings important psychological benefits. It can boost your sense of well-being and improve your ability to cope with the stresses of being a new parent.

If you exercised before and during pregnancy and had an uncomplicated vaginal delivery, it's generally safe to resume activity as soon as you feel ready. Start with gentle walking and increase as your body allows. Kegel exercises can be started in these early weeks after birth as well. Try doing three sets of 10 per day.

As you begin to be more active again, be forgiving of yourself, and don't expect to return immediately to your pre-pregnancy level of exercise. Some new moms take part in and enjoy exercise classes designed especially for women who have just had a baby. The key is to listen to your body. Decrease the intensity of your exercise if you have pain, an increase in bleeding or other physical concerns.

Here are some tips for exercising after giving birth:

▶ Exercises to tone and strengthen your abdominal and pelvic floor muscles

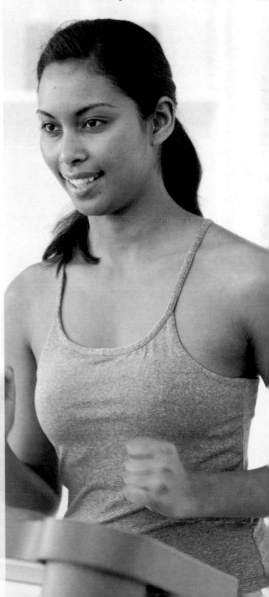

are important after either a vaginal or cesarean birth. The exercises help restore abdominal strength, tone and flatten the abdomen, and help you maintain good posture. Exercise can also help heal an episiotomy or tear, prevent incontinence, and re-establish control of the anal muscles.

- Start with a series of small, achievable fitness goals — aim for moderate rather than high-intensity workouts. Exercise a few times a day in brief sessions rather than for one long period.
- Choose activities you can do with your baby, such as walking with a stroller or baby carrier, dancing with the baby, and jogging with a jogging stroller.
- Wear a supportive bra and comfortable clothing.
- If you're breast-feeding, you'll probably feel more comfortable if you feed your baby shortly before you exercise.
- Avoid jumping and jerky, bouncy or jarring motions during the first six weeks after childbirth. It's also a good idea to avoid certain floor exercises: deep flexion or extension of joints, knee-to-chest exercises, full sit-ups and double leg lifts.

- Don't overdo it. Stop before you feel tired, and skip your workout if you're feeling particularly exhausted. Stop exercising immediately if you experience pain, faintness, dizziness, blurred vision, shortness of breath, heart palpitations, back pain, pubic pain, nausea, difficulty walking or a sudden increase in vaginal bleeding.
- Drink plenty of liquids — ideally water — before, during and after exercising.
- Stick with it. Even after you lose your pregnancy weight, regular physical activity brings many physical and mental health benefits, and it sets a great example for your little one.

THE BABY BLUES

Many new moms feel depressed to some degree after giving birth, a phenomenon known as the baby blues. The abrupt drop in levels of the hormones estrogen and progesterone after childbirth, compounded by a loss of sleep, likely causes the baby blues and contributes to postpartum depression.

DEALING WITH THE BLUES

If you find yourself struggling with the baby blues, try these tips:

- *Keep in mind that your feelings are very normal.* Up to 80 percent of women feel mood changes in the first two weeks after birth.
- *Sleep and rest when you can.* It can be more difficult to cope with anything when you are sleep deprived.
- *Reach out to your support people.* Let friends and family know you need and would appreciate extra help around the house or with baby care.
- *Eat well.* Good nutrition helps your body to heal and gain strength.
- *Get fresh air.* If you're able, try to get out for short walks, by yourself for some alone time or with the baby.

Causes Hormonal changes, however, aren't the only factor. If you're feeling overwhelmed, it's natural to feel depressed. Other possible contributing factors include the many physical changes your body goes through after delivery, difficulties during your pregnancy or labor, the letdown after an exciting event, changes in your family's finances, unrealistic expectations of childbirth and parenting, inadequate emotional support, and relationship and identity adjustments.

Some men also experience symptoms of depression after their babies are born. Men whose partners have postpartum depression are at particular risk of experiencing depression themselves.

Signs and symptoms The baby blues, a mild form of depression, is common among new mothers. Signs and symptoms include episodes of anxiety, sadness, crying, headaches and exhaustion. You may feel unworthy, irritable and indecisive. After the initial excitement of having the baby wears off, you may find that the reality of motherhood seems difficult to cope with. The baby blues usually occur in the first two weeks after birth.

You can help recover more quickly if you get extra rest, eat a healthy diet and get regular exercise. In addition, try to express your feelings by talking about them, particularly with your partner.

Is it more than the blues? If your signs and symptoms seem to be lasting longer than the first two weeks, you may have a more severe form of mood disorder, such as postpartum anxiety or postpartum depression. For more information on this, see page 476. Talk with your care provider if your symptoms are severe or persisting beyond a few weeks after your delivery.

BABY BONDING

As soon as babies are born, they need and want you to hold, cuddle, touch, kiss, talk and sing to them. These everyday expressions of love and affection promote bonding. They also help your baby's brain develop. Just as an infant's body needs food to grow, his or her brain benefits from positive emotional, physical and intellectual experiences. Relationships with other people early in life have a vital influence on a child's development.

Some parents feel an immediate connection with their newborn, while for others the bond takes longer to develop. Don't worry or feel guilty if you aren't overcome with a rush of love at the very

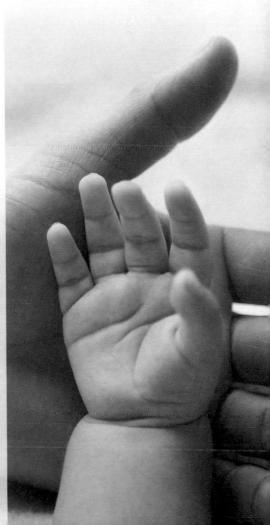

beginning. Not every parent bonds instantly with a new baby. Your feelings will become stronger with time.

Give it time At first, most of your time with your new son or daughter is likely to be spent feeding him or her, changing diapers, and helping your little one sleep. These routine tasks present an opportunity to bond. When babies receive warm, responsive care, they're more likely to feel safe and secure. For example, as you feed your baby and change diapers, gaze lovingly into his or her eyes and talk gently to him or her.

Babies also have times when they're quietly alert and ready to learn and play. These times may last only a few moments, but you'll learn to recognize them. Take advantage of your baby's alert times to get acquainted and play.

To bond with and nurture your baby:

- *Don't worry about spoiling your newborn.* Respond to your child's cues and clues. Among the signals babies send are the sounds they make — which will be mostly crying during the first week or two — the way they move, their facial expressions and the way they make or avoid eye contact. Pay close attention to your baby's need for stimulation as well as quiet times.
- *Talk, read and sing to your baby.* Even infants enjoy music and being read to. These early "conversations" encourage your baby's language capacity and provide an opportunity for closeness. Babies generally prefer soft, rhythmic sounds.
- *Cuddle and touch your baby.* Newborns are very sensitive to changes in pressure and temperature. They love to be held, rocked, caressed, cradled, snuggled, kissed, patted, stroked, massaged and carried.

- *Let your baby watch your face.* Soon after birth, your newborn will become accustomed to seeing you and will begin to focus on your face. Allow your baby to study your features, and provide plenty of smiles.
- *Play music and dance.* Put on some soft music with a beat, hold your baby's face close to yours and gently sway and move to the tune.
- *Establish routines and rituals.* Repeated positive experiences provide children with a sense of security.

Be patient with yourself in these first weeks. Caring for a new child can be daunting, discouraging, thrilling and perplexing — all in the same hour! In time, your skills as a parent will grow, and you will come to love this little one far more than you could have imagined.

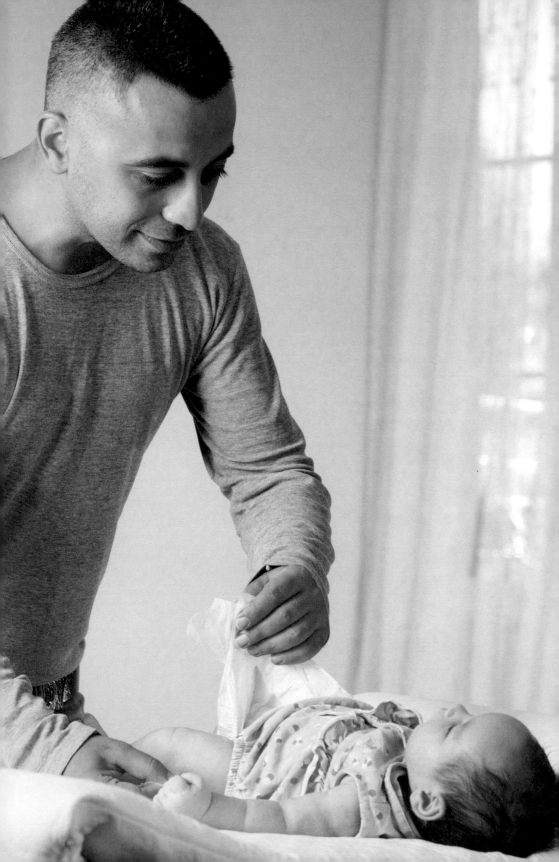

CHAPTER 19

Managing as parents

You've made it home from the hospital. The car seat probably seemed enormous, but you got your little one tucked in and buckled up. The drive was slow and careful, savoring your baby's first entrance into the big outside world. Then you settle in at home and it hits you — your baby is here. So now what?

For some new parents, along with the joy and elation of bringing home a first baby, comes the further realization that this baby is solely in your care. Rest assured that feeling anxious or nervous about your new responsibilities is completely normal. Unless you've taken care of an infant in the past, being around a young child so reliant on you may be a new experience. If you're wondering, "How do I do this?" you're not alone.

The transition to parenthood, as experts like to call it, is one of the biggest changes to take place in a person's life cycle. Bringing a newborn into the family has a way of producing profound alterations in the way you live, the way you look at the world and in how you relate to others. Becoming a parent is a transition so profound, in fact, that it often requires you to develop new dimensions to your identity to accommodate the transition.

EARLY SURVIVAL TIPS

Don't be surprised if the first few weeks, or even months, with your newborn are full of chaos. During pregnancy, and even in the hospital, it's easy to imagine your blissfully content family sitting down for a wonderful home-prepared meal while everyone laughs and coos at the baby. Unfortunately, reality more frequently plays out to the tune of takeout food wolfed down while you and your partner take turns trying to figure out why your baby is unhappy at the moment, amid a clutter of diapers and wipes and blankets and burp cloths. Add a big dose of sleep deprivation to the situation, and it's quickly apparent that all may not go as planned. And by the way, why didn't anyone tell you it would be this hard?

Tackling transitional stress Now that you've been warned — transitioning to parenthood is stressful — consider these suggestions for easing the transition and making life a little simpler for all parties involved, including baby:

- *Reach out to friends and family.* OK, so you don't necessarily want your mother-in-law to move in and set up shop, but it does help to remain open-minded to accepting help from others. Family members and friends can perform important household functions — such as cooking a meal, loading the dishwasher, doing laundry, taking the dog for a walk — that may allow you and your partner to get some rest, spend time with the baby or with each other. It's OK to set limits on outside sources of help, but it's OK to accept help, too.
- *Find what works for you.* Family and friends will almost certainly offer suggestions and advice for life with a little one. That's to say nothing of online communities, where strangers freely (and often fervently) share opinions. Perhaps you'll welcome any ideas for calming fussiness, but don't hesitate to set aside others' opinions or advice that aren't helpful. As your child's parents, you get to decide what is best for your baby.
- *Keep your strength up.* You're less help to your baby and the rest of your family if you're not good to yourself. That means eating right, exercising regularly and taking time to relax. Make sleep a priority. Lack of sleep is cumulative, and constant fatigue can be a trigger for depression and anxiety.
- *Protect your time.* If you feel overwhelmed, eliminate activities that aren't absolutely necessary. Just because the gutters don't get cleaned or the lawn mowed right now doesn't mean you won't ever do it again. Your days will eventually fall into a more routine schedule. But for the first few weeks or months after the baby is born, you can reserve the right to say no to certain tasks or events.
- *Simplify your goals.* It may be more difficult to cope with everyday demands while you're adjusting to a life change, such as parenting a newborn. Keep things simple by working on one task at a time. Make bathing the baby the main event for the afternoon and proclaim the day a productive one.
- *Practice forgiveness.* No parent is perfect, and no new parent is going to get everything right on day one. Try to be more tolerant of yourself and of your partner. Successful parenting takes practice, which means making mistakes and moving on to the next strategy. Be realistic with your expectations of how you should feel or not feel. It's normal to feel uncomfortable or disoriented during a transition period. Some days will always be better than others.
- *Accept change as a constant.* Certainly this is true when it comes to newborns. If a pacifier works today, it may not work tomorrow. And the swaddling technique you've worked so hard to master may become completely unnecessary the moment you've finally perfected it. Resiliency, the ability to adapt to changes and overcome obstacles, is key here. In general, people who can roll with the punches generally come out of transitions more successfully than those who refuse to be flexible.
- *Maintain a sense of humor.* Babies can make you do things you've never

dreamed of before, like cleaning poop off your hands. The ability to find humor in yourself and your circumstances can play a key role in helping you adapt to your new role. Laughter in itself relieves tension and relaxes your muscles as well as your mind.

Getting enough sleep The premium placed on sleep generally skyrockets in every newborn's household. While newborns can sleep up to 16 or 17 hours a day, they usually do it in spurts of a few hours at a time. And sometimes it may feel as if all the baby's sleep is taking place during the day and none of it at night. Where does that leave you? Exhausted. But babies' sleep patterns evolve rapidly during the first few months, and eventually your baby will consistently sleep for longer stretches at night, allowing you to get more sleep, too.

Volumes have been written on how to get infants to sleep at night, and many experts have important and helpful advice to share. But your baby is unique, and so are you as parents. So try different strategies, but don't be too disappointed if a particular method — even your friend's "fail-safe" trick — doesn't work out exactly as you hoped. Eventually, you will find a schedule that works for you and your baby. In the meantime, some of these suggestions may help:

▶ *Sleep (or just relax) when you can.* Turn off the ringer on the phone, hide the laundry basket and ignore the dishes in the kitchen sink. But if you're grabbing a daytime nap, try to make sure it's quality sleep. In other words, don't lie on the couch in the midst of household traffic. Aim for a dark, quiet spot with a comfortable surface to stretch out on.

▶ *Don't nap if it makes you feel worse.* Some evidence indicates that for relieving fatigue, a more severe form of tiredness experienced by many new parents, daytime napping or dozing is less likely to help than a few hours of solid, undisturbed sleep. If you prefer not to nap while your baby naps, it may be more helpful to catch up on some necessary tasks, so you can use evening hours for sleep.

▶ *Set aside your social graces.* When friends and loved ones visit, don't offer to be the host. Let them care for the baby while you excuse yourself for some much-needed rest or personal time (even if it's just to take a shower).

▶ *Don't share a bed during sleep.* It's OK to bring your baby into your bed for nursing or comforting — but return

---

WHEN SLEEP BECOMES A STRUGGLE

Sometimes, you may feel so weary that sleep eludes you and you're unable to relax. If you have trouble falling asleep, make sure your environment is suited for sleep. Turn off the TV and keep the room cool and dark. Avoid nicotine, caffeine and alcohol because they can disturb your sleep cycle, making your rest incomplete. Don't agonize over falling asleep, though. If you don't nod off within 30 minutes, get up and do something else that you know will help you relax, such as reading a book, sipping a cup of decaf tea or listening to soft music.

your baby to the crib or bassinet when you're ready to go back to sleep.

▶ *Share nighttime duties.* Work out a schedule with your partner that allows both of you to rest and care for the baby. If you're breast-feeding, perhaps your partner can bring you the baby and handle nighttime diaper changes. If you're using a bottle, take turns feeding the baby.

▶ *Postpone the inevitable.* Sometimes, middle-of-the-night fussing or crying is simply a sign that your baby is settling down. Unless you suspect that your baby is hungry or uncomfortable, it's OK to wait a few minutes to see what happens.

Negotiating household chores By now, you've probably gotten the message that once your baby arrives, attending to household chores may need to give way to more important matters such as tending to your baby's needs and getting some sleep.

It's not always easy to let these things go, however. Closing your eyes to your surroundings offers temporary relief but doesn't solve the problem. In addition, maintaining some control over your environment can be helpful when you don't necessarily feel a comfortable grasp on other aspects of your life, such as breast-feeding or managing a colicky baby. To help you cope with basic household tasks, think about these tips:

▶ *Embrace the chaos.* Often, becoming a parent means more stuff, more clutter, more chaos around the house. And while there are a variety of ways of sorting, storing and organizing, you're generally going to have more disorder and more-frequent messes than you had before becoming a parent.

▶ *Refresh your household organizational chart.* Divisions of labor between you and your partner that worked before may need to be revisited as a result of new responsibilities. For example, if one partner is taking on more infant care duties, the other can step in to fill gaps, such as making dinner or doing the laundry. If you and your partner are able to establish clear expectations and a goal of working as a team, there's likely to be less resentment on either side about who does what when it comes to household chores.

▶ *Get help.* If friends or loved ones offer to help with meals or household chores, accept it. It leaves you with a few less tasks to accomplish. If this type of help isn't available and you're overwhelmed by other duties, you might consider hiring a cleaning company or a handyman to help you. Many parents attest that this is money well spent.

Paying for baby Raising a child can be one of the biggest financial investments you'll ever make. The U.S. Department of Agriculture (USDA) estimates that the cost of raising a child from birth through the age of 17 in a middle-income, married-couple family with two children is more than a quarter of a million dollars, or $233,610. And this doesn't even include college.

Still, you don't have to be a millionaire to raise a family. There are ways to trim this number and get around assumptions made by the USDA. Following are the main spending categories measured by the USDA and tips for saving in each.

Housing Housing accounts for the biggest expense in raising a child, about 30 percent. The USDA includes in its estimate the average cost of an additional bedroom for each additional child, either

INTRODUCING YOUR PET TO A NEW BABY

If your family already includes a pet, adding a new baby can be just as life-changing for your pet as it is for you! By planning ahead, you can help minimize the stress of the introduction, maximize safety and ensure that everyone, animals included, stays happy and comfortable with each other. The Humane Society of the United States has these tips for ensuring a successful integration of furry and nonfurry family members.

Before baby is born

▶ Gradually introduce your pet to circumstances that will be similar to having a baby around, especially new noises in your home. Play a recording of a baby crying, rock in the rocking chair and offer your pet a treat to create positive associations.

▶ Encourage friends with infants to visit your home so that your pet can become more familiar with babies. Closely supervise all interaction between your pet and any infants.

▶ Accustom your pet to your baby's things and nursery furniture, but discourage your pet from jumping up on the crib, the changing table or other places your baby will lie. If the nursery is off-limits to your pet, install a sturdy gate or screen door, so that your pet can still see and hear what's going on.

▶ Play act with a baby doll. Carry around a swaddled doll so that your pet gets used to routine baby activities. Take the doll in a stroller on a walk with the dog.

▶ Make sure your pet's vaccinations are up to date.

▶ Consult a veterinary doctor or animal-behavior specialist about any concerns you may have about interactions between your pet and your baby. Resolving problems before the baby is born can help smooth the transition for your pet and put your mind at ease.

After baby is born

▶ Have your partner or a friend take an item with your baby's scent on it to your home, so your pet can become familiar with it.

▶ Ask someone else to hold the baby when you walk in your home, so that you can have your hands free to warmly greet your pet.

▶ Allow, but don't force, your pet to sit near you and your baby. Reward good behavior with treats to reinforce the positive nature of the baby's arrival.

▶ Always supervise any interaction between your pet and your baby.

▶ Try to maintain routines, such as daily walks, as much as possible.

by moving to a bigger house or renovating. For some families, additional space is a necessity, but you can also get around this cost if you're able to maximize the space you already have.

Food Food costs are the second largest expenditure for middle-income families. If you choose to formula-feed, food costs can begin to accumulate early. However, it's only a matter of months before your baby needs more than just breast milk or formula to thrive. One way to cut costs on baby food, cereals and other bulk items is to join a warehouse club such as Costco, Sam's Club or BJ's. And if you can't use up all the items yourself, or you don't have the storage space, consider dividing up the goods with friends. Shopping online for bargains or taking advantage of coupons also may trim your food expenses.

Child care and education This is the next biggest cost, and is typically highest in the first few years of a child's life. But not every family carries this expense. If one parent stays home to care for the kids, there are no child-care expenses. However, the income that parent may lose to stay at home isn't counted in the USDA cost estimate, nor is the potential income growth lost during the years spent out of the workforce. For schooling, education in public schools is less expensive than is private tuition.

Transportation Transportation comes next in the lineup of expenses, and it includes monthly car payments and down payments, car insurance, fuel, repairs and public transportation. This expense is on a lot of new parents' minds as they consider the kind of vehicle they want for transporting their little one. Keep in mind that while new cars are great, their value drops considerably once you drive them off the sales lot. To save money, consider buying a gently used car, maybe one that's just been returned from a lease and still has some of its warranty left. Also, shop around for an auto insurance policy to find the best rate.

Health care This cost includes medical and dental expenses not covered by insurance, and health insurance premiums not paid by an employer. If you purchase your own health insurance, covering your family's premiums can be a substantial cost. Shop around to compare different plans and to find a reasonable rate. You might consider finding an insurance agent who can help you find the best plan for your budget and circumstances. Health insurance premiums that you pay for yourself are also tax-deductible.

Clothing When you have your first baby, it can be hard to resist buying all those cute baby clothes. But this budget item represents another opportunity for savings. Many parents are happy to give away clothing that their kids have outgrown, and with any luck, your baby will be six to 12 months behind the fashionable toddler next door. Depending on where you live, you may also find local hand-me-downs for a steal through online communities and platforms. Consignment shops, outlet stores and end-of-season sales offer additional ways to save. Warehouse clubs and online grocery stores frequently offer discount prices on items such as diapers and wipes.

Miscellaneous This category includes personal care expenses for the child, such as toothbrushes and haircuts, and toys and entertainment. As your little one grows, this category will consume a greater share of your income.

PARENTING AS A TEAM

What sort of impact does a baby have on a couple? A pretty big one, as it turns out. Up until your baby's birth, you and your partner may have enjoyed a very equitable relationship, perhaps with dual careers, a healthy work-life balance, shared household tasks, and a relationship of sexual equals. If you're not consciously prepared for your new roles as parents (and who is, really?), you may be surprised when a new baby upsets the harmonious precedent you've set.

Marital relationships often suffer following the arrival of a newborn, in part because roles are suddenly unclear and work and home life expectations become unbalanced. Frequently, couples will revert, if unintentionally, to more traditional gendered divisions of labor, with one taking on most of the household maintenance and child care and the other becoming a more distant caregiver.

In essence, new parents tend to emulate their own parents because their parents are their role models, and this is what they know. But in an era of modern expectations, resentment and conflict can quickly brew, spilling over into all areas of the marriage.

In addition, disagreements that may have lived primarily in the background — about life goals, for example, or how to handle finances and other family affairs — may now be brought to the forefront. Couples also tend to spend less time together after the baby arrives, and both are likely to be sleep deprived, setting frayed nerves even further on edge.

Still, the arrival of your newborn doesn't have to be followed by lasting marital conflict. Keeping a clear-eyed view of the challenges that lie ahead can help you stay alert to negative attitudes that can corrode a relationship, yet optimistic about developing complementary new roles together as parents. In the end, you may be surprised at the strengths you and your partner uncover.

The transition to parenthood Research has repeatedly confirmed that bringing home a baby for the first time begins a transformative period in a couple's relationship — the transition to parenthood. Efforts to reorganize the family structure and adapt each person's role to new needs constitute a significant, often stressful challenge. Amid changing roles at home, new parents may also experience shifts in their friendships and their professional identities. And recent research indicates that the difficulty of managing these shifts isn't limited to traditional gender roles. Many of these challenges also appear to apply to same-sex couples experiencing the transition to parenthood.

Both parents typically feel an overwhelming range of emotions during this time, some overlapping with their partner and some different. In one extensive review of parenthood experiences during the child's first year, common feelings expressed by new parents included:

- Amazement and enjoyment
- Complete love for the child
- Unpreparedness
- Powerlessness and inadequacy
- Loss of a previous lifestyle
- Disappointment
- Frustration with lack of personal time
- Resentment of partners who don't seem as tied down by the baby
- Fatigue
- Sense of closeness as a family
- Strain due to new demands
- Confusion resulting from lack of guidelines or role models
- Fear of being isolated or left out
- A strong need to protect and provide

The importance of support As you can see, it's not unusual to have mixed feelings while adapting to your new role as a parent. But when a parent perceives a high level of support for his or her role, it tends to have a positive influence on the parent's feelings. For example, greater reported empathy among partners has been associated with better adjustment to parenthood and higher sexual satisfaction. Similarly, parents who perceive greater fairness of household labor tend to feel more satisfied in their relationship while raising an infant.

Other studies have looked at couples' perceptions and expectations of marriage and parenthood during pregnancy, before the birth of their first child. Couples who had realistic expectations of both marriage and parenthood were able to weather the stress of first-time parenthood better than others. In other words, knowing that marriage could be difficult and required maintenance — especially in times of transition — led to a more cooperative and positive transition.

In one study, partners who had unrealistic expectations after the baby's arrival tended to be less supportive of the other's parenting style, perhaps because they unwittingly blamed their spouses for their unfulfilled hopes. Recognizing that the road ahead might be a bit bumpy seemed to better prepare them for the transition to parenthood.

Setting the tone Parents' marital satisfaction is closely linked to the parenting experience. For example, a new mother who is overloaded with the new responsibilities and tasks of caring for a baby is likely to filter that stress down to her marriage. If she invests herself in the baby at the expense of her husband, he may begin to feel left out and less satisfied with the marriage.

On the other hand, the more fathers are involved in caring for their babies, the more marital satisfaction the mothers generally feel. Husbands, in turn, are more involved in infant care when wives feel more autonomous and allow their husbands to share in child-care duties — even if a husband's methods differ from his wife's.

A marriage also sets the tone for the rest of the family. When parents engage each other with respect and mutual appreciation, are attentive to their relationship, and are sensitive to sharing the tasks of parenthood, they create an optimal environment for a child to grow into a mature, confident and responsible adult.

In general, a couple who was satisfied with their marriage before the baby's

---

WHAT MAKES A STRONG, HEALTHY FAMILY?

Regardless of their structure, healthy families tend to share certain key qualities. According to the American Academy of Pediatrics, successful, functional families are typically supportive and respectful, cohesive (fostering a sense of belonging), loving, communicative, mutually appreciative, and resilient.

In addition, families often function best if they follow routines, participate in their communities, and honor each family member's individuality and needs. Parents model their values as well as discuss them with their children. And of course, sharing fun and meaningful time together also is key to a healthy, happy family life.

birth is more likely to have a higher level of marital satisfaction after the baby's arrival than a couple who wasn't satisfied prior to baby's birth.

FINDING TIME FOR YOURSELF AND EACH OTHER

Part of the stress involved in early parenting comes from the nearly constant demand placed on your energy and resources. Burning yourself out, however, is no way to be a good parent or a good partner. It's important to regularly take time to recharge on your own and also to invest in your relationship with your partner.

Getting away on your own It's not always easy to get away from your new parent duties, but one way to do this is to swap brief interludes of personal time with your partner. Allowing your partner some time off, even if begrudgingly at first, can help your partner refresh his or her reserves and come back feeling renewed and ready to get back in the fray. Getaways don't have to be long; in fact, you may not even need to leave the house. Here are some suggestions to get you inspired:

- Go out for a cup of coffee or tea. It will make you feel like a regular adult again.
- Take a walk at a nearby park. Nature has a way of soothing away stress.
- Ask your partner to take the baby out so that you'll have time at home alone.
- Make a quick trip to your local driving range or gym. If it's something you enjoy, it might help release some stress.
- If you like to cook and it relaxes you, ask your partner to watch the baby while you prepare a favorite meal.

- Stake out a remote corner of the house and do some stretches or deep breathing.

The important thing is to have a few minutes all to yourself so that you can relax and regroup.

Getting away together It takes time and effort to invest in your marriage, but it's worth it, both for you and your child. You don't have to book a trip to Tahiti to renew your relationship, but find something to do together that you enjoyed previously and that you share a common bond over, something you can both laugh or talk about easily.

This can be as simple as watching your favorite show together at an opportune moment. Or sitting outside together for a few moments after the baby's been fed and put down to sleep, even if it is late at night. If you do want to get out of the house, most grandparents are more than willing to watch their new grandchild for a few hours. If grandparents aren't available, ask a family member or friend, who most likely will be glad to help out.

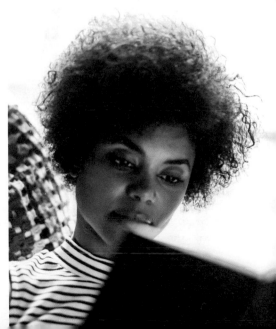

Sex after pregnancy Yes, sex does occur after pregnancy. While sex may not be foremost on your mind right away, in time it will become important again.

For one thing, it takes time for your body to heal after giving birth, whether your baby was delivered vaginally or by C-section. Many care providers recommend waiting four to six weeks before having sex. This allows time for the cervix to close, postpartum bleeding to stop, and any tears or repaired lacerations to heal, although your body may need longer.

The other important timeline is your own. Some women feel ready to resume sex within a few weeks of giving birth, while others need a few months or more. Factors such as fatigue, postpartum blues and changes in body image all can take a toll on your sex drive.

Caring for a newborn is exhausting. If you're too tired to have sex at bedtime, say so. This doesn't mean your sex life has to end, however. Consider making love early in the morning or while your baby naps.

And don't forget there's more to an intimate relationship than sex, especially when you're adjusting to life with a new baby. If you're not feeling sexy or you're afraid sex will hurt, share your concerns with your partner. Until you're ready, you can maintain intimacy in other ways. Most couples are ready to resume sexual intercourse six months after childbirth.

When you are ready to have sex again, take it slow. Due to hormonal changes, the vagina may be dry and tender, especially if you're breast-feeding. Start with cuddling, kissing or massaging. Gradually build the intensity of stimulation. If vaginal dryness is a problem, use a lubricating cream or gel. Try different positions to take pressure off any sore areas and control penetration. Be sure to tell your partner what feels good — and what doesn't.

If sex continues to be painful, talk to your care provider. Low doses of estrogen cream applied to the vagina can help, but the estrogen could possibly decrease your milk production if you're breast-feeding. Ask your care provider to help you weigh the pros and cons.

SINGLE PARENTHOOD

If you're a single parent, you're likely to face many of the same challenges as any other new parent, married or otherwise. In fact, many of the sections discussed earlier in the chapter may apply just as well to single parents as to married ones. But parenting a newborn on your own presents its own set of challenges, not the least of which is the fact that nearly all parenting responsibilities rest ultimately on the physical, mental, emotional and financial resources of one person: you.

Many children, both young and old, can attest to the monumental love and support provided to them by a parent who happened to be single. Whatever your specific circumstances may be, creating a positive family experience without the help of a partner is doable, and is a wonderful testament to a parent's resilience.

To cope with some of the particular challenges of single parenthood, consider the following suggestions:

▶ *Gather support.* Support for your role as a parent is critical as you navigate the ups and downs of learning how to be a parent. This may mean cultivating and drawing on sources of support such as the baby's grandparents, aunts and uncles, friends, a religious or spiritual community, or a network of other parents who are in a similar situation.

- *Seek out good child care.* Most single parents are also working parents, so finding child care that promotes your child's well-being and accommodates your schedule is critical. Get recommendations from family, friends and other parents. Visit the location and talk to the person who will supervise your child's care before committing.
- *Provide worthy role models.* As your child grows, it's helpful to have role models of both sexes for your child to learn from. Incorporate activities with adults you trust and admire into your child's life. You are an important role model for your child, as he or she sees you succeed both in the workplace and at home.
- *Make time for your child.* Single parents are often busy managing the demands of work and baby care, and time with your child may not be as much as you'd like. Still, take the opportunity to interact with your baby whenever possible. Sing in the car on the way to child care, spend a lazy Saturday morning together perusing magazines (or keeping your baby from eating them), or take a long walk around a park.
- *Make time for yourself.* Single parents need breaks, too — perhaps even more so than couples. Plan dinner and a movie for yourself after the baby has gone to sleep. Find a fitness center that offers baby-sitting services while you work out. Gather the phone numbers of prized baby sitters from your parent friends or take up your mom's offer to watch the baby while you dine out with a friend or see a movie on your own.
- *Be part of a community.* Feeling connected to the world around you is important for anyone, but can be especially helpful for a single parent. Get to know your neighbors, join a church or spiritual community, or connect with groups dedicated to single parents. Being connected to a larger community can also be beneficial if a crisis arises.

HANG IN THERE

Becoming a parent, no matter what your situation, is an intense and life-changing experience. Those first few weeks can be confusing, exhilarating, exhausting and amazing. Learning the ins and outs of successful parenting is an ongoing challenge, even for experienced parents. But as you begin your parenting journey, remember that it's also likely to be one of the most rewarding aspects of your life.

For all the challenges raising a child brings, it can also bring unimaginable love, raucous fun and deep satisfaction. What's more, billions of others around the world have managed to do it. So read as much as you can, learn as you go and listen to others. Doing these things will help you understand what's normal and what's not and when to get help. But most of all, listen to yourself and your child. Taking the time to get to know your baby over the next few months will set the stage for a lifelong relationship of the most intimate sort, parent and child.

PART 4

Important decisions of pregnancy

CHAPTER 20

Genetic screening

Genetic screening is one of those topics that parents might prefer to avoid because it may seem frightening and complicated. No parent wants to read or hear about things that could go wrong with a child. Don't be frightened, though, if this topic comes up during your pregnancy. Your care provider may address the issue of genetic screening during one of your early prenatal appointments. Keep in mind that most babies are born healthy without genetic problems.

WHAT IS IT?

Genetic screening tests offer expectant and new parents an opportunity to explore whether their child may be at risk of a genetic disorder. This is done by screening either the parents or the child for inherited genetic diseases. For some couples, there may be a family history of a genetic disorder, while for others, disease is found with no family history.

Different types of genetic screening tests are available before conception, during pregnancy and immediately after birth. Family-history-based screening, ethnic-based screening and expanded carrier screening (ECS) are typically done before conception or early in pregnancy. Prenatal screening is done in the first trimester or early second trimester (see Chapter 21). Newborn screening is often done when an infant is a day old (see Chapter 16).

ECS and genetic screening tests based on family history or ethnicity are designed to identify people who don't have signs and symptoms of a specific disease, but who carry a copy of an altered gene or chromosome that could be passed on to their children, possibly leading to disease.

Prospective parents worried about possible genetic disorders in their children can undergo genetic screening before or shortly after a baby is conceived. With this information, potential parents can weigh their risk of having a child with a genetic disease and make decisions accordingly.

If you're planning to become pregnant or are already pregnant and you or your partner has a family history of a genetic disorder, you might consider family-history-based screening. You might consider ethnic-based screening if you identify with a racial or ethnic group in which a genetic disease is known to be more common (see page 303).

ISSUES TO CONSIDER

The decision to pursue genetic screening is a personal one. Consider these questions as you make your decision.

9 key questions
1. Is there a family history of a certain disorder?

DIFFERENT TYPES OF GENETIC TESTS

The process is often the same, but genetic testing is done for different reasons.

Diagnostic testing. If you have symptoms of a disease that may be caused by a genetic abnormality, diagnostic testing can confirm that you have the suspected disorder. Genetic testing is available for an ever-increasing number of diseases. Some disorders for which genetic testing may be used to confirm a diagnosis include polycystic kidney disease, Marfan syndrome and neurofibromatosis.

Presymptomatic screening for adult disorders. If you have a family history of a genetic condition, undergoing genetic testing before you develop symptoms may show if you're at risk of developing that condition. Examples include testing for inherited breast and ovarian cancers (BRCA 1 and 2) and Huntington's disease.

Carrier testing. If you or your partner has a family history of a genetic disorder, such as cystic fibrosis or spinal muscular atrophy, you may choose to have genetic testing before you have children. Carrier testing can determine if you carry a copy of an altered gene that would put a child at risk of developing the disorder. Ethnic-based screening and expanded carrier screening are types of carrier testing.

Prenatal testing. If you're pregnant, tests are available that can detect abnormalities in your fetus. Spina bifida and Down syndrome are two congenital abnormalities that are common enough that many mothers consider such testing. Prenatal tests for fetal abnormalities are discussed in Chapter 21.

Newborn screening. This is the most common type of genetic screening. Newborn screening is performed in all 50 states and the District of Columbia. The tests screen for specific conditions, such as congenital hypothyroidism and phenylketonuria. Newborn testing is important because if a disorder is found, treatments that may prevent symptoms can begin immediately. These tests are discussed in Chapter 16.

2. Are you from a racial or ethnic group that puts you at higher risk of being a carrier for a certain disorder?
3. Are you and your partner interested in learning about the risk of genetic disorders independent of your family history or ethnicity?
4. How will you use the information if you find that you and your partner are carriers of the same genetic condition?
5. Do your religious or spiritual beliefs affect your view of genetic testing?
6. How might you respond emotionally to the testing process?
7. Will the test be covered by your insurance? If not, will you be able to afford the testing? Many genetic tests are relatively expensive. Be aware that tests used for purposes other than diagnosing a condition may not be covered by insurance.
8. Will the time it takes to complete the test give you adequate time to make decisions regarding beginning or continuing a pregnancy?
9. Would discussing the options and issues related to genetic carrier screening with a genetic counselor, geneticist or other care provider benefit you? These individuals are specially trained in human genetics and genetic counseling.

TYPES OF GENETIC DISORDERS

Genetic disease can result from a number of different types of problems within the genetic material that parents pass on to a child.

Autosomal recessive diseases Autosomal recessive diseases occur when both parents are carriers of an abnormal gene. Carriers have one normal and one abnormal gene. The normal gene is able to compensate for the abnormal gene, so carriers generally have no symptoms. However, if both you and your partner contribute an abnormal gene for the same disease to the fetus, the baby will be affected with the disease. Testing for autosomal recessive diseases may be done for specific ethnic groups in which certain recessive diseases are more common or if there's a family history of an autosomal recessive disease. Examples include cystic fibrosis and Tay-Sachs disease.

Adult-onset autosomal dominant diseases These disorders occur when a person has one abnormal copy of a gene. Some autosomal dominant diseases don't cause symptoms until adulthood, and occasionally not until after the person carrying such a gene has had children. If a person is found to carry such a disease, each of his or her children has a 50 percent risk of inheriting the disease. Examples include Huntington's disease and some inherited cancers.

X-linked disorders These disorders result from an altered gene located on the X chromosome. With rare exceptions, a woman carries two X chromosomes and a man an X and a Y chromosome. A woman may be a carrier of an X-linked recessive disorder, but have no symptoms or mild symptoms because the normal gene on her other X chromosome provides most of the needed gene function. However, the woman has a 50 percent chance of passing the altered chromosome on to her child. If she does, and if the child is a boy, he will develop the disease because boys have only one X chromosome. If the altered chromosome is passed on to a girl, she, like her mother, will be a carrier.

AUTOSOMAL RECESSIVE DISORDER can result when both parents carry a single altered gene for the same disease. If both parents pass the altered gene to the child, the child is affected by the disease. Most disorders included in ethnic-based and expanded carrier screening are autosomal recessive.

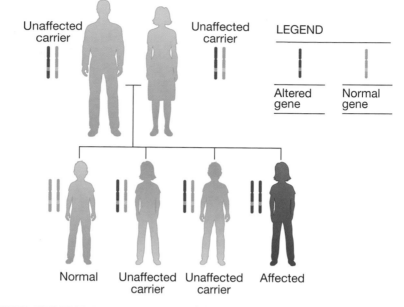

X-LINKED RECESSIVE DISORDERS result from an altered gene carried on one of the mother's X chromosomes.

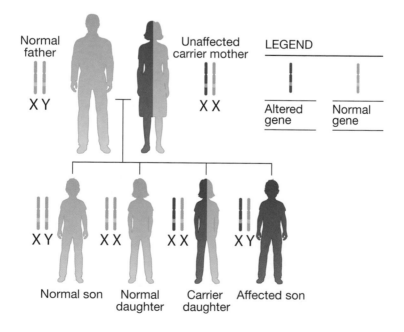

Examples of X-linked disorders include Duchenne type muscular dystrophy, hemophilia A and fragile X syndrome.

Chromosome structural abnormalities In some families, babies are born with birth defects caused by missing or duplicated pieces of a chromosome. This can happen if a parent carries a structural chromosome arrangement that's different from normal. If the parent passes on an abnormal arrangement in which the genetic structure is unbalanced, it could result in severe problems. A chromosome rearrangement can also lead to more miscarriages than expected in a family. If you have a family member who's experienced a high number of miscarriages, mention this to your care provider.

Mitochondrial disorders Some disorders are caused by errors in a separate set of genes found in the energy-producing organs of the cell (mitochondria). Since mitochondria are inherited only from the mother, most of these diseases are passed from mother to child. Mitochondrial disorders can have many different signs and symptoms, such as low blood sugar, muscular problems, blindness and seizures.

FAMILY HISTORY SCREENING

If a certain genetic disorder runs in your family, you may wish to be tested to determine whether you carry the genetic abnormality that may put your future children at risk of inheriting the disorder.

An inherited genetic disorder may result from a problem with a single gene. This includes autosomal recessive diseases, X-linked diseases, autosomal dominant

ETHNIC-BASED SCREENING

Certain racial and ethnic groups are at higher risk of specific disorders than are others. If you belong to one of these groups, talk to your care provider or a genetic counselor about your risks of being a carrier and the screening process.

Racial or ethnic group	Genetic disorder
Ashkenazi Jew	Tay-Sachs disease, cystic fibrosis, Canavan disease, Niemann-Pick disease (types A and B), Fanconi anemia (group C), Bloom syndrome, Gaucher disease, familial dysautonomia, mucolipidosis IV
French Canadian, Cajun	Tay-Sachs disease, cystic fibrosis
Black	Sickle cell disease, beta-thalassemia, glucose-6-dehydrogenase deficiency
Mediterranean	Beta-thalassemia, glucose-6-phosphate dehydrogenase deficiency
Chinese, Southeast Asian (Cambodian, Filipino, Laotian, Vietnamese), Mediterranean	Alpha-thalassemia, beta-thalassemia, glucose-6-dehydrogenase deficiency
White (European)	Cystic fibrosis

GENETIC DISEASES

The following genetic diseases can be identified with genetic testing.

Alpha-thalassemias result in a deficiency of red blood cells (anemia). The most severe form results in fetal or newborn death. Most forms are much less severe.

Beta-thalassemias also result in anemia. In its most severe form (thalassemia major), children require regular blood transfusions. With proper treatment, most people with this condition live into adulthood.

Sickle cell disease causes red blood cells to have an abnormal shape (sickle shape), which can keep them from moving smoothly through the body. Affected people have an increased susceptibility to infection, anemia and episodes of pain. Severe episodes can result in damage to vital organs. With early and consistent medical treatment, complications can be minimized.

Cystic fibrosis affects the respiratory and digestive systems, causing severe chronic respiratory disease, diarrhea, malnutrition and exercise limitation. Recent treatments enable many affected people to live into adulthood.

Duchenne type muscular dystrophy is the most common form of muscular dystrophy affecting children. It affects the muscles of the pelvis, arms and legs, and in later stages of the disease, it may also affect the diaphragm and heart. Because it's an X-linked disease, it occurs primarily in young boys. Females may have milder symptoms. In severe forms, muscle weakness can lead to death in the late teenage years or early adulthood.

Fragile X syndrome is the most common genetically inherited cause of intellectual disability. It results from problems with a gene on the X chromosome. Female carriers may have infertility, while male and female carriers may have movement problems (ataxia). The genetics of fragile X should be discussed with a specialist.

Canavan disease is a severe condition of the nervous system that's usually diagnosed soon after a child's birth. Death usually occurs in early childhood.

Spinal muscular atrophy affects nerves in the spinal cord and brainstem, causing the breakdown of muscle tissue and general weakness. In the most severe form, symptoms may be lethal in early childhood.

Tay-Sachs disease is a condition in which the enzyme needed to break down certain fats (lipids) in nerve cells is missing. These lipids build up in cells of the brain and spinal cord, leading to nerve cell destruction and, usually, death in early childhood.

disorders and mitochondrial disorders. Symptoms of some disorders may not occur until adulthood, while other disorders may have more-severe symptoms in children than in the parents. Some of these problems are discussed in more detail later in this chapter.

EXPANDED CARRIER SCREENING

While screenings based on family history or ethnicity are focused on individual conditions, newer technologies in genetic testing have made it possible to screen for a wide array of disorders with one test. Known as expanded carrier screening (ECS), this type of testing offers the same screening for anyone, regardless of family or ethnic background.

ECS can provide parents with information about many potential genetic conditions that may affect their child, though most are rare. A genetic counselor can talk you through the types of conditions being screened and also discuss the limitations of the screening.

While ECS provides a more comprehensive picture, this method of testing is not as accurate as others in screening for certain conditions. If you have a family history of a genetic disease, a genetic counselor may recommend specific screenings or diagnostic tests.

HOW IT'S DONE

Often, genetic screening requires only a blood sample. A needle is inserted into a vein in your arm and blood is drawn. Occasionally, a swab sample from the inside of your cheek may be used. Rarely, a skin or muscle biopsy is needed. For newborn screening, blood is collected via a heel prick. Umbilical cord blood also can be collected immediately after delivery if there is concern that the infant may have a genetic disorder. Cord blood is easy to collect, has no risk to mother and infant, and avoids a needle stick to the infant. The sample is sent to a lab for analysis.

With some genetic tests — those screening for autosomal recessive disorders, in which both parents need to be carriers for the disorder to occur — testing may be done initially for just one parent. If the results are normal, the second partner doesn't need to be tested. If testing in the first partner finds an abnormality, it's recommended the other partner consider being tested.

UNDERSTANDING THE RESULTS

If carrier test results are normal, no special precautions are necessary. However, don't take the results as a guarantee that your child will be healthy. Genetic carrier screening doesn't identify all carriers or test for all diseases. Some diseases have many mutations, and the test may focus only on the most common mutations.

If testing reveals an increased risk of a genetic disorder, your care provider, a geneticist or a genetic counselor can help you understand the implications of the disease and assess your options.

The technology of genetic testing is evolving quickly, and more-detailed testing options will likely be available in the years to come. For the most up-to-date information, consult with a specialist who can confer with your obstetrician or primary care provider.

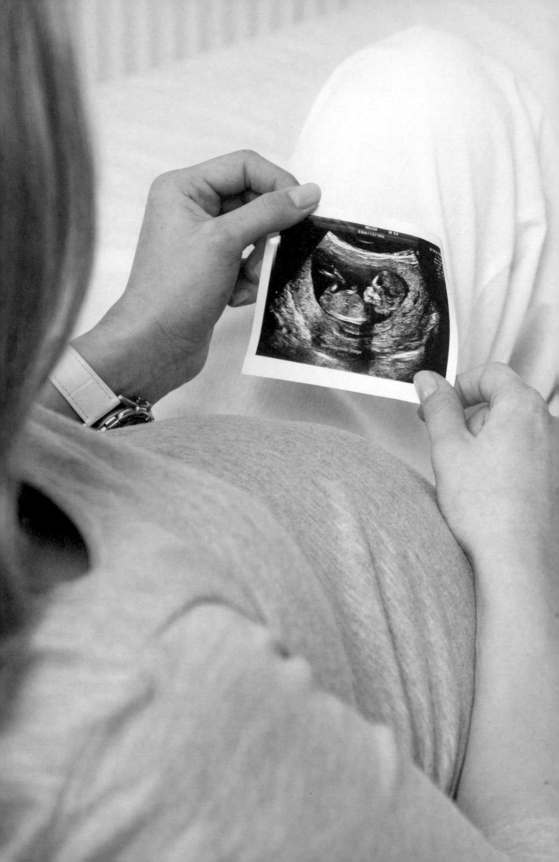

CHAPTER 21

Prenatal testing

As you look forward to your baby's arrival, you may be wondering about a number of things. Will you have a girl or a boy? Will he have blue eyes or brown eyes? Will she be funny like her dad, smart like her mom? How will it feel to finally hold your baby in your arms?

Along with feelings of excitement and joy, you may have moments of doubt and anxiety. What if something goes wrong with the pregnancy? Will your baby be healthy? These are completely normal feelings experienced by most pregnant women. It may reassure you to know that most pregnancies — more than 95 percent — are healthy and result in the safe delivery of a healthy baby.

Still, in some instances you may wish to know specific information about your baby's health before his or her birth. Perhaps because of your age or family history you may be at increased risk of carrying a baby with a chromosomal problem or some other genetic disorder. Whatever the reason, certain tests can help determine the health of your baby while he or

she is still in your womb. These are called prenatal tests.

Two types of prenatal tests are used during pregnancy:

- *Screening tests.* These are noninvasive tests that are offered to all pregnant women. Screening tests are meant to identify a pregnancy with a higher risk of certain conditions. If a screening test indicates an increased risk, a diagnostic test is offered to determine more clearly whether a condition is present. Screening tests aren't required, but your care provider will probably ask whether you are interested in genetic screening.
- *Diagnostic tests.* Diagnostic tests are usually offered when a pregnancy is at increased risk of a specific condition based on family history, ultrasound findings or screening results. These tests can provide enough information to diagnose a medical condition while the baby is in the uterus. They are generally more invasive and may carry a slight risk to the pregnancy.

ISSUES TO CONSIDER

Prenatal tests are voluntary, and each test has its own risks and benefits. It's worthwhile to know about screening options so that you can make informed decisions about them. Before you undergo a prenatal test, think about what information the test will provide and how you will use the information. Many women choose to undergo basic ultrasounds and blood tests. Most women don't undergo the more detailed diagnostic tests because most pregnancies don't carry a high risk of complications.

6 key questions Before scheduling a prenatal test, you might consider these questions:

1. What will you do with the information once you have it? How will it affect decisions regarding your pregnancy? Most results from prenatal testing come back normal, which can help ease any anxiety you may be feeling. If a test indicates that your baby may have a birth defect or another health condition, how will you handle it? You may be faced with decisions you never expected to have to make, such as whether to continue the pregnancy. On the other hand, knowing about a problem ahead of time may give you the option of planning for your baby's care in advance.

If you feel a test won't provide you with useful information or it won't affect the way you handle your pregnancy, it's OK to say no to it.

2. Will the information provide better care or treatment during pregnancy or delivery? At times, prenatal testing can provide information that affects your care. Testing may uncover a problem with your baby that doctors can treat while you're pregnant. It may alert your care provider to a problem that requires a specialist to treat your baby right after he or she is born.

3. How accurate are the results of the test? Prenatal tests aren't perfect. Even if the result of a screening test is normal (negative), indicating that your baby is at low risk of having a certain condition, there's still a small chance that the condition is present. If it is, this is known as a false-negative result.

On the other hand, an abnormal (positive) screening test result may place the baby at higher risk for a genetic condition when none exists. This is a false-positive result. The proportion of false-negative and false-positive results varies from test to test. Be sure to discuss the accuracy of each test with your care provider.

4. Will undergoing a test be worth the anxiety it may cause? Screening tests identify women at risk of certain conditions. Even if a test indicates a risk, the majority of women will have a healthy baby. Thus, a screening test may cause unnecessary anxiety.

5. What are the risks of the procedure? You may want to weigh the risks of the tests, such as pain or possible miscarriage, against the value of having the information.

6. How much does the test cost? Is it covered by your health insurance? Tests that aren't medically necessary may not be covered by insurance. A genetics professional may be able to help you get information about insurance coverage or financial assistance for genetic testing. If financial help isn't available, are you willing and able to cover the cost of the test?

ULTRASOUND IMAGING

The ultrasound exam is probably the prenatal test you've heard the most about. Your care provider uses ultrasound imaging to see a picture of your unborn baby and determine how your pregnancy is progressing. Usually, you're able to see images of your baby while the test is being done. Ultrasound can also be used to diagnose some types of birth defects, such as a spinal abnormality (neural tube defect), heart defects or other abnormalities.

As with other prenatal tests, talk with your doctor about the ultrasound and what information you might get from it.

The ultrasound exam uses sound waves as energy. The transducer, which is placed on your abdomen, produces high-frequency sound waves that humans cannot hear. The sound waves bounce off tissues in your body, including the baby, and back to the transducer. They return to the transducer at different times with different qualities, depending on the density of the tissue and its distance from the transducer. As the signals return, they're converted into an image, which is viewed on a monitor. Several different types of ultrasound examinations are available:

▶ *Basic ultrasound.* This type of ultrasound creates two-dimensional (2-D) images that can give your care provider information about your pregnancy. It can be used to determine the age of your baby, how he or she is developing, the location of the placenta, information about your baby's brain, face, chest, neck, spine and limbs, and the relationship between your body and the baby. It usually lasts about 20 minutes.

▶ *Detailed ultrasound.* This type of testing is often used to explore a suspected abnormality found during a standard

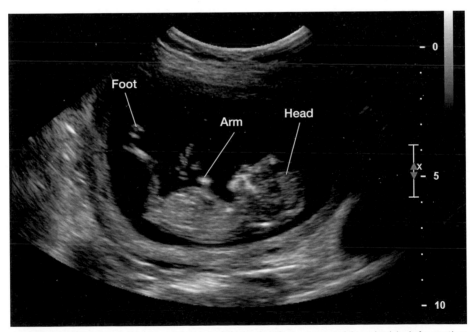

An ultrasound image creates a picture of the baby that can provide valuable information about your pregnancy.

ultrasound or a screening test. It may also be used if your baby has a suspected growth problem, problem with the amniotic fluid level or possible infection. The exam is more thorough and may use more sophisticated equipment. It's also longer, taking from 30 minutes to over an hour. Your care provider also may recommend this type of ultrasound if you have a high-risk pregnancy.

▸ *Transvaginal ultrasound.* In early pregnancy, your uterus and fallopian tubes are closer to your vagina than to your abdominal surface. If you have an ultrasound during your first trimester, your care provider may opt for a transvaginal scan. It provides a clearer picture of your baby and the structures around your baby. This type of ultrasound may also be used to detect problems with your cervix during pregnancy. A transvaginal ultrasound uses a slender, wandlike device that's placed inside your vagina.

▸ *3-dimensional (3-D) and 4-dimensional ultrasound.* Three-D ultrasound involves the collection of a series of 2-D image "slices" that can be reconstructed to produce a 3-D picture of your baby. Four-dimensional ultrasound is 3-D imaging viewed in real time. The 3-D ultrasound is not routinely used. However, it may be useful for more detailed evaluation of certain fetal abnormalities.

▸ *Doppler ultrasound.* Doppler imaging measures changes in the frequency of the ultrasound waves as they bounce off moving objects, such as blood cells. It can measure the speed and direction at which blood circulates. With it, care providers can determine how much resistance there is to the flow of blood through various tissues. If you have complications of pregnancy, such as high blood pressure or preeclampsia, a Doppler ultrasound may help determine if there are problems with blood flow to the baby or the placenta.

▸ *Fetal echocardiography.* This type of exam uses ultrasound waves to provide a more detailed picture of your baby's heart. It focuses on the heart's anatomy and function and may be used to confirm or rule out a congenital heart defect.

When and how it's done An ultrasound exam can be done at any time during your pregnancy. An ultrasound during the first trimester is generally performed to identify how many babies you're carrying, to verify that the baby is alive and well, and to determine his or her age. It can also be used as part of screening performed in the first trimester.

Most often an ultrasound is performed between the 18th and 20th weeks of pregnancy. At this stage in pregnancy, an ultrasound can often identify the sex of the baby in addition to verifying baby's age, and it can detect structural abnormalities. Your baby has developed enough at this point so that his or her skeletal structure and organs can be identified, and all four chambers of the heart and the major arteries can be seen.

It's important to note that ultrasound determination of your baby's age is most accurate when done in the first trimester. So if a first trimester ultrasound confirmed your due date, the date will not be changed based on measurements of the baby's growth in the second trimester.

In some situations, such as a high-risk pregnancy, ultrasounds may be repeated throughout the pregnancy. They can be used to monitor the health of both the mother and the baby and to track the baby's growth.

Once in the exam room, you will be asked to lie on your back and a gel will be applied to your abdominal area. The gel acts as a conductor for sound waves and helps to eliminate air bubbles between the transducer and your skin. The transducer is a small plastic device that sends out the sound waves and records them as they bounce back.

During the exam, the person administering the test moves the transducer back and forth over your abdomen, directing sound waves into the uterus. Depending on your baby's age and position, you may be able to make out a face, tiny hands and fingers, or arms and legs. Throughout the exam, your care provider will measure your baby's head, abdomen and long bones. These measurements help your care provider determine your baby's growth. Pictures may also be taken of important structures such as the baby's heart.

Unlike an X-ray, an ultrasound examination doesn't involve radiation. Forty years of use has not raised any concerns that ultrasound causes harm to mothers or babies.

What the results may tell you Based on the images produced by the exam, your care provider can determine a number of things about your pregnancy and your baby, including:

▶ That you are indeed pregnant.
▶ How far along your pregnancy is (baby's gestational age).
▶ The number of babies you're carrying.
▶ Your baby's growth and development.
▶ Your baby's movement, breathing and heart rate.
▶ The location of the pregnancy. Sometimes a pregnancy develops outside the uterus (ectopic pregnancy), usually in the fallopian tube. This can be a medical emergency.

▶ Structural variations or abnormalities in your baby.
▶ The location and development of the placenta.
▶ Whether you've had a miscarriage.
▶ Assessment of the cervix and the possible risk of preterm delivery.
▶ Measures of fetal well-being such as the volume of fluid around the baby, muscle tone and activity.
▶ The sex of your baby. Being able to determine what sex your baby is depends on the baby's position in the uterus and the position of the umbilical cord. Decide in advance if you want to know this information. You can ask in advance that the sex of the baby not be revealed to you.

Reasons to have it done For most pregnant women, an ultrasound exam basically confirms assumptions regarding baby's due date and health. But because it's an important screening test for identifying inaccurate dating, multiple pregnancies and placental disease, most care providers wouldn't do without it.

If concerns do develop, however, ultrasound is often the best tool to address those concerns. If you're not sure when you became pregnant, an ultrasound can determine the baby's gestational age. If screening tests indicate an abnormality, an ultrasound may be able to identify it. If there's any bleeding or a concern about the baby's growth rate, an ultrasound is the best initial test. In addition, ultrasound imaging can be used to guide your care provider while performing other prenatal tests, such as amniocentesis or chorionic villus sampling.

Many parents-to-be look forward to an ultrasound because it gives them a first glimpse of the baby or a chance to find out the baby's sex. However, having an ultrasound solely for a nonmedical reason — such as to learn the sex of your baby — generally isn't recommended.

Accuracy and limitations of the test Although ultrasound is a useful imaging tool, it can't detect all fetal abnormalities or genetic disorders. If an ultrasound can't offer an explanation for a perceived problem, your care provider may recommend other diagnostic imaging or testing, including magnetic resonance imaging (MRI), amniocentesis or chorionic villus sampling (CVS).

PRENATAL SCREENING

Following is a detailed list of the screening tests you might encounter during your pregnancy. This guide gives basic information on each test. But be sure to talk with your care provider about the tests you're considering. He or she can best assess the risks and benefits, based on your individual circumstances.

All prenatal screening has limitations in pregnancies with twins or other multiples. If test results are abnormal, it may not be possible to determine if one or more of the babies is at increased risk of chromosomal problems. In some cases, abnormal ultrasound findings may provide additional information. If you are pregnant with twins or other multiples, and are interested in prenatal screening, you will likely be referred to a genetics professional for a discussion of the benefits and limitations of prenatal screening.

Prenatal screening and testing is changing as technology advances. Talk with your care provider to find out about recent updates in prenatal test offerings.

First trimester combined screening First trimester screening involves a two-

step process that offers early information on your baby's health:

▶ *Blood test.* It measures levels of two pregnancy-specific substances, pregnancy-associated plasma protein-A (PAPP-A) and beta-human chorionic gonadotropin (beta-HCG).

▶ *Ultrasound exam.* This test is done to measure the size of the clear space in the tissue at the back of a baby's neck (nuchal translucency, or NT). A vaginal ultrasound is often used for this assessment.

Your care provider uses the results of these tests to screen for:

▶ *Down syndrome (trisomy 21).* This is a genetic condition that causes intellectual disability, congenital heart problems, other medical problems and characteristic facial features. In the vast majority of cases, the fetus has three copies of chromosome 21, instead of two copies.

▶ *Trisomy 18.* This is a chromosomal abnormality characterized by an extra copy of chromosome 18. Trisomy 18 typically causes severe deformity and intellectual disability. Most babies with trisomy 18 die before birth or within their first year. The risk of having a baby with trisomy 18 is very low.

▶ A first trimester screen may heighten suspicion regarding a potential heart defect or skeletal problem, but the test isn't done for this purpose.

When and how it's done First trimester screening is done between weeks 11 and 14 of pregnancy. For the blood test, a sample of blood is taken from a vein in your arm and sent to a lab for analysis.

During the ultrasound, your care provider or a technician uses the images to measure the size of the clear space in the tissue at the back of your baby's neck (NT). This test may take up to an hour.

First trimester screening poses no risk of miscarriage and isn't known to cause other pregnancy complications.

What the results may tell you Your care provider will use the test results to help gauge your risk of carrying a baby with Down syndrome or trisomy 18. Other factors, such as your age and personal or family health history, also may affect your risk.

First trimester screening results are given as positive or negative and also as a probability, such as a 1 in 5,000 risk of carrying a baby who has Down syndrome. Generally, the test is considered positive for Down syndrome if the risk is 1 in 230 or greater (the exact number may vary slightly with different laboratories). For trisomy 18, the test is considered positive if the risk is 1 in 100 or greater.

Reasons to have it done Because first trimester screening can be done earlier than most other prenatal screening tests, you'll have the results early in your pregnancy. This gives you more time to make decisions about further diagnostic tests, the need for expert counseling and the course of your pregnancy. If your baby is diagnosed with a genetic condition, you'll also have more time to prepare for the possibility of caring for a child with special needs.

If you do undergo first trimester screening, you may be faced with the decision of whether to undergo further testing based on the results. Before the screening, consider what level of risk would be enough for you to choose additional testing. Follow-up diagnostic tests provide more information, but they're more invasive.

Accuracy and limitations of the test First trimester screening correctly identifies about 85 percent of women who are carrying a baby with Down syndrome. About 5 percent of women have a false-positive result, meaning that the test result is positive, but the baby doesn't actually have Down syndrome. For trisomy 18, the detection rate is approximately 90 percent with a 2 percent false-positive rate.

Second trimester quadruple screening The quadruple screening test, also known as the quad screen, measures levels of four substances in a pregnant woman's blood:
▶ Alpha-fetoprotein (AFP), a protein made by the baby's liver
▶ Human chorionic gonadotropin (HCG), a hormone made by the placenta
▶ Estriol, a hormone made by the placenta and the baby's liver
▶ Inhibin A, another hormone made by the placenta

The quad screen evaluates the risk of carrying a baby with developmental or chromosomal conditions, such as:
▶ *Down syndrome (trisomy 21).* See previous page for more information.
▶ *Trisomy 18.* See previous page.
▶ *Neural tube defect.* This rare condition occurs when tissue doesn't form properly around an embryo's spinal cord or brain, most often resulting in spina bifida or anencephaly, respectively. Spina bifida is often associated with excess brain fluid (hydrocephalus), mobility problems and intellectual disability. Anencephaly is more severe. A baby born with anencephaly may be stillborn or die within a few hours or days after birth.
▶ *Abdominal wall defect.* This occurs when the abdominal wall does not close properly early in pregnancy. This problem may be isolated or part of a syndrome. Babies with abdominal wall defects will require surgery and other treatments after delivery.

When and how it's done Ideally, the quad screen is performed between weeks 15 and 18 of your pregnancy, but may be done as late as 22 weeks. Levels of the chemicals measured change substantially as your baby continues to develop, so it's critical that the calculated age of your baby is correct. The AFP test is most accurate when done between the 16th and 18th weeks of pregnancy. For the screen, a member of your health care team takes a sample of blood from a vein in your arm, which is sent to a lab for analysis.

The quad screen doesn't pose any risk of miscarriage or other pregnancy complications. The biggest issue for most mothers is the anxiety caused by waiting for the test results. In a small percentage of cases, results will be positive, and additional, more invasive and riskier tests will be offered. Still, most women within this positive group have unaffected babies.

What the results may tell you A positive quad screen simply means that levels of some or all of the substances measured in your blood were outside the normal range. This can indicate a potential problem that may need follow-up testing. However, positive results can occur for various reasons, including:

▶ Inaccurate dating (miscalculation of how long you've been pregnant)
▶ Pregnancy with multiples
▶ In vitro fertilization
▶ The presence of other medical conditions, such as diabetes
▶ Maternal smoking

Reasons to have it done If you didn't have the first trimester screening, the quad screen offers another chance to assess your risk of carrying a baby with chromosomal or anatomical abnormalities. Negative results may give you peace of mind. If you receive positive results,

you can talk to your care provider or a genetic counselor about your options.

Accuracy and limitations of the test The quad screen correctly identifies about 80 percent of women who are carrying a baby who has Down syndrome. Approximately 6 to 7 percent of women have a false-positive result, meaning that the test result is positive but the baby doesn't actually have Down syndrome.

Screening tests combined across first and second trimesters You may also have the option for a screening test that combines aspects of both first trimester and second trimester (quad) screening.

The integrated test, one type of combined screening, uses the first trimester ultrasound (NT) and blood test from the first and second trimester screening. A single result is provided when results are completed in the second trimester.

The serum integrated test is similar to the integrated test but does not include the ultrasound. It may be a helpful option if an ultrasound (NT) measurement is not available. Results are provided in the second trimester.

The stepwise sequential test starts with the first trimester screen. If results indicate a high risk of Down syndrome or trisomy 18, you'll be referred for chorionic villus sampling (see page 316). If the first trimester screening portion of the test does not indicate increased risk, you'll then go on to complete the second trimester portion of the screening test. Final results are provided in the second trimester.

Reasons to have it done If you can wait beyond the first trimester to find out your results, some of the combined screening tests can give slightly better accuracy in screening than the first or second trimester test alone can.

Accuracy and limitations of the test The integrated test correctly identifies 85 percent of pregnancies with Down syndrome, with a false-positive rate of only 0.8 percent. The serum integrated test also detects about 85 percent of Down syndrome cases, while the stepwise sequential test identifies about 95 percent of cases. Both have a similar false-positive rate of about 4 or 5 percent. As with the other screening tests, an abnormal result does not mean that the baby is affected, but that there is an increased risk of the condition.

Cell-free DNA (cfDNA) screening

Also known as noninvasive prenatal testing (NIPT), cell-free DNA screening is a newer method to screen for specific chromosomal abnormalities during pregnancy. Like the first trimester screen and the quad screen, it also uses a sample of your blood. However, this test looks at fragments of DNA from the placenta that are floating in your blood. This genetic material from the placenta typically matches the genetic makeup of your baby, so the DNA sample can be used to analyze for chromosomal problems in the baby. This test can also determine the sex of the baby by checking for the presence or absence of Y chromosome DNA in the sample.

When and how it's done Cell-free DNA screening can be done as early as week 10 of pregnancy. A routine blood draw takes a sample of your blood, which is sent to a lab for analysis.

What the results may tell you Prenatal cell-free DNA screening can be used to screen for your baby's sex, as well as:

- ***Down syndrome (trisomy 21).*** See page 312 for more information.

- ***Trisomy 18.*** See page 312.
- ***Trisomy 13.*** As with trisomy 18, this condition causes severe intellectual disability and physical defects. It is often fatal for the baby during pregnancy or in early infancy.

Other cell-free DNA screening tests are available, but the accuracy and sensitivity of certain tests are still being analyzed and evaluated. These tests include screening for increased risk of:

- ***Trisomy 16 and trisomy 22.*** Trisomies 16 and 22 are rare chromosomal problems that usually result in miscarriage.
- ***Triploidy.*** This is a rare chromosomal condition that causes severe physical defects. This condition usually leads to miscarriage or death of the baby during the early second trimester.
- ***Sex chromosome aneuploidy.*** Sex chromosome aneuploidy is any of several abnormalities in the number of sex chromosomes. Some of these conditions have no symptoms, while others are associated with risk of infertility, mild intellectual disability or cardiac abnormalities.
- ***Specific microdeletion syndromes.*** These are rare chromosomal disorders caused by a small segment of chromosome that's missing (a deletion) or by an extra copy of a small segment of a chromosome (a duplication). One of the more familiar microdeletions is 22q11.2 deletion syndrome, also known as DiGeorge syndrome. Its symptoms vary widely among affected people.
- ***Certain single-gene disorders.*** Some laboratories are offering cell-free DNA screening for specific disorders caused by mutations in a single gene. This screening may be prompted by specific ultrasound findings. However, the accuracy of cell-free DNA screening for detection of single-gene disorders has not yet been established.

As with first and second trimester screenings, cell-free DNA screening is not a diagnostic test. If results show an increased risk of a genetic disorder, your provider will talk with you about additional testing.

Reasons to have it done Cell-free DNA screening is one of the most accurate methods to screen for common chromosomal conditions such as Down syndrome and trisomies 13 and 18. It can be used whether risk of the conditions is high or low.

Accuracy and limitations of the test Cell-free DNA screening can identify 99 percent of babies with Down syndrome, with a false-positive rate of less than 1 percent.

One limitation of this screening is the possibility of a "no call" result. This occurs when the amount of placental DNA in the maternal bloodstream is too low for the test to be reliably completed. Because this result has been associated with a high maternal body mass index (BMI), cell-free DNA screening is generally not recommended in women whose BMI is over 35. A low amount of placental DNA in mom's blood has also been associated with fetal chromosome problems. Your provider may discuss additional testing if the amount of baby's DNA in your blood is low.

Until more data is available on how well cell-free DNA screening can detect other genetic conditions, this screening should be used primarily to screen for Down syndrome and trisomies 13 and 18.

PRENATAL DIAGNOSTIC TESTS

If a screening test indicates a higher risk of a genetic condition, or if you know from personal or family history that your baby has an increased risk of a condition, you may consider diagnostic testing. The following tests can provide more information about your baby's health.

Chorionic villus sampling Chorionic villus sampling (CVS) is a diagnostic test often used to follow up on abnormal results obtained from a screening test. This test can detect chromosomal and other genetic abnormalities in your baby by examining DNA from a small amount of tissue from the placenta. Part of the placenta is made up of a membrane layer called the chorion. Tiny, hairlike projections called villi extend out of the chorion and act as routes for nutrients, oxygen and antibodies from you to your baby. These chorionic villi contain fetal cells complete with your baby's chromosomes and DNA.

When and how it's done CVS is usually performed between the 11th and 14th weeks of gestation. If you wish to have a diagnostic test early on to help inform your management of the pregnancy, your doctor may recommend CVS.

During the procedure, your doctor takes a sample of chorionic villus cells from the placenta by inserting a thin, hollow tube (catheter) through your vagina and cervix or by inserting a needle through your abdomen. The sample is then sent to a laboratory for analysis. Which approach your doctor uses depends on the position of the placenta and his or her experience. In general, placentas on the back side of the uterus are easier to sample through the cervix. Placentas in the front allow for either approach.

An ultrasound is done before the procedure to determine the position of the placenta, and ultrasound guidance is used throughout the procedure.

CVS requires an experienced obstetrician to perform the procedure. Although it is a relatively safe test, it carries a few risks:

▶ *Miscarriage.* The risk of pregnancy loss from CVS is about 1 in 455. If the baby is small for its gestational age, the risk may be higher.

▶ *Post-procedural complications.* Up to 1 in 3 women experience spotting or bleeding after CVS, although persistent bleeding is less common. Other complications, such as infection or leakage of amniotic fluid, occur in very few cases.

▶ *Red cell antigen (protein) incompatibility.* Rarely, CVS may cause fetal cells to cross into the maternal bloodstream. If your blood type is different from your baby's in certain ways — for example, if yours is rhesus (Rh) negative and your baby's is Rh positive — you can develop red cell antibodies that may be harmful to your baby or a subsequent baby. If you are Rh negative, your doctor will treat you with medication to prevent this.

What the results may tell you Analysis of fetal cells in the sample can tell you whether your baby has a chromosomal abnormality, such as Down syndrome. In pregnancies at risk of specific genetic disorders, DNA obtained from CVS can be used to test for the specific disease.

Reasons to have it done The decision to have CVS can be difficult. Talk to your care provider or a genetic counselor about your options. The advantage of

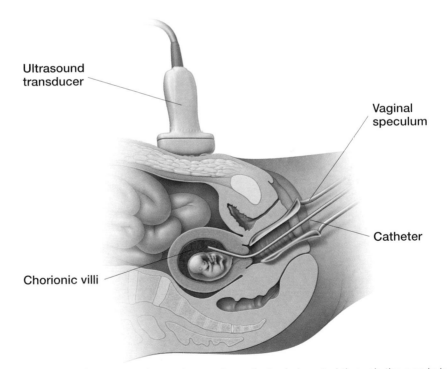

Ultrasound transducer

Vaginal speculum

Catheter

Chorionic villi

A vaginal speculum opens the vagina, and a catheter is inserted through the cervix into the chorionic villi during a transcervical chorionic villus sampling (CVS). A sample is gently removed by suction for testing in a laboratory. As with amniocentesis, the doctor uses an ultrasound image to check the position of the fetus and guide the catheter into position.

CVS over other diagnostic tests is that results are available earlier in pregnancy. Reasons to consider the test may include:

▶ You received abnormal results from a screening test, such as the first trimester screen or cfDNA screen.

▶ You have a family history of a specific genetic condition.

▶ Either parent is a known carrier of a genetic condition, including a single-gene disorder such as Tay-Sachs disease or cystic fibrosis.

▶ You'll be 35 or older when you have the baby. The older you are, the higher your baby's risk of having a chromosomal abnormality.

▶ A previous pregnancy was complicated by a chromosomal abnormality or genetic condition.

Accuracy and limitations of the test CVS has less than a 1 percent chance of yielding false-positive results — indicating the baby has an abnormality when there really is none. If you get negative results, you can be almost certain that no chromosomal abnormalities are present in your baby. But CVS can't be used to check for all conditions. For example, it can't be used to test for neural tube defects, such as spina bifida.

Amniocentesis Like CVS, amniocentesis is a diagnostic test often used to follow up on screening results. You may also choose amniocentesis to learn more detailed information about your pregnancy or to learn if your baby is affected by a genetic condition previously identified within the family.

With amniocentesis, a small sample of amniotic fluid is withdrawn from the sac surrounding your baby. (Your body quickly replaces the small amount sampled.) The amniotic fluid is a clear liquid that envelops your baby in the uterus and provides a cushion. Amniotic fluid consists mostly of urine from your baby but also contains cells that your baby has shed and proteins made by the baby. These cells can provide genetic and other information about your baby.

There are two common types of amniocentesis:

▶ *Genetic amniocentesis.* The cells taken from the amniotic fluid sample can be collected and sent to a genetics laboratory for analysis. This may include studies of the chromosomes or study of a single gene abnormality. For some tests, the cells will need to be grown (cultured) to obtain an adequate amount of genetic material for testing. In those cases, test results may not be ready for three to four weeks.

The alpha-fetoprotein (AFP) level in the amniotic fluid sample can also be tested for signs of neural tube defects, such as spina bifida. In families with certain known genetic disorders, amniotic fluid may also be collected for other highly specialized tests.

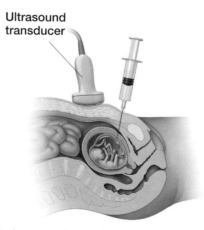

Ultrasound transducer

During genetic amniocentesis, an ultrasound transducer shows on a screen the positions of your fetus and the needle, enabling your doctor to safely withdraw a sample of amniotic fluid for testing.

▶ *Maturity amniocentesis.* With this test, the fluid is analyzed to find out if the baby's lungs are mature enough to function normally at birth.

When and how it's done Genetic amniocentesis can be done at any time during pregnancy, but is usually performed between the 15th and 20th weeks of gestation. At this point, your uterus generally contains enough amniotic fluid, and there's decreased likelihood of fluid leakage. Amniocentesis performed earlier than this carries more risk.

Maturity amniocentesis is done when there may be a reason to deliver the baby before the due date, usually between 34 and 39 weeks of gestation.

The test can be performed in your doctor's office. Ultrasound is used to determine the position of the fetus. Guided by the ultrasound images, your doctor inserts a thin, hollow needle through your abdomen and into your uterus. About 2 to 4 teaspoons of amniotic fluid are withdrawn into a syringe and sent to a laboratory for analysis. The procedure is over when the needle is removed.

WHEN THE RESULTS INDICATE A PROBLEM

The unthinkable is happening: Your prenatal test results suggest that your baby has a problem. Amid the shock and worry, one question surfaces: What now?

Your care provider will likely refer you to certain specialists to discuss results and implications for your pregnancy and your baby. These specialists may include a maternal-fetal medicine specialist, a genetics professional, a neonatologist and other pediatric specialists, and a social worker. Here are some questions you might consider asking your care providers during your appointments:

▶ How accurate are the test results? Is it possible there's a mistake?

▶ Can my baby survive this condition? If so, how long is he or she likely to live?

▶ What problems might be caused by this condition? How might the baby be affected physically? How might the baby be affected mentally?

▶ Are there additional tests that can provide more information about the baby's condition?

▶ Is it likely that my child will need surgeries or other medical treatments to manage the condition?

▶ Are there other health care professionals who can give us more information?

▶ What is involved in caring for a child with this condition?

▶ Is there a support group in our community for families who have a child with this condition? How can we contact parents of children who have a similar condition?

▶ What are the chances that this condition will affect future pregnancies?

▶ What resources are available if we decide to end the pregnancy? What counseling services or support groups are available?

The information you gather can help you make decisions based on your personal circumstances.

GENETIC STUDIES AFTER CVS OR AMNIOCENTESIS

The samples obtained after chorionic villus sampling or amniocentesis can be sent to the genetics laboratory for several types of testing.

Chromosome analysis Also called karyotype analysis, this test examines a baby's chromosomes. It can detect conditions of chromosomes that are duplicated or missing, including Down syndrome, trisomy 13 and trisomy 18. This testing may be recommended if one of the parents is known to carry a specific chromosome problem.

This test typically requires that the cells obtained are cultured prior to the analysis, so it may take one to three weeks for the laboratory to return results.

Fluorescence *in situ* hybridization (FISH) This test uses cells retrieved during chorionic villus sampling or amniocentesis. The test can identify certain chromosomal abnormalities such as Down syndrome, trisomies 13 and 18, and monosomy X (Turner syndrome) in as little as one or two days. FISH is highly accurate in identifying specific chromosomal defects. Because it is targeted, both positive and negative results are usually followed up with karyotype or microarray analysis.

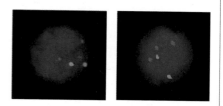

The red color in these FISH test images identifies three copies of chromosome 21, indicating Down syndrome.

Cells do not need to be grown for the FISH test, allowing for test results to be completed in two to three days.

Chromosomal microarray (CMA) This type of testing provides a higher resolution look at a baby's chromosomes. It may detect small segments of a chromosome that are deleted (microdeletions) or duplicated (microduplications), which may be associated with specific genetic syndromes.

Chromosomal microarray testing may be considered if you've had abnormal results from genetic screening, certain abnormalities detected in an ultrasound, or amniocentesis or chorionic villus sampling. You may also consider it if you've previously experienced a miscarriage or stillbirth.

Single-gene testing This test is performed when the family history or carrier screening shows that the baby is at risk of a single-gene disorder. DNA is extracted from placental cells (after CVS) or amniocytes (after amniocentesis). The lab may need to culture the cells to obtain an adequate amount for testing. The DNA is then analyzed for the mutation(s) previously identified in family members. This testing may take one to four weeks to complete.

Many women find that the procedure isn't as painful as they had anticipated. You'll notice a prick when the needle enters your skin and some menstrual-like cramping during the procedure.

The risks of amniocentesis are similar to those of CVS. The risk of all complications, including minor complications, is approximately 1 to 2 percent.

- *Miscarriage.* Amniocentesis done before 24 weeks of gestation carries a risk of miscarriage of about 1 in 900. Amniocentesis to check maturity has almost no risk of pregnancy loss.
- *Complications.* You may have cramping or spotting after the procedure, and approximately 1 to 2 percent of women may have amniotic fluid leakage. In most cases, the leakage stops within a week, and the amniotic fluid returns to a normal level.
- *Needle injury.* There's a slight chance the baby may be punctured by the needle, though use of the ultrasound for guidance makes this rare. Usually no long-term problems are associated with a needle stick to the baby.
- *Red cell antigen incompatibility.* As in CVS, this occurs in very few cases. See page 431 for more information.

What the results may tell you Genetic amniocentesis can tell you if your baby has a chromosomal abnormality, such as Down syndrome; a genetic disorder, such as cystic fibrosis; or a neural tube defect, such as spina bifida. However, most cases of spina bifida are detected by ultrasound.

In addition to testing lung maturity, another use of amniocentesis is testing for anemia in a pregnancy with rhesus (Rh) incompatibility or another form of red cell antigen incompatibility. Or if your doctor thinks you and your baby have been exposed to an infection, a sample of amniotic fluid can be taken for testing. The sample will be sent to a lab where it will be analyzed for the suspected infection.

Reasons to have it done Genetic amniocentesis may be considered for many of the same reasons as CVS (see page 318). In addition, your care provider might recommend amniocentesis if a previous pregnancy was affected by a neural tube defect or if you have abnormal ultrasound findings.

Accuracy and limitations of the test Although amniocentesis is accurate in identifying certain genetic disorders, it can't identify all birth defects. For example, it can't detect a heart defect, intellectual disability, or cleft lip and palate.

Fetal blood sampling In rare situations, sampling of your baby's blood from the umbilical cord may be recommended. This is also known as percutaneous umbilical blood sampling (PUBS) or cordocentesis. This type of sampling is most often recommended when there is concern for severe anemia in the baby. However, the sample can also be used to study the baby's chromosomes or to analyze for infectious disease.

When and how it's done Fetal blood sampling is usually done later in the pregnancy, after 18 weeks. Before this point, the umbilical vein is still fragile and the procedure is much more difficult. Similar to an amniocentesis, you lie on your back with your abdomen exposed. Gel is spread over your abdomen, and advanced ultrasound is used to locate the umbilical cord. Your doctor inserts a thin needle through your abdomen and uterus into the umbilical cord vein and withdraws a sample of blood. The sample is then sent to the lab for analysis. You and your baby will be monitored for a short period after the procedure to make sure that the baby is doing well.

PUBS carries a higher risk of miscarriage — about 1 to 2 percent — than that of CVS or amniocentesis. Other risks include bleeding from the needle entry site, which usually goes away on its own, temporary slowing of the baby's heart rate, infection, cramping and fluid leakage.

What the results may tell you Most often, umbilical cord sampling is used to evaluate for fetal anemia, and to provide red cells or platelets to your fetus. In rare situations, fetal blood sampling may be used to evaluate for genetic conditions or for fetal infection. Having an experienced care provider perform the procedure is critical to the test's success.

FETAL SURVEILLANCE OR LATE PREGNANCY TESTS

Under certain circumstances, your care provider may recommend tests to check on your baby's health late in your pregnancy. These include fetal nonstress and stress tests, biophysical profile testing, and Doppler ultrasound.

Fetal nonstress and stress tests
A nonstress test is a simple, noninvasive test. It's called nonstress because it avoids putting stress on the baby, such as through induced contractions. During the test, baby's movement and heart rate are monitored for about 20 to 40 minutes. If the baby doesn't move, that doesn't necessarily indicate there's a problem; the baby may just be in a sleep cycle.

This test may be used to check on your baby's oxygen supply if there are concerns about how the placenta is functioning or the blood flow through the umbilical cord.

A contraction stress test is also used to evaluate the baby's well-being, but it monitors baby's reaction to the stress of contractions. To induce uterine contractions, you may be given the hormone oxytocin through an IV, or you may be asked to rub your nipples, which tells your body to release oxytocin. If your baby's heart rate slows down (decelerates) in a certain pattern after a contraction, your baby may not be receiving adequate oxygen and may not tolerate labor and vaginal delivery.

When and how they're done These tests are generally performed after 28 weeks of pregnancy, or after a time when the baby could survive outside of the womb if delivery was necessary. The tests are performed as follows:

▶ *Nonstress test.* For this test, monitors that measure your baby's heart rate, movements and spontaneous contractions are attached to your abdomen. Your provider will look for changes in baby's heart rate pattern during the test. Most of these changes occur in association with your baby's movement.

▶ *Contraction stress test.* The contraction stress test is performed in much the same manner as the nonstress test, but baby's fetal heart rate is measured while you're having mild contractions. The contractions may have to be induced.

What the results may tell you A normal (reactive) result generally suggests that baby is getting enough oxygen. If one or both tests have an abnormal (nonreactive) result, it may not mean that your baby is in danger. These tests have a high false-positive rate, suggesting there's a problem when there really isn't one. Certain patterns in your baby's heart rate may warrant further evaluation.

Reasons to have the tests done Your provider may recommend a nonstress test or a contraction stress test in specific situations, such as if you notice a marked decrease in your baby's movement or if your baby's growth rate seems abnormally slow. The tests may also be recommended if you have one of the following conditions:

▶ Diabetes
▶ Kidney or heart disease
▶ High blood pressure
▶ A history of stillbirth
▶ A postterm pregnancy
▶ A multiple birth pregnancy

Accuracy and limitations of the tests Both tests have high false-positive rates. A false-positive means the test indicates a problem when there actually is none. Thus, your care provider may recommend additional testing or monitoring if the results are abnormal. On the other hand, results indicating that baby is healthy are more reliable.

Biophysical profile testing Biophysical profile testing combines an ultrasound examination with a nonstress test. In some situations, the ultrasound portion of the test alone will be used to evaluate your baby. The tests generally assess five different aspects of your baby's health, including his or her:

▶ Heart rate
▶ Breathing movements
▶ Body movement
▶ Muscle tone
▶ Amniotic fluid level

Each of these factors is given a score of 0 or 2, and the scores are added together to achieve a total from 0 to 10. Biophysical profile testing helps you and your care provider keep track of your baby's health before delivery, particularly if you have a high-risk pregnancy.

When and how it's done This test may be used as early as the 26th week of pregnancy, but it more typically is started at 28 to 32 weeks.

Your baby's heart rate is measured using a nonstress test. The other four factors — breathing, movement, muscle tone and amniotic fluid — are evaluated with ultrasound. If a factor is normal, it receives an individual score of 2. If it's absent or less than expected, it receives a score of 0. (All scores are even numbers.)

What the results may tell you A score of 6 or lower may indicate your baby is getting less than adequate oxygen. The lower the score, the greater the cause for concern. Depending on the baby's age and the circumstances, your care provider may recommend delivery.

Accuracy and limitations of the test The false-positive rate for any individual factor of the biophysical profile is high, but when all factors are combined, the false-positive rate decreases. Having a low score doesn't necessarily mean that your baby must be delivered. It may just mean that you need special care throughout the rest of your pregnancy.

Doppler ultrasound Doppler ultrasound (see page 310) is another method to evaluate your baby's health late in pregnancy. This test is most often used when your pregnancy is complicated by maternal hypertension or growth problems with your baby. It monitors blood flow through the umbilical cord and your baby's blood vessels. Doppler studies are also used for babies at risk of fetal anemia, characterized by abnormally low levels of blood or red blood cells in baby's bloodstream.

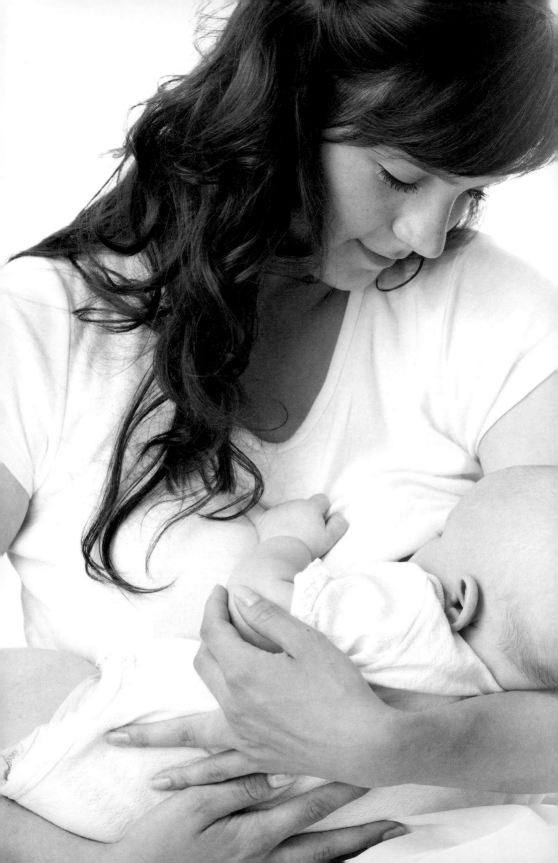

CHAPTER 22

Breast-feeding

Do you plan to feed your baby with breast milk or formula? Some women know the answer to this question right away; others struggle.

Breast milk is best, and the benefits of breast-feeding are well-established. Breast milk contains the right balance of nutrients for your baby, and the antibodies in breast milk boost your baby's immune system to help fight disease. But sometimes breast-feeding isn't possible. Feeding your baby formula instead of breast milk shouldn't lead to feelings of guilt. Feeling guilty isn't good for you or your baby.

For almost every new mom, the first few weeks with a newborn are likely to be demanding and exhausting. Both you and your baby are adapting to an entirely new reality, and that takes time.

Throughout this adjustment, remember that feeding your newborn is about more than just nourishment. It's a time of cuddling and closeness that helps build the connection between you and your baby. You want to make every feeding a

time to bond with your baby. Find a quiet place to feed the child, where you're both less likely to be distracted. Cherish the time before your baby is old enough to start feeding himself or herself. That time will come soon enough.

Many women have misconceptions about breast-feeding. Learn as much as you can about feeding your baby. Seek out expert advice if needed. Your care provider will be very supportive of breast-feeding unless you have specific health issues, such as a certain disease or disease treatment, that make formula-feeding a better choice.

BREAST-FEEDING

The American Academy of Pediatrics recommends that infants be fed breast milk exclusively for the first six months of life. Breast-feeding gives complete nutrition, and it's highly encouraged because it has many known health benefits for your little one — and for you. The longer you breast-feed, the greater the chances that your baby will experience these benefits.

Milk production Breast-feeding is really quite amazing. Early in your pregnancy, your milk-producing (mammary) glands prepare for nursing. By about the sixth month of pregnancy, your breasts are ready to produce milk. In some women, tiny droplets of yellowish fluid (colostrum) appear on the nipples at this time. Protein-rich colostrum is what a breast-fed baby gets the first few days after birth. It's very good for the baby because it contains infection-fighting antibodies from your body and very little milk sugar (lactose).

Your milk supply gradually increases between the third and fifth days after your baby's birth. Your breasts will be full and sometimes tender. They may feel lumpy or hard as the glands fill with milk. When a baby nurses, breast milk is released from the milk-producing glands and is propelled down milk ducts, which are located just behind the dark circle of tissue that surrounds the nipple (areola). The sucking action of the baby compresses the areola, forcing milk out through tiny openings in the nipple.

Your baby's sucking stimulates nerve endings in your areola and nipple, sending a message to your brain to release the hormone oxytocin. Oxytocin acts on the milk-producing glands in your breast, causing the ejection of milk to your nursing baby. This release is called the let-down (milk ejection) reflex, which may be accompanied by a tingling sensation.

The let-down reflex makes your milk available to your baby. Although your baby's sucking is the main stimulus for milk let-down, other stimuli may have the same effect. For example, your baby's cry — or even thoughts of your baby — may set things in motion.

Regardless of whether you plan to breast-feed, your body produces milk after you have a baby. Your milk production is then based on supply and demand. If you don't breast-feed, your milk supply will eventually stop. If you do breast-feed, the more frequently your breast is emptied, the more milk your breasts produce.

Benefits for baby Breast milk provides babies with:

Ideal nutrition Breast milk has just the right nutrients, in the right amounts, to nourish your baby completely. It contains the fats, proteins, carbohydrates, vitamins and minerals that a baby needs for growth, digestion and brain development. Breast milk is also individualized; the composition of your milk changes as your baby grows.

Protection against disease Research shows that breast milk may help keep your baby from getting sick. Breast milk provides antibodies that help your baby's immune system fight off common childhood illnesses. Breast-fed babies tend to have fewer colds, ear infections and urinary tract infections than do babies who aren't breast-fed. Breast-fed babies may also have fewer problems with asthma, food allergies and skin conditions, such as eczema. They may be less likely to experience low levels of red blood cells (anemia). Research suggests that breast-feeding might also help to protect against sudden infant death syndrome (SIDS), and it may offer a slight reduction in the risk of childhood leukemia.

Breast milk may even protect against disease long term. As adults, people who were breast-fed may have a lowered risk of heart attacks and strokes — due to lower cholesterol levels — and may be less likely to develop diabetes. Breast milk may also help protect against bowel disorders such as celiac disease or inflammatory bowel disease.

Protection against obesity Studies indicate that babies who are breast-fed are less likely to become obese as adults.

Easy digestion Breast milk is easier for babies to digest than is formula or cow's milk. Because breast milk doesn't remain in the stomach as long as formula does, breast-fed babies spit up less. They have less gas and less constipation. They also have less diarrhea, because breast milk appears to kill some diarrhea-causing germs and helps a baby's digestive system grow and function.

Other benefits Nursing at the breast helps promote normal development of your baby's jaw and facial muscles. It may even help your baby have fewer cavities later in childhood.

Benefits for you For mothers, the benefits include:

Faster recovery from childbirth The baby's suckling triggers your body to release oxytocin, a hormone that causes your uterus to contract. This means that the uterus returns to its pre-pregnancy size more quickly after delivery than it does if you use formula.

Suppresses ovulation Breast-feeding delays the return of ovulation and therefore your period, which may help extend the time between pregnancies. However, additional birth control is recommended to avoid unintended pregnancy.

May protect long-term health Breast-feeding may reduce your risk of getting breast cancer before menopause. Breast-feeding also appears to provide some protection from uterine and ovarian cancers. It's thought to reduce your risk of diabetes and heart disease, too.

Pros vs. cons Aside from infant and maternal health, other issues to consider include:

▶ *Convenience.* Breast-feeding can be done anywhere, at any time, whenever your baby shows signs of hunger. Plus, no equipment is necessary. Breast milk is always available — and at the perfect temperature. Because you don't need to prepare a bottle and you can nurse lying down, nighttime feedings may be easier.

▶ *Cost savings.* Breast-feeding can save money because you don't need to buy formula, and you may not need bottles. It's also environmentally friendly.

▶ *Bonding.* Breast-feeding can promote intimacy and closeness between mom and baby. It can be extremely rewarding and fulfilling for you both.

▶ *Rest time for mom.* Breast-feeding allows for rest time every few hours while you feed your baby.

Breast-feeding, however, can present some challenges and inconveniences. These may include:

▶ *Exclusive feeding by mom.* In the early weeks, parenting can be physically demanding. At first, newborns nurse every two to three hours, day and night. That can be tiring for mom, and the other parent may feel left out of feedings. Eventually, you can express milk with a breast pump, which will enable others to take over some feedings. It may take about a month before your milk production is well-established so that you can use a pump to express and collect breast milk.

▶ *Restrictions for mom.* Drinking alcohol isn't recommended for mothers who are breast-feeding, because alcohol can pass through breast milk to the baby. In addition, you may not be able to take certain medications while nursing. Talk with your care provider for personalized guidance.

▶ *Sore nipples.* Some women may experience sore nipples and even breast infections. These can often be avoided with proper positioning and technique. Ask for guidance from a lactation consultant or your care provider.

WHEN BREAST-FEEDING MAY NOT BE AN OPTION

Almost any woman is physically capable of breast-feeding her baby. The ability to do so has nothing to do with the size of your breasts; small breasts don't produce less milk than do large breasts. Women who've had breast reduction surgery or breast implants may still be able to breast-feed.

In rare situations, a woman may be encouraged to bottle-feed her baby instead of breast-feed. Your care provider may suggest formula-feeding if:

▶ You have untreated, active tuberculosis; HIV; human T-cell lymphotropic virus; or active herpes lesions on the breast. These infections can be transmitted to your baby either through breast milk or close contact. Note that if you develop chickenpox (varicella) while breast-feeding, your breast milk is still recommended and is safe for your baby. But your contact with baby may need to be limited, so bottle-feeding breast milk may be an option.

▶ You drink heavily or use illicit drugs. Breast milk can pass alcohol and other drugs to your baby.

▶ You're receiving treatment for cancer (chemotherapy, hormone therapy, targeted therapy or radiation) or HIV (antiretroviral therapy).

▶ Your newborn has certain health conditions. Some rare metabolic conditions, such as phenylketonuria (PKU) or galactosemia, may require using specially adapted formulas.

▶ Your newborn is premature or isn't growing well. Some infants with poor growth may need to have measured amounts of milk and nutritional supplements. Breast milk may be possible, but you may need to give it by bottle, tube or cup until growth improves.

▶ Your baby has a mouth deformity, such as a cleft lip or cleft palate. If so, he or she may have difficulty breast-feeding, necessitating that you use a bottle to feed. However, you do have the option of expressing breast milk and putting it in a bottle for your baby.

Keep in mind also that certain medications can pass into your breast milk and could pose some harm to or side effects for your baby. Before you begin or continue any medication, talk with your baby's care provider or a lactation consultant about whether you need to discontinue or change any prescription or nonprescription medications you're taking. If there are concerns with anything you're taking, alternative medications that are safer for breast-feeding may be available.

▶ *Other physical side effects.* When you're lactating, your body's hormones may keep your vagina relatively dry. Using a water-based lubricating jelly can help treat this problem. It may also take time for your menstrual cycle to establish a regular pattern.

Vitamin D supplementation If you exclusively or partially feed your infant breast milk, talk to your baby's doctor about vitamin D supplements for your baby. Breast milk may not provide enough vitamin D, which is essential to help your baby absorb calcium and phosphorus — nutrients necessary for strong bones. In rare cases, too little vitamin D can cause rickets, a softening and weakening of bones. The American Academy of Pediatrics and the Institute of Medicine recommend that during their first year of life infants receive 400 international units (IU) of vitamin D daily.

Getting started If this is your first experience with breast-feeding, you may be nervous, which is normal. If it goes easily for you from the first feeding, that's wonderful. If not, be patient. Starting to breast-feed requires practice. It's a natural process, but that doesn't mean it comes easily to everyone. It's a new skill for both you and baby. It may take a few attempts before you've both gotten the hang of it.

The time to begin breast-feeding is right after the baby is born. If feasible, put the baby to your breast within the first hour after delivery. Early skin-to-skin contact has been shown to improve breast-feeding outcomes. Arrange to have baby in your room at the hospital or birthing center, if possible, to facilitate nursing. To help your baby learn to breast-feed, request that he or she not be given any supplementary bottles of water or formula. Preferably, baby also shouldn't receive a pacifier, unless medically necessary, until breast-feeding is well-established.

Seek help if you need it While you're in the hospital, ask your doctor, midwife,

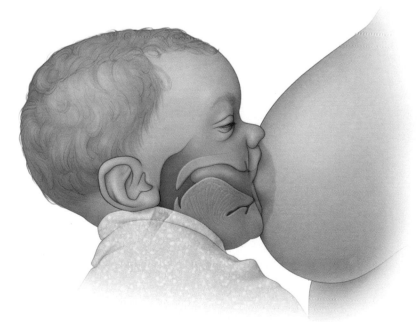

nurse or a lactation consultant to assist you. These experts can provide hands-on instruction and helpful tips. If you have questions after you go home, consider seeking out a lactation consultant in your area. Look for someone with an International Board Certified Lactation Consultant (IBCLC) credential. Explore other local breast-feeding support resources, too. These may include a public health nurse visit and support groups led by experienced volunteers who are trained and certified by prominent organizations such as La Leche League International.

A good first step, before baby arrives, is to take a class on breast-feeding. Information on breast-feeding may be part of childbirth classes, or you may need to sign up for a separate class. Most hospitals and birthing centers offer these classes.

Have your supplies on hand You'll want to invest in a couple of nursing bras.

They provide important support for lactating breasts. What distinguishes nursing bras from regular bras is that both cups open to the front, usually with a simple maneuver that you can manage unobtrusively while you hold your baby.

You'll also need nursing pads, which can absorb milk that leaks from your breasts. Slim and disposable, they can be slipped between the breast and bra to soak up milk leakage. Avoid those with plastic shields, which prevent air circulation around the nipples. You can also buy reusable pads that can be washed. Nursing pads can be worn continuously or as needed. Some women don't bother with the pads, but most find them helpful.

Try to relax When it's feeding time, find a quiet location. Have a glass of water close at hand, as it's common to feel thirsty when your milk lets down. You may want to have the phone nearby, or turn it off.

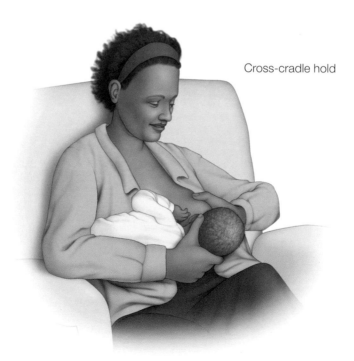

Cross-cradle hold

You might also want a book or the TV remote within reach, but take advantage of this time with your baby.

Get into a comfortable position Both you and baby should be comfortable. Choose supportive furniture, such as a chair or a couch with low arm rests, and sit up straight. You may want a pillow behind the small of your back or under your arms for additional support.

Feeding positions Move your baby across your body so that he or she faces your breast, with his or her nose near your nipple. Make sure your baby's whole body is facing you — tummy to tummy — with ear, shoulder and hip in a straight line. Begin by placing your free hand up under your breast to support it for breast-feeding. Support the weight of your breast in your hand while squeezing lightly to point the nipple straight forward.

Different women find different nursing positions most comfortable. Experiment with these positions to see which works best for you:

Cross-cradle hold Bring your baby across the front of your body, tummy to tummy. Hold your baby with the arm opposite to the breast you're feeding with. Support the back of the baby's head with your open hand. This hold allows you especially good control as you position your baby to latch on. With your free hand, support your breast from the underside in a U-shaped hold to align with baby's mouth.

Cradle hold Cradle your baby in an arm, with your baby's head resting comfortably in the crook of the elbow on the same side as the breast you're feeding with. Your forearm supports your baby's back. Use your free hand to support your breast.

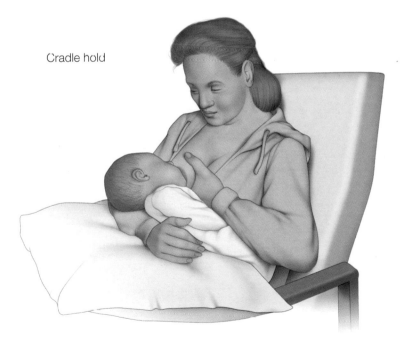

Cradle hold

Football (clutch) hold In this position you hold your baby in much the same way a running back tucks a football under the arm. Hold your baby at your side on one arm, with your elbow bent and your open hand firmly supporting your baby's head faceup at the level of your breast. Your baby's torso will rest on your forearm. Put a pillow at your side to support your arm. A chair with broad, low arms works best. With your free hand, support your breast from the underside in a C-shaped hold to align with baby's mouth.

Because the baby isn't positioned near the abdomen, the football hold is popular among mothers recovering from C-sections. It's also a frequent choice of women who have large breasts or who are nursing premature or small babies.

Side-lying hold Although most new mothers learn to breast-feed in a sitting position, at times you may prefer to nurse while lying down. Use the hand of your lower arm to help keep your baby's head positioned at your breast. With your upper arm and hand, reach across your body and grasp your breast, touching your nipple to your baby's lips. After your baby latches on firmly, you can use your lower arm to support your own head and your upper hand and arm to help support your baby.

Nursing basics If your baby's mouth doesn't open immediately to accept your breast, stroke your baby's cheek or lip with the nipple. If your baby is hungry and interested in nursing, his or her mouth should open. As soon as your baby's mouth is opened wide, like a yawn, move his or her mouth onto your breast. You want your baby to receive as much nipple and areola as possible. It might take a few attempts before your baby opens his or her mouth wide enough to latch on

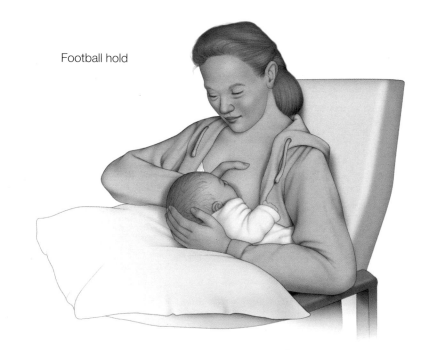

Football hold

Side-lying hold

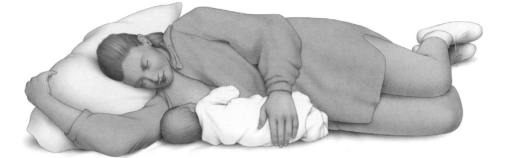

KEEPING YOURSELF HEALTHY

If you're like most new mothers, your attention may be focused intently on the needs of your baby. Although this commitment is completely reasonable, don't forget about your needs. If your baby is to thrive, he or she needs a healthy mother.

Nutrition The best approach to nutrition while breast-feeding is like the best approach at other times in your life: Eat a healthy, balanced diet. There are no special foods to avoid when you're breast-feeding. In addition, drink 6 to 8 cups of fluids each day. Water, milk and juice are good choices. Small amounts of coffee, tea and soft drinks are fine.

As a new mother, it can be hard to prepare healthy meals each day. You may find it easier to snack on healthy foods throughout the day. Partners can help support a breast-feeding mother by bringing her refreshments while she's nursing.

Rest Try to get rest as a new parent, as hard as that may seem at times. You'll feel more energetic, you'll eat better and you'll enjoy your new baby best when you're rested. Rest promotes the production of breast milk by enhancing the production of milk-producing hormones. The soothing effect of breast-feeding can make you feel sleepy, so try to sleep on baby's schedule.

Don't be afraid to ask others to help out with daily chores so that you can rest. Younger children may appreciate being able to help out mother and baby by pitching in around the house.

properly. You can also express some milk, which may encourage baby to latch on.

As your baby starts suckling and your nipple is being stretched in your baby's mouth, you may feel some surging sensations. After a few suckles, those sensations should subside a bit. If they don't, sandwich the breast more and draw the baby's head in more closely. If that doesn't produce comfort, gently remove the baby from your breast, taking care to release the suction first. To break the suction, gently insert the tip of your finger into the corner of baby's mouth. Push your finger slowly between baby's gums until you feel the release. Repeat this procedure until your baby has latched on properly. You want your baby to create a firm bond of suction.

You'll know that milk is flowing and your baby is swallowing if there's a strong, steady, rhythmic motion visible in your baby's cheek. If your breast is blocking

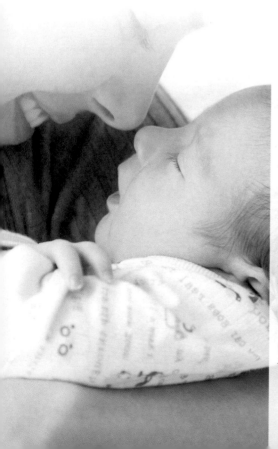

your baby's nose, elevating your baby slightly, or angling the baby's head back and in, may help provide a little breathing room. If your baby attaches and sucks correctly — even if the arrangement feels awkward at first — the position is correct. Once nursing begins, you can relax the supporting arm and pull your baby's lower body closer to you.

Offer your baby both breasts at each feeding. Allow your baby to end the feeding on the first side. Then, after burping your baby, offer the other side. Alternate which side you start with to equalize the stimulation each breast receives.

In general, let your baby nurse as long as he or she wants. The length of feedings may vary considerably. However, on average, most babies nurse for about half an hour, usually divided between both breasts. Ideally, you want the baby to finish one breast at each feeding before switching to the other side. Why? The milk that comes first from your breast, called the foremilk, is rich in protein for growth. But the longer your baby feeds at that breast, the more he or she gets the hindmilk, which is rich in calories and fat and therefore helps your baby gain weight and grow. So wait until your baby seems ready to quit before offering him or her your other breast.

Because breast milk is easily digested, breast-fed babies usually are hungry every two to three hours at first. During those early days and weeks, it may seem that all you do is breast-feed! A baby's need for frequent feeding isn't a sign that the baby isn't getting enough; it reflects the easy digestibility of breast milk. If your baby is satisfied after feeding and is growing, you can be confident that you're doing well.

Breast care Once your milk supply is well-established and you and your baby are comfortable with breast-feeding, you should be able to work through most problems. However, as you start to breast-feed, you may experience:

Fullness A few days after your baby is born, your breasts may become full, firm and tender, making it challenging for your baby to grasp your nipple. This swelling, called engorgement, also causes congestion within your breasts, which makes your milk flow slower. So even if your baby can latch on, he or she may be less than satisfied with the results.

To manage engorgement, express some milk by hand before trying to breast-feed. Support with one hand the breast you intend to express. With your other hand, gently stroke your breast inward toward your areola. Then place your thumb and forefinger at the top and bottom of the breast just behind the areola. As you gently compress the breast between your fingers, milk should flow or squirt out of the nipple. Taking a warm shower also may result in let-down of milk and provide some engorgement relief. You can also use a breast pump to express some milk.

As you release your milk, you'll begin to feel your areola and nipple soften. Once enough milk is released, your baby can comfortably latch on and nurse. Frequent, lengthy nursing sessions are the best means to avoid engorgement. Nurse your baby regularly and try not to miss a feeding. Wearing a nursing bra both day and night will help support engorged breasts and may make you feel more comfortable.

If your breasts are sore after nursing, apply an ice pack to reduce swelling. Alternatively, some women find that a warm shower relieves breast tenderness. Fortunately, the period of engorgement is usually brief, lasting no more than a few days following delivery.

Sore nipples At the beginning, you may experience some nipple discomfort as baby latches on. This is quite common and is due to tender or cracked nipples. Sore nipples are usually caused by incorrect positioning and latching. At each feeding, you want to make sure that the baby has the areola and not just the nipple in his or her mouth. You also want to be certain that the baby's head isn't out of line with his or her body. This position causes pulling at the nipple.

To care for your nipples, express milk onto your nipples and let them air-dry after each feeding. Over-the-counter products such as lanolin also can be soothing and healing for cracked nipples. You don't need to wash your nipples after nursing. There are built-in lubricants around the areola that provide a natural salve. When you're bathing, use water alone to wash your nipples, and let them air-dry.

Blocked milk ducts Sometimes, milk ducts in the breast become clogged, causing milk to back up. Blocked ducts can be felt through the skin as small, tender lumps or larger areas of hardness. Because blocked ducts can lead to an infection, you should treat the problem right away. The best way to open up blocked ducts is to let your baby empty the affected breast, offering that breast first at each feeding. If your baby doesn't empty the affected breast, express milk from it by hand or by breast pump. It may also help to apply a warm compress before nursing and to massage the affected breast. If the problem doesn't go away with self-treatment, call a lactation consultant or your care provider for advice.

Breast infection This is a more serious complication of breast-feeding. Infection (mastitis) may be caused by a failure to empty your breasts at feedings. Germs may also gain entry into your milk ducts from cracked nipples and from your baby's mouth. These germs are not harmful to your baby; everyone has them. They just don't belong in your breast tissues.

Mastitis starts with flu-like signs and symptoms such as a fever, chills and body aches. Redness, swelling and breast tenderness then follow. If you develop such signs and symptoms, call your care provider. You may need antibiotics, in addition to rest and more fluids. Keep nursing if you're taking antibiotics. Treatment for mastitis doesn't harm your baby, and emptying your breasts during feedings will help to prevent clogged milk ducts, another possible source of the condition. If your breasts are really painful, express some milk by hand as you soak your breasts in a bath of warm water.

Pumping your breasts There may be times when you're unable to breast-feed and you want to express your breast milk so it can be fed to your baby when you're away. You can do this either with a breast pump or by hand. However, most breast-feeding mothers find using a breast pump easier than expressing milk manually.

Whether you're going back to work or simply want the flexibility a breast pump can offer, you'll have many choices. Ask yourself these questions to decide which type of breast pump — manual or electric — is best for you. If you're still not sure, ask for help. A lactation consultant or your baby's care provider can help you make the best choice, and offer help and support if problems arise.

How often will you use the breast pump? If you'll be away from the baby only occasionally, a simple hand pump may be all you need. These pumps are small and inexpensive. You simply squeeze the handle to express the milk. If you're returning to work full time or you're planning to be away from your baby for more than a few hours a day, you'll want to invest in an electric pump, which stimulates the breasts more effectively than a hand pump. This helps empty your breasts and protect your milk supply.

Will you need to pump as quickly as possible? A typical pumping session lasts about 15 minutes for each breast. A double electric pump can pump both breasts at once for efficient pumping at work or in other time-crunched situations. If you want to multitask, you may also need a hands-free pumping bra. Certain pumps or accessories can even fit inside a nursing bra for more discreet, faster pumping.

How much can you afford to spend on the pump? You can purchase breast pumps from medical supply stores, as well as most drugstores, baby stores, many big-box stores and online retailers. While manual models generally cost less than $50, electric pumps that include a carrying case and insulated section for storing milk may cost $200 to $300 or more. Some hospitals or medical supply stores rent hospital-grade breast pumps, although the equipment that attaches your breast to the pump (pumping kit) must be purchased. Because there's a small risk of contamination, borrowing a personal-use pump or buying a used personal-use pump isn't recommended.

Check with your health insurance about coverage for a breast pump. Most plans cover the cost of buying or renting a pump, but policies differ on covering a manual or electric pump, the length of a rental, and other details.

Is the pump easy to assemble and transport? If the breast pump is difficult to assemble, take apart or clean, it's bound to be frustrating, which may reduce your enthusiasm for pumping. If you'll be toting the pump to work every day or traveling with the pump, look for a lightweight model. Some breast pumps come in a carrying case with an insulated section for storing expressed milk. Also keep noise level in mind. Some electric models are quieter than others.

Is the suction adjustable? What's comfortable for one woman may be uncomfortable for another. Choose a pump that allows you to control the degree of suction. With some manual models, you can adjust the pump handle position.

Are the breast shields the correct size? Every pump has a cone-shaped cup called a shield to place over your breast. If you're concerned that the standard breast shield is too small, check with individual manufacturers about other options. Larger shields are often available. If you want to pump both breasts at once, make sure the pump is equipped with two breast shields.

Storing breast milk Once you start pumping, it's important to know how to safely and properly store your expressed breast milk. Consider these do's and don'ts for breast milk storage.

What kind of container should I use to store expressed breast milk? Store expressed breast milk in capped glass or plastic containers that have been cleaned in a dishwasher or washed in hot, soapy water and thoroughly rinsed. Consider boiling the containers after washing them if the quality of your water supply is questionable.

If you store breast milk for three days or less, you can also use a plastic freezer bag designed specifically for human milk storage. While economical, plastic bags aren't recommended for long-term breast milk storage because they may spill, leak and become contaminated more easily than hard-sided containers. Also, certain components of breast milk may adhere to the soft plastic bags during long-term breast milk storage, which could deprive your baby of essential nutrients.

BREAST-FEEDING MULTIPLES

A mother can certainly breast-feed more than one baby. If you have twins, you can breast-feed one baby at a time. Or you can nurse them simultaneously, once breast-feeding is established. To accomplish this feat, you can position both babies in the football (clutch) hold. Or you can cradle them both in front of you with their bodies crossing each other. Use pillows to support the babies' heads and your arms.

With triplets, it's possible to breast-feed, although it takes a little more creativity. You might nurse two babies at the same time while a third waits his or her turn. You may also choose to give a bottle to the third. At the next feeding, use the bottle for a different baby. The goal is that all three babies have a chance to feed at the breast.

If you're the parent of multiples, you may want to discuss a breast-feeding plan with your care provider or a lactation consultant before you leave the hospital. Ask them if they know of a mother who has successfully breast-fed her twins or triplets and who would be willing to offer support and practical advice.

What's the best way to store expressed breast milk? You can store expressed breast milk in the refrigerator or freezer. Using waterproof labels and ink, label each container with the date and time of your pumping. Place the containers in the back of the refrigerator or freezer, where the temperature is the coolest. Use your oldest pumped milk first.

To minimize waste, fill individual containers with the amount of milk your baby will need for one feeding. Also consider storing smaller portions — 1 to 2 ounces — for unexpected situations or delays in regular feedings. Keep in mind that breast milk expands as it freezes, so don't fill containers to the brim.

Can I add freshly expressed breast milk to already stored milk? You can add freshly expressed breast milk to refrigerated or frozen milk you expressed earlier in the same day. However, be sure to cool the freshly expressed breast milk in the refrigerator or a cooler with ice packs for at least one hour before adding it to previously chilled milk. Don't add warm breast milk to frozen breast milk, because it will cause the frozen milk to partially thaw. Keep milk expressed on different days in separate containers.

How long does expressed breast milk keep? The length of time you can safely keep expressed breast milk depends on the storage method.

▶ *Milk stored at room temperature.* Freshly expressed breast milk can be kept at room temperature — up to 77 F — for six to eight hours. If you won't use the milk that quickly, store it in the refrigerator or freezer.

▶ *Milk stored in an insulated cooler.* Freshly expressed breast milk can be stored in an insulated cooler with ice packs for up to 24 hours. Then use the

milk, or transfer the containers to the refrigerator or freezer.

▶ *Milk stored in the refrigerator.* Breast milk can be stored in the refrigerator at 39 F for up to five days.

▶ *Milk stored in the freezer.* Breast milk can be stored in a freezer compartment inside the refrigerator at 5 F for two weeks. If your freezer has a separate door and a temperature of 0 F, breast milk can be stored for three to six months. If you have a deep freezer that's opened infrequently and has a temperature of -4 F, breast milk can be stored for six to 12 months.

The sooner you use the milk, the better. Some research suggests that the longer you store breast milk — whether in the refrigerator or in the freezer — the greater the loss of vitamin C in the milk. Other studies have shown that refrigeration beyond two days may reduce the bacteria-killing properties of breast milk and long-term freezer storage may lower the quality of breast milk's healthy fats.

How do I thaw frozen breast milk? Thaw the oldest milk first. Simply place the frozen container in the refrigerator the night before you intend to use it. You can also gently warm the milk by placing it under warm running water or in a bowl of warm water. Avoid letting the water touch the mouth of the container.

Don't thaw frozen breast milk at room temperature, which enables bacteria to multiply in the milk. Also, don't heat a frozen bottle on the stove or in the microwave. These methods can create an uneven distribution of heat and destroy the milk's antibodies. Use thawed breast milk within 24 hours. Discard any remaining milk. Don't refreeze thawed or partially thawed breast milk.

Thawed breast milk may smell different from freshly expressed milk or taste soapy due to the breakdown of milk fats, but it's still safe for your baby to drink.

What else do I need to know about breast milk storage? During storage, expressed breast milk will separate — causing thick, white cream to rise to the top of the container. Before feeding your baby, gently swirl the contents of the container to ensure that the creamy portion of the milk is evenly distributed. Don't vigorously shake the container or stir the milk. Also be aware that the color of your breast milk may vary, depending on your diet.

Going back to work With a little planning and preparation, you can do both — breast-feed and return to work. Many women do this with the help of a breast pump.

Some mothers work at home, while some arrange to have their babies brought to them for feedings, or they go to the babies. Most mothers, though, use breast pumps to pump their breasts. You can provide your baby with bottled breast milk by expressing milk at work and saving the milk for the next day. Using a double breast pump is the most effective. A double breast pump requires about 15 minutes of pumping every three to four hours. If you need to increase your milk supply, nurse and pump more often.

If you choose not to express your milk while at work, you may pump milk at other times to provide breast milk for the next day. For example, pump after the morning feeding and after the feeding when you return home. As long as all of your milk produced in 24 hours is removed either by your baby or from pumping, you'll maintain a good supply.

You may decide to have your child-care provider give your baby infant formula. This will decrease your milk supply but allow enough to remain for nursing at home. To prevent overly full breasts at

---

INTRODUCING A BOTTLE

During the first several weeks of your child's life, it's best to nurse exclusively to help you and your baby learn how to breast-feed and to be sure your milk supply becomes well-established. Once your milk supply is established and you feel confident that you and your baby are doing well with breast-feeding, you may give your baby an occasional bottle of breast milk. This allows others, such as your partner or a grandparent, an opportunity to feed the baby. If your baby receives a bottle of milk, you may want to pump your breasts for your comfort and to maintain your milk supply.

The feel of a bottle nipple in a baby's mouth is different from that of the breast. The way a baby sucks from a bottle nipple also is different. It may take practice for your baby to be comfortable with a bottle nipple. A baby may initially be reluctant to take a bottle from mom because he or she associates mother's voice and scent with breast-feeding.

When you give your baby a supplementary bottle, follow your baby's cues as to the amount to give. There's no set amount that's right. Your baby may be satisfied with a few ounces.

work, some mothers find they need to give thawed breast milk or formula to their baby on days off from work at the same times the child care provider feeds the baby.

Once in a while, your baby may take a bottle, then later reject the breast. If this happens, hold your baby skin to skin and give baby extra cuddling and attention before feeding.

Donor milk If you've adopted your baby or can't provide your own milk to breast-feed your baby, donor milk may be an option. This is breast milk that has been purchased from a reputable milk bank, ideally a member of the Human Milk Banking Association of North America. Lactating women who are pre-screened for infectious diseases, medications and healthy lifestyle choices provide their milk as a donation. This milk is then pasteurized, tested for bacteria, packaged, and sold to private parties or hospitals.

Donor milk is an excellent and safe way to provide the benefits of breast milk in situations where it is otherwise unavailable. It can also be used with babies who are premature or have formula intolerance.

Be aware that purchasing breast milk online or through milk-sharing communities is not recommended. These venues have little to no control over the milk collection process, packaging, mailing or screening for infectious diseases. Because of this, the milk may pose serious risks to your baby's health.

BOTTLE-FEEDING

If you can't breast-feed or choose not to, be assured that your baby's nutrition can be met with the use of infant formula.

A wide variety of infant formulas are on the market. The majority of them are based on cow's milk. However, never use regular cow's milk as a substitute for formula. Although cow's milk is used as the foundation for formula, the milk has been changed dramatically to make it safe for babies. It's treated by heat to make the protein in it more digestible. More milk sugar (lactose) is added to make the concentration similar to that of breast milk, and the fat (butterfat) is removed and replaced with vegetable oils and animal fats that are more easily digested by infants.

Infant formulas contain the right amount of carbohydrates and the right

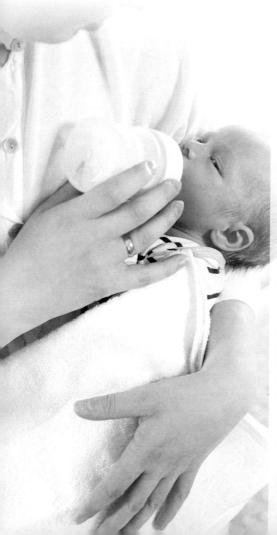

BREAST OR BOTTLE: FEEDING TIPS

At first, it may seem that all you do is feed your baby. How often you feed your baby depends on how often your baby is hungry, and one feeding may seem to blur right into the next. Breast-fed babies likely will want to be fed between eight and 12 times in 24 hours — about every two to three hours. And formula-fed babies probably will want to be fed between six and nine times in 24 hours — about every three to four hours — for the first few months of life.

Your baby won't always feed this often. As your baby matures, he or she will gradually need fewer daily feedings and eat more at each feeding. A feeding pattern and routine will begin to emerge after the first month or two. Expect that a newborn will wake routinely one or more times at night for feeding and that your baby may demand more milk during growth spurts.

Feed on cue The size of your infant's stomach is very small, about the size of his or her fist, and the time it takes to become empty varies from one to three hours. Feeding on cue requires you to watch for signs that a baby is ready to eat: Your baby makes sucking movements with his or her mouth or tongue (rooting), sucks on his or her fist, makes small sounds, and, of course, cries. The sensation that hunger produces often makes babies cry. You will soon be able to distinguish between cries for food and those for other reasons, such as pain, fatigue or illness. It's important to feed your baby promptly when he or she signals hunger. This helps your baby learn which kinds of discomfort mean hunger and that hunger can be satisfied by sucking, which brings food. If you don't respond promptly, your baby may become so upset that trying to feed at this point may prove more frustrating than satisfying.

Let baby set the pace Try not to rush your baby during a feeding. He or she will determine how much and how fast to eat. Many babies, like adults, prefer to eat in a relaxed manner. In fact, it's normal for an infant to nurse, pause, rest, socialize a bit and then return to feeding. Some newborns are speedy, efficient eaters, consistently whizzing through feedings. Other babies are grazers, preferring snack-sized feedings at frequent intervals. Still others, especially newborns, are snoozers. These babies may take a few vigorous sucks and blissfully doze off, then wake, feed and doze again intermittently throughout a typical feeding session.

Your baby will also let you know when he or she has had enough to eat. When your baby is satisfied, he or she will stop sucking, close his or her mouth, or turn away from the nipple. Your baby may push the nipple out of his or her mouth with his or her tongue, or your baby may arch his or her back if you try to continue feeding. If, however, your baby needs burping or is in the middle of a bowel movement, his or her mind may not be on eating. Wait a bit and then try offering the breast or bottle again.

percentages of fats and protein for babies. The Food and Drug Administration monitors the safety of commercially prepared infant formula. Each manufacturer must test each batch of formula to ensure it has the required nutrients and is free of contaminants.

Infant formula is designed to be an energy-dense food. More than half its calories are from fat. Many different types of fatty acids make up that fat. Those that go into infant formula are specifically selected because they're similar to those found in breast milk. These fatty acids help in the development of your baby's brain and nervous system, as well as in meeting his or her energy needs.

Pros vs. cons Parents who bottle-feed feel the main advantage of a bottle is:

- *Flexibility.* Using a bottle with formula allows more than one person to feed the baby. For that reason, some mothers feel they have more freedom when they're bottle-feeding. Partners may like bottle-feeding because it allows them to share more easily in the feeding responsibilities.

Bottle-feeding can also present some challenges, such as:

- *Time-consuming preparation.* Bottles must be prepared for each feeding. You need a steady supply of formula. Bottles and nipples need to be washed. If you go out, you may need to take formula with you.
- *Cost.* Formula is costly, which is a concern for some parents.
- *Formula intolerance.* It may take time to find a formula that works well for some infants.

Bottle-feeding basics The first time you purchase infant formula, you may be surprised by how many different types are available. Consult your baby's care provider for advice about choosing the right formula. For most babies, an iron-fortified, cow's-milk-based formula is the best choice.

Several special formulas also are available, such as those containing soy protein and protein hydrolysates. These formulas are made for specific digestive problems and should be used only under a care provider's direction.

Iron-fortified formula is important for preventing anemia and iron deficiency, which can cause slow development. In general, iron deficiency isn't a risk in the

---

BE FLEXIBLE

Don't expect your baby to eat the same amount every day. Babies vary in how much they eat, especially if they're experiencing a growth spurt. At these times, your baby will need and demand more milk and more-frequent feedings. It may seem like your baby can't get full. During these times, you may need to put your baby to your breast or offer a bottle more often.

Most babies don't eat at precise intervals throughout the day, as you might first expect. Most babies bunch (cluster) their feedings at various times of the day and night. It's common for a baby to eat several times within a few hours and then sleep for a few hours.

first few months of a baby's life. However, it can occur later in the first year. Iron deficiency in 6- to 10-month-old infants was common before iron supplementation became routine.

Infant formulas come in three forms: powder, liquid concentrate and ready-to-feed liquid. Both the powder and concentrate liquid formulas must have a specific amount of water added to them. Dry powder formulas generally are the least expensive. Ready-to-feed brands offer great convenience.

If you decide to bottle-feed your baby with infant formula, you'll need the right supplies on hand when you bring your baby home from the hospital. Let the medical staff assisting your birth know of your plans to bottle-feed. The staff at the hospital or birthing center can provide bottle-feeding equipment and formula during your recovery and show you how to bottle-feed your newborn. But you will still need to stock up on your own supplies.

The equipment needed for bottle-feeding typically includes:

▶ A variety of bottle sizes
▶ Eight to 10 nipples of different flow rates
▶ A measuring cup
▶ A bottle brush
▶ Infant formula

In addition to buying the right equipment, consider requesting instruction about formula preparation and bottle feeding in the hospital. If you've never bottle-fed a baby before, hands-on instruction will help you feel more comfortable when you bring your baby home.

Getting started The bottles for feeding your baby can be glass, plastic or plastic with a soft plastic liner. Bottles generally come in two sizes: 4 ounces and 8 ounces. The amount the bottle holds isn't an indication of how much your baby needs to drink in a feeding. Your baby may need less or more for any given feeding.

Many types of nipples are on the market, which have openings sized according to a baby's age. For many babies, it makes little difference which nipples you use. But for a full-term baby, don't select overly soft nipples designed for use by a premature baby. A full-term baby should use a regular nipple. Use the same kind of nipple for all the bottles.

Nipples come in sizes for a newborn, 3-month-old, 6-month-old and so on, making the flow rate appropriate for the baby's age.

It's important that formula flows from the nipple at the correct speed. Milk flow that's either too fast or too slow can cause your baby to swallow too much air, leading to stomach discomfort and the need for frequent burping. Test the flow of the nipple by turning the bottle upside down and timing the drops. One drop per second is about right.

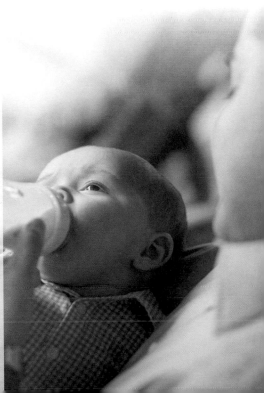

Preparing formula Commercial infant formulas are regulated by the Food and Drug Administration. Three major types are available:

- *Cow's milk formulas*. Most infant formula is made with cow's milk that has been altered to resemble breast milk. This gives the formula the right balance of nutrients and makes the formula easier to digest. Most babies do well on cow's milk formula. But some babies, such as those allergic to the proteins in cow's milk, need other types of infant formula.
- *Soy-based formulas*. Soy-based infant formulas may be an option for babies who can't tolerate or allergic to cow's milk formula or to lactose, a sugar naturally found in cow's milk. However, babies who are allergic to cow's milk may also be allergic to soy milk. Babies who are born pre-term should not be given soy-based formula, as it

has lower availability of the nutrients calcium and phosphorous.
- *Protein hydrolysate formulas.* These are meant for babies who have a family history of milk or soy allergies. Protein hydrolysate formulas are easier to digest and less likely to cause allergic reactions than are other types of formula. They are also called hypoallergenic formulas.

In addition, specialized formulas are available for premature infants and babies who have specific medical conditions.

Whatever type and form of formula you choose, proper preparation and refrigeration are essential, both to ensure the appropriate amount of nutrition and to safeguard the health of your baby.

Wash your hands before handling formula or the equipment used to prepare it. All equipment that you use to measure, mix and store formula should be washed with hot, soapy water and then rinsed and dried before every use. Sterilizing bottles and nipples isn't necessary as long as you wash and rinse them well. Use a bottle brush to wash bottles. Brush or rub the nipples thoroughly to remove any traces of formula. Rinse well. You can also clean bottles and nipples in the dishwasher.

Whether using powder formula or liquid concentrate formula, always add the exact amount of water specified on the label. Measurements on bottles may be inaccurate, so pre-measure the water before adding it to the formula. Using too much or too little water can be harmful to your baby. If formula is too diluted, your baby won't get enough nutrition for his or her growth needs and to satisfy his or her hunger. Formula that's too concentrated puts strain on the baby's digestive system and kidneys, and could dehydrate your baby. Generally, you can store all prepared formula or liquid concentrate in

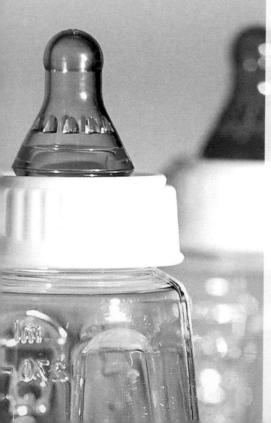

the refrigerator for up to 48 hours. After that, throw away all unused formula.

Warming formula isn't necessary for nutritional purposes, but your baby may prefer it warm. To warm formula, set the bottle in a pan of warm water for a few minutes. Shake the bottle and test the temperature of the milk by dropping a few drops of formula on the top of your hand. Don't microwave formula, because this can cause hot spots that can burn your baby's mouth. Once you warm formula, don't refrigerate the leftovers. Discard the unused portions of formula.

In general, it's best to make up formula when you need it, not in advance. However, you may prefer to make up a bottle or two in the evening and store them in the refrigerator for use that night. This can help make nighttime feedings easier.

Getting into position The first step to bottle-feeding is to make sure you and baby are both comfortable. Find a quiet place where you and your baby won't be distracted. Cradle your baby in one arm, hold the bottle with the other and settle into a comfortable chair, preferably one with broad, low armrests. You may want to put a pillow on your lap under the baby for support. Pull your baby in toward you snugly but not too tightly, cradled in your arm with his or her head raised slightly and resting in the bend of your elbow. This semi-upright position makes swallowing much easier.

Now that you're ready to start feeding, help your newborn get ready. Using the nipple of the bottle or a finger of the hand holding it, gently stroke your baby's cheek near the mouth, on the side nearest you. The touch will cause your baby to turn toward you. Then touch the nipple to your baby's lips or the corner of the mouth. Your baby will open his or her mouth and gradually begin sucking.

When feeding your baby, position the bottle at about a 45-degree angle. This angle keeps the nipple full of milk. Hold the bottle steady as your baby feeds. If your baby falls asleep while bottle-feeding, it may be because he or she has had enough milk, or gas has made your baby full. Take the bottle away and burp your baby, then start to feed again.

Always hold your baby while feeding. Never prop a bottle up against your infant. Propping may lead to overeating and is also a choking hazard. In addition, never give a bottle to your baby when he or she is lying on his or her back. This may increase your baby's risk of developing an ear infection.

Although your baby doesn't have teeth yet, they're forming beneath the gums. Don't develop a habit of putting your baby to sleep with a bottle. Formula lingers in the mouth when a baby falls asleep while sucking a bottle. The prolonged contact of sugar in milk can cause tooth decay.

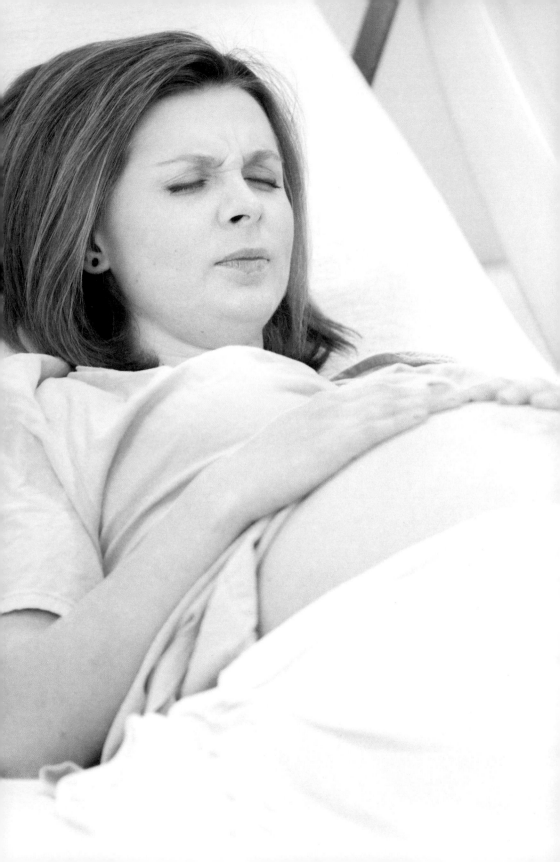

CHAPTER 23

Pain relief during childbirth

What type of pain management is best during labor? The answer to that question largely depends on your preferences and on how your labor progresses. No two women have the same tolerance for pain. No two labors are exactly the same, either. Some women need little or no pain medication. Others find that pain relief gives them a better sense of control over their labors and deliveries. Ultimately, you need to choose what's right for you.

The decision of whether to use medication during labor and delivery is yours. However, it should take into account your care provider's recommendations, and it will depend in part on what's available where you give birth and the specific character of your labor.

Sometimes you won't know what kind of pain relief you want until you're in labor. Your capacity to deal with pain during childbirth can be affected by factors such as the length of your labor, the size and position of your baby, and how rested you are as labor begins. No one can predict how you'll cope with the pain

of your first labor, and subsequent labors often don't follow the same pattern.

Before that first contraction kicks in, it's a good idea to think about the method, or methods, of pain relief you might prefer. It may also be helpful to discuss your preferences with your care provider. Whatever birth plan you ultimately devise, keep an open mind about it. Labors often don't go according to plan.

In addition, when making your decision, keep in mind that birth isn't a test of endurance. You won't have failed if you ask for pain medication.

ISSUES TO CONSIDER

To help you choose the pain relief method or methods that are right for you, keep these questions in mind as you review your options. Ask yourself:

▶ What's involved in the method?
▶ How will it affect me?
▶ How will it affect my baby?

- How quickly will it work?
- How long will the pain relief last?
- Do I need to organize or practice the method in advance?
- Can I combine it with other pain relief methods?
- Can I use it at home before I go to the hospital?
- When during labor is the method available?

YOUR OPTIONS

Women have more options for managing the discomforts of childbirth than ever before. These options generally fall into two broad categories: pain medications and natural pain relief methods. Learning about your options ahead of time will help you make an informed decision about pain relief during labor and delivery.

When it comes to childbirth, education itself may be a form of pain relief. Fear has been shown to worsen the pain of labor. If you know what to expect during labor and delivery and you've reviewed your pain relief choices, you'll likely get through childbirth more smoothly than if you were tense and fearful.

Pain medications Medications to relieve pain are called analgesics. Anesthetics, another type of pain medication, work by more fully blocking any feeling. Both types of pain medications are commonly used during labor, particularly local anesthetics and opioids (a type of analgesic). In expert hands, these medications are very useful and quite reliable.

Depending on the types of drugs and doses used, pain medications during childbirth can either lessen the pain of labor and delivery (analgesia) — without affecting consciousness — or they can remove sensation (anesthesia). Two examples of anesthetic techniques used in childbirth are epidural blocks and spinal blocks. With these pain relief options, local anesthetic may be injected near nerves of the spinal cord, helping to block feeling in the whole lower region. In a cesarean birth, a higher dose of anesthesia or general anesthesia can be used for complete loss of feeling in the area (see page 229).

Natural methods Natural methods refer to labor and delivery techniques that don't involve the use of pain medications. Natural pain relief methods take many forms, some dating back centuries. Some natural methods are most effective if practiced regularly before your labor. Relaxation and massage are two examples of pain relief options of natural childbirth.

PAIN MEDICATIONS

Pain medication can be a valuable tool during your labor and delivery. It helps reduce your discomfort and allows you to rest during your labor.

You're free to request or refuse pain medications during your labor and delivery, but remember that medications may have different benefits and risks at different times during labor. You always need to take into account the course and progress of your labor when choosing a pain relief method.

The stage of labor at which you take certain medications is as important as the type of drug taken. A baby can be affected by medication you take, but the extent of that effect depends on the type of medication, the dose and how close to delivery it's administered. For example, if enough time passes between when you receive an opioid pain medication intravenously and

WHAT'S A DOULA?

A doula is someone who is specifically trained to be a labor coach. Women have been assisting one another through labor for centuries, but the role of the doula is a more formal and modern interpretation of assisted birth. For some women, as they prepare for labor and childbirth, hiring a doula becomes part of their over-all birth plan.

What do doulas do? A doula's main role is to help pregnant women through childbirth. A doula won't take the place of your labor coach or the medical experts caring for you during your labor and delivery. She is there to offer additional sup-port and expertise. Most doulas are mothers themselves. Many doulas also un-dergo training in childbirth.

Some doulas become involved early on in your pregnancy, helping to educate you on what to expect during labor and delivery and to create a birth plan. If you request it, your doula can come to your home during early labor to coach you through your beginning contractions.

But the real work of doulas becomes evident at the hospital or birthing center. A doula can offer you — and your partner — continuous support once your labor has started. She can lend an extra hand, bringing you ice chips or massaging your back. She can help you with your breathing and relaxation techniques. She can advise you on labor positions. Most important, doulas provide both you and your partner with welcome words of encouragement and reassurance.

A doula can also serve as a mediator, helping you make educated decisions during labor. She can explain medical terms and procedures. She can indicate your wishes to your care provider for you. However, doulas don't perform medical exams or assist in the actual birth, and they can't give or deny your consent for a medical procedure.

Doulas provide expectant parents with extra attention and care as they bring their new babies into the world. Doulas give emotional support, which may be important to women during childbirth. Some studies indicate that women who have the support of doulas tend to have fewer complications in childbirth.

A doula, however, is not essential or commonplace. Doulas can be most help-ful for first-time mothers, especially single mothers who have no other long-term support. For many pregnant women, the functions offered by a doula may be more comfortably provided by a partner or family member. In addition, most labor and delivery units have very high nurse-to-patient ratios — often one-to-one — so many of the services a doula provides may be redundant with those that a nurse is ready to offer.

How do you find a doula? Your doctor or the hospital or birthing center where you plan to deliver may be able to provide you with a list of names. Some hospitals and birthing centers offer doula services. Most doulas charge a one-time fee for their services, and many base their fees on a sliding scale. The cost of a doula may not be covered by your insurance, so check with your insurance provider.

when your baby is born, your body will process the drug, and your baby will have minimal effects from the medication at birth. If not, the baby may be sleepy and have trouble latching and feeding if you try to nurse soon after delivery. Less frequently, the baby may experience breathing difficulties. Any such effects on the newborn are short-lived and can be treated, if necessary.

The care provider with you during labor and delivery is there to ensure that your baby arrives safely and in good health. He or she is familiar with each medication option and can share this knowledge with you. Trust him or her to tell you when it's safe — or not — to take medications. Understand that you may not always be able to have a medication when you feel you need it.

Epidural block An epidural block is a regional analgesic or anesthetic (or a combination) that can be used during labor or before a cesarean section. The medication is administered into the lower back, just outside the bag of fluid surrounding the spinal cord, through a thin tube (catheter) that remains in place. It takes about 10 to 20 minutes to administer an epidural block and another 10 to 20 minutes for the medication to take effect.

Pros An epidural block alleviates most pain in your lower body without significantly slowing labor, and it's safe for your baby. Medication slowly flows from the epidural pump through a catheter to provide continuous pain relief. You remain awake and alert while receiving the medication. By pressing a button, you may be able to give yourself small, additional doses of medication, if needed.

Cons An epidural may decrease your blood pressure, which can slow the baby's

heart rate. Your care providers will monitor your blood pressure after epidural placement and treat low blood pressure, if necessary. Rarely, you may have a severe headache when you're upright in the days after delivery. If an epidural is used during cesarean birth, the numbness it causes may affect your chest wall and for a while you may feel as if you're having difficulty breathing. Because epidural anesthesia may block the ability to empty your bladder, you may need a urinary catheter.

Approximately 7 to 10 percent of epidurals do not adequately relieve labor pain. For example, it may work on one side of your body more than the other. You may want another procedure if the epidural doesn't work as well as expected.

Spinal block Spinal anesthesia is a regional anesthetic used shortly before a C-section or during active labor if delivery is expected very quickly. The medication is injected directly into the fluid surrounding the spinal cord in the lower back and takes effect quickly.

Pros A spinal block provides complete pain relief from the chest down for up to two hours. The medication is usually given only once. You'll remain awake and alert.

Cons Similar to an epidural block, a spinal block may decrease your blood pressure — which can slow the baby's heart rate — and cause a headache in the days after delivery. If the anesthesia affects your chest wall, you may temporarily experience a sensation of difficulty breathing, and because spinal anesthesia blocks the ability to empty your bladder, you may need a urinary catheter.

Combined spinal epidural This technique offers the rapid pain relief of a spi-

RECEIVING AN EPIDURAL BLOCK

To receive an epidural block:

1. You sit on the bed with your back rounded, or lie on your side in a curled-up position.
2. The doctor numbs an area of your back with a local anesthetic.
3. The doctor inserts a needle into the epidural space just outside the membrane that encloses the spinal fluid and spinal nerves.
4. A thin, flexible tube (catheter) is threaded through the needle, and the needle is removed. The catheter is taped in place.
5. The medication is injected through the catheter. The medication flows through the catheter to surround the nerves, blocking the pain.

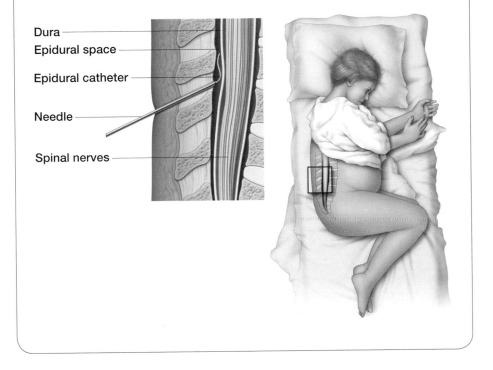

Dura
Epidural space
Epidural catheter
Needle
Spinal nerves

nal block and the continuous relief of an epidural.

An anesthesiologist or nurse anesthetist carefully guides an epidural needle into your lower back. He or she places the narrower spinal needle inside the epidural needle (so you only need to be stuck once), guides it through the membrane surrounding your spine and injects a small dose of medication into your spinal fluid. The spinal needle is then removed, but the epidural catheter remains in place.

In early labor, you rely primarily on the opioids in the spinal injection for pain relief for the first hour or two. Then the anesthetic given through the epidural catheter provides pain control to the area.

Opioids Various opioids may be injected into a muscle in your thigh or buttock or given through an intravenous (IV) catheter. If you have an IV, you may be able to control your dosage. The medication takes effect in minutes.

Pros Opioids decrease the perception of pain for two to six hours. They promote rest without causing muscle weakness.

Cons Opioids may cause sleepiness and temporarily depress breathing for you or the baby. Your baby may experience temporarily slowed reflexes as well.

Local anesthetic A local anesthetic is typically the main medication used in epidurals to provide regional pain relief. It also may be used to numb the vaginal area if you need an incision to extend the opening of the vagina (episiotomy) or repair a tear after delivery. When used for this purpose, the medication is injected into tissue at the vaginal opening and takes effect quickly.

Pros Local anesthetics temporarily relieve pain in a specific area. Negative effects for mother or baby are rare.

Cons Local anesthetics don't relieve the contraction pain. An allergic reaction is possible. Rarely, injecting the medication into a vein may decrease your blood pressure.

Nitrous oxide Commonly known as laughing gas, nitrous oxide is a gas that can be inhaled to reduce labor pain. It is typically self-administered by holding a mask over your face and breathing in a mixture of nitrous oxide and oxygen from a portable tank. A growing number of birthing centers in the United States are making it available to women in labor.

Pros While it provides limited pain relief, nitrous oxide is associated with high maternal satisfaction, is extremely safe for you and your baby, and can be used off and on throughout labor as you want.

Cons The actual pain relief provided by nitrous oxide is much less than with an epidural. Common side effects can include nausea, drowsiness and dizziness.

NATURAL METHODS

Although many women choose to have pain medication during labor, women give birth all of the time without it. If you want to accomplish it, you can do it!

With natural methods of pain management, you forgo the use of drugs for pain relief and instead rely on other methods to lessen pain. Natural (nonmedicinal) methods of pain relief work in a variety of ways. They may stimulate your body to release its own natural painkillers (endorphins). These substances distract you from your pain, and they can soothe and relax you, allowing you to stay more in control.

Natural pain relief methods will help you manage pain, but they won't stop it entirely. Before considering pain relief medications, many women will try nondrug measures first to relieve pain during labor.

Natural methods to manage the discomfort of labor can be used throughout the entire process of labor and birth. They are also useful for women who know they will eventually choose to have pain medications or an epidural, to bridge the gap until that time.

Natural pain relief options include breathing and relaxation techniques and many other methods.

Breathing techniques Breathing techniques, like other natural pain relief options, don't involve drugs or require medical supervision. You're in control. They involve the use of practiced, paced breathing during contractions.

Concentrating on your breathing helps distract you from the pain and relaxes your muscles so that tension, which heightens pain, is eased. Deep, controlled, slow breathing can also reduce nausea and dizziness. Perhaps most important, concentrated breathing helps bring oxygen to you and your baby.

It's best to learn about and practice breathing techniques before you go into labor. Breathing methods are taught in most childbirth classes. Take your labor coach with you to class so that he or she can help you with the techniques during labor. The more you practice, the more natural it will be to use these methods once contractions begin.

Breathing exercises can work immediately, should you choose to use them. However, these methods aren't always successful because they depend on your reaction to labor pain, which can't be predicted, and on your ability to concentrate on something other than your contractions. Breathing techniques can be combined with other types of pain relief.

Lamaze method The Lamaze philosophy holds that birth is a natural, normal, healthy process, and women can be empowered through education and support to approach childbirth with confidence. Lamaze is known for a technique of conscious breathing used in labor.

Lamaze classes focus on relaxation techniques, but they also encourage you to actively help your body progress through labor. For example, you're taught different movements to try and controlled breathing exercises, which are more constructive ways to deal with pain and help your birth progress naturally than are holding your breath and tensing your muscles.

As your contractions intensify, you might take a deep, cleansing breath to begin and end each one: Inhale through your nose, imagining cool, pure air. Exhale slowly through your mouth, imagining tension blowing away. The deep breath signals your body to relax, pulls in oxygen and helps you focus.

Different levels of Lamaze breathing are available to use in labor and delivery, as outlined below. Try the first breathing technique and use it as long as it works for you, then move on to the next level. Find a variation or pattern that feels right to you at each stage of your labor.

Lamaze level 1: Slow-pace breathing. This is the type of breathing you use when you're relaxed or sleeping. Take in slow, deep breaths through your nose and exhale through your mouth at about half the speed of your normal rate. If you like, repeat a phrase with the breathing: "I am (inhaling) relaxed (exhaling)," or "In one-two-three (inhaling), out one-two-three (exhaling)." Or breathe in rhythm while walking or rocking.

Lamaze level 2: Modified-pace breathing. Breathe faster than your normal rate but shallowly enough to prevent hyperventilation: "In one-two (inhaling), out one-two (exhaling), in one-two (inhaling), out one-two (exhaling)." Keep your body, particularly your jaw, relaxed. Concentrate on the rhythm, which may be faster at the height of the contraction, then slower as it fades.

Lamaze level 3: Pattern-pace breathing. Use this type near the end of labor or at the height of strong contractions. The rate is a little faster than normal, as with modified-pace breathing, but now you use a pant-blow rhythm such as "ha-ha-ha-hoo" or "hee-hee-hee-hoo" that forces you to focus on the breathing rather than the pain. Repeat the pattern. Start slowly. Increase the speed as each contraction peaks and decrease as it fades. Keep in mind that when you increase the rate, the breathing should become shallower so that you don't hyperventilate — if your hands or feet tingle, slow down. It's possible to remove too much carbon dioxide from your body, which can lead to these symptoms. If moaning or making other noises helps, go ahead. Keep your eyes open and focused and your muscles relaxed.

Breathing to prevent pushing. You may feel the urge to push before your cervix is fully dilated. If that happens and you must hold back, blow out tiny puffs with your cheeks — as if you're blowing out birthday candles, or a rapid "pa-pa-pa" — until the urge to push passes.

Breathing for pushing. When your cervix is fully dilated and your care provider tells you to go ahead and push, take a couple of deep breaths and bear down when you feel the urge. Push for about 10 seconds. Exhale. Then take in another breath and push again. Some women will feel more power if they hold their breath while pushing, while others will naturally let the air out slowly during the push. Do what feels right to you. Contractions at this stage will last for a minute or more, so take time to rest fully and gain strength between your pushing efforts.

Your personal preferences and the nature of your contractions will guide you in deciding when to use breathing exercises in your labor. You can choose breathing techniques or invent one on your own. Even if you plan on having pain medication during labor, it's still important to learn breathing and relaxation techniques.

Relaxation techniques Relaxation is the release of tension from the mind and body through conscious effort. By reducing muscle tension during labor and delivery, you can short-circuit a cycle of fear, tension and pain. Relaxation allows your body to work more naturally, helping you conserve energy for the work ahead. Relaxation and patterned breathing are mainstays of the self-comforting measures women use for labor. These methods and others are usually taught in childbirth classes.

Relaxation doesn't mean fighting the pain, which would actually create more tension. Instead, it means allowing the pain to roll over you while you concentrate on exercises to relieve tension and distract you from sensations of pain.

Relaxation is actually a learned skill and one that will be most effective if you practice it before the onset of labor. The more proficient you become at it, the more self-confident you'll be during labor. Here are some tips for mastering self-relaxation:

- Choose a quiet environment in which to practice.
- Turn on soft music, if you want.
- Assume a comfortable position with pillows to support you.
- Use slow, deep abdominal breathing. Feel the coolness of the air as you breathe in. Feel the tension carried away as you breathe out.
- Become aware of areas of tension in your body and concentrate on relaxing them.

Progressive relaxation With this technique, you relax groups of muscles in a series between or during your contractions or at periodic times during labor when you feel yourself becoming tense. Beginning with your head or feet, relax one muscle group at a time, moving toward the other end of your body. If you have trouble isolating the muscles, first tense each group for a few seconds, then release and feel the tension melt away. Pay particular attention to relaxing your jaw and hands.

Touch relaxation This is similar to progressive relaxation, but your cue for releasing each muscle group is when your labor coach presses on that area of your body. He or she should apply firm pressure or rub using small circular movements for five to 10 seconds, then move on to the next spot. For example, your labor coach could start by rubbing your temples and move on to touching the base of your skull, and then points on your back and shoulders, your arms and hands, and finally, your legs and feet.

Massage During labor, various massage techniques may help relax you. These techniques may include light or firm rhythmic stroking over your shoulders, neck, back, abdomen and legs; firm kneading, friction or pressure on your feet and hands; or a fingertip massage of your scalp.

Massage can soothe aching and tense muscles, as well as stimulate your skin and deeper tissues. It can be used at any time during labor. In addition to encouraging relaxation, massage blocks pain sensations. Some women feel most of the pain of labor in their backs, and for them, a back massage given by a labor coach can really help. You may find yourself requesting that your labor coach push hard on your lower back, because

counterpressure can be a very effective natural pain relief method for back labor.

Before labor, you and your labor coach may want to establish the kinds of massage you prefer. But keep in mind that you'll both want to remain flexible when the time comes.

Guided imagery This technique helps laboring mothers create an environment with a feeling of relaxation and well-being. Sometimes called visualization, this method can be used anytime during your labor to help you relax. It involves imagining yourself in a comfortable and peaceful place. For example, you may picture yourself sitting on a warm, sandy beach or walking through a lush, green forest. Your chosen place can be real or imaginary. Sometimes you can enhance the imagery by playing tapes of surf, rain, waterfalls, birds in the woods or any soft music you enjoy.

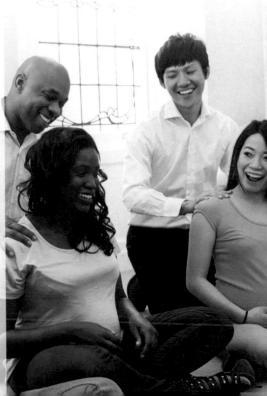

Hypnotherapy "Hypnobirthing" is a birthing method that teaches you self-hypnosis and relaxation techniques to help you achieve a peaceful and empowering birth. In a hypnobirthing class, taught by a certified instructor, you learn to focus your thoughts and trust your body, and you are always in control. Hypnobirthing is typically most successful with a partner and when practiced during the pregnancy. Search your area for classes or instructors.

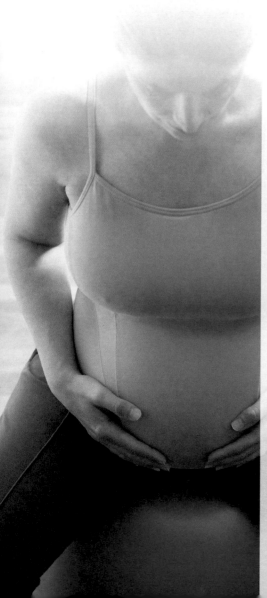

Meditation Focusing on a calming object, image or word can help relax you during labor and reduce the amount of pain you experience. Focus on a single point. This can be something in the room, such as a picture you have brought along, or it can be a mental image or a word you repeat to yourself over and over. When distracting thoughts come into your consciousness, allow them to pass by without dwelling on them and bring your focus back to your chosen focal point.

Aromatherapy To trigger relaxation and ease pain naturally during labor, try using comforting smells. When you're at home, light a scented candle or burn incense. When you're at the hospital or birthing center, bring along a pillow scented with your favorite fragrance. Or, if allowed, have your labor coach use a lightly scented oil or lotion during massage. Aromatherapy may relax you and reduce stress and tension. However, being in labor may make you sensitive to certain smells.

Music Music allows you to focus your attention on something other than your pain and helps you relax during childbirth. If you've been practicing relaxation techniques or breathing methods to music at home, bring the same technology with you to the hospital or birthing center. Music can be an excellent distraction.

Other techniques These natural techniques can help you manage the discomfort of labor beyond general relaxation.

Mindfulness This practice focuses on purposefully and nonjudgmentally paying attention to what you're experiencing in the present moment. Mindfulness practice has been shown to help people reduce stress and manage chronic pain, and in recent years, interest is growing in its potential to improve the childbirth experience for parents. Training in mindfulness teaches skills to help parents weather difficult and painful moments with less fear and stress — in labor and in life. Look for Mindfulness-Based Childbirth and Parenting programs near you, or the childbirth-focused Mind in Labor course (see page 151). Mindfulness is another method you'll want to practice beforehand to reap the benefits in labor.

Changing positions Moving about freely during labor allows you to find the most comfortable positions. So change positions often if you're able, experimenting to find the ones most comfortable for you. Be upright when possible to utilize gravity. Frequent position changes also can help the baby adjust his or her head to find the perfect position within the pelvis. Moving helps improve your circulation, too. Try a new position whenever you feel like it. Some women find that rhythmic movements, such as rocking in a chair or rocking back and forth on their hands and knees can be a soothing distraction from pain.

Heat and cold Applying heat or cold during labor may help make you more comfortable so that you can better relax. You may want to use a combination of both.

Heat relieves muscle tension. It can be applied through a heating pad, a warm towel, a hot compress, a hot water bottle, or a heated rice-filled pack or sock. You can apply heat to your shoulders, lower abdomen or back to relieve pain.

Cold can be applied with a cold pack, a chilled soda can or a baggie filled with ice. Some women like a cold pack on the lower back to help relieve back pain. You may find that a cool, moistened washcloth on your face helps ease tension and cools you during labor. Sucking on ice chips also can help cool you and create a distracting sensation in your mouth.

Hydrotherapy Most hospitals and birthing centers have showers, bathtubs or whirlpool baths in their labor rooms to help ease the discomforts of labor. The soothing, warm water helps relieve pain naturally by blocking pain impulses to your brain. Warm water is also relaxing. You can try this method of pain relief at home, too.

If you use a shower, you may want to sit in a chair and direct water onto your back or abdomen with a hand-held showerhead. Ask your labor coach to bring a bathing suit and join you.

Birthing ball Leaning or sitting on a large rubber ball (birthing ball) can decrease the discomfort of your contractions, relieve the pain of back labor and aid in the descent of your baby into the birth canal. Your hospital or birthing center may provide one for you. Or you may need to bring one with you. Have someone on your care team show you how to get the most out of a birthing ball. Its use can be combined with other techniques, such as massage and touch relaxation.

Sterile water injections To ease low back pain in labor, your care provider may inject a small amount of sterile water just under your skin on the low back. Ideally the sterile water is given in four injection sites, but even two can give relief. You'll feel an immediate sting that goes away in about 60 seconds. The majority of women who try water injections gain significant relief from their back pain. The relief lasts for about 90 minutes, and the injections can be repeated. Experts think this method works by fooling pain receptors in the affected area, in addition to causing a release of local endorphins.

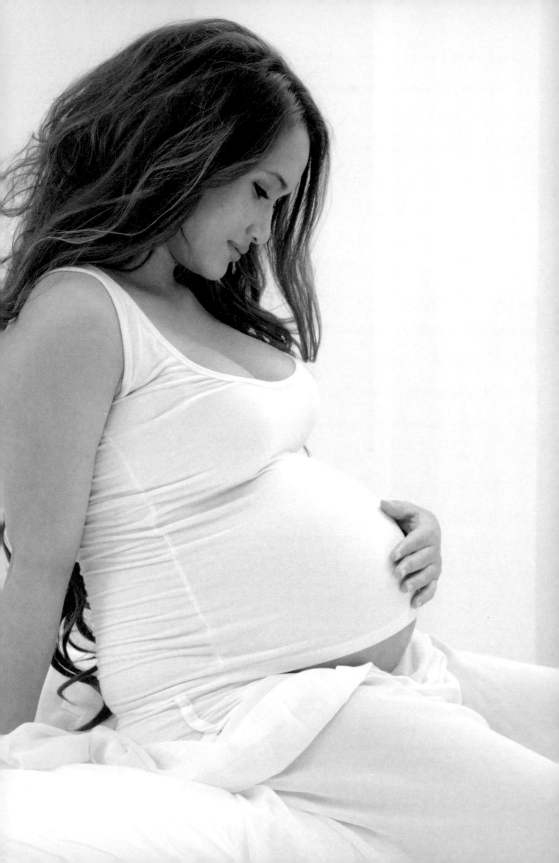

CHAPTER 24

Elective cesarean birth

Some women who are enjoying a healthy pregnancy will request a cesarean delivery — even when there are no pregnancy complications or problems with the baby. Some of these women want the convenience of scheduling the birth, to avoid waiting for an unknown date. For other women, their preference for a cesarean birth (C-section) is driven by fear:

▶ Fear of labor and delivery and the pain associated with both
▶ Fear of damage to the pelvic floor
▶ Fear of sexual problems after birth

If this is your first baby, labor and delivery is an unknown, and that can be scary. You may have heard frightening stories about childbirth, or about women leaking urine when they laugh or cough after having a baby. If you had a previous vaginal delivery and it didn't go well, you may be afraid of a repeat experience.

If you're considering an elective C-section, talk candidly with your care provider. If fear is your major motivation, a frank discussion of what to expect might help, along with childbirth education classes. When someone starts to tell you about a difficult birth experience, politely but firmly say that you'll be glad to listen after your baby is born.

If you had a previous vaginal delivery that was especially difficult, remind yourself that no two labors are alike and that giving birth this time may be a much different experience. Examine what made the last birth so bad, and then discuss it with your care provider or a support person. There may be things you can do to help ensure a more positive birth experience this time.

If your care provider supports your request for an elective C-section, the decision is up to you. However, it should generally be scheduled for no earlier than 39 weeks into your pregnancy, to help ensure your baby's safety. If your provider is not able to support your request — he or she will not perform an elective C-section — you can ask your provider to refer you to another medical professional who will do the procedure. Educate yourself about the risks and benefits of both ways of delivery, and discuss the pros and cons with your health care team — but don't let fear be the deciding factor.

ISSUES TO CONSIDER

Elective cesarean birth is controversial. Those in favor of it say that a woman has a right to choose how she wants to deliver her child. Those against it say that the risks of cesarean birth outweigh any potential benefits. To date, there's no convincing evidence in the medical liter-

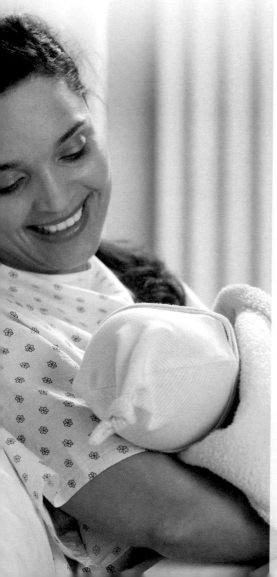

ature indicating an advantage to elective cesarean deliveries. Good medical practice generally resists doing procedures — especially surgical ones — that have no clear advantage to a person's health. Only a few studies have addressed the issue.

Because the procedure is controversial, you might find that care providers' opinions on this subject are quite varied. Some are willing to consider it. Others will not perform the procedure, believing that an elective cesarean birth could potentially be harmful and, therefore, against their medical pledge to do no harm.

The best way to make a decision is to be as informed as possible. Ask yourself why this approach is attractive to you. Research the issue thoroughly, talk to your health care team, and carefully weigh the pros and cons of the procedure.

BENEFITS VS. RISKS

Most health professionals believe that with the advances in surgical techniques, elective cesarean births are virtually as safe as vaginal deliveries if this is your first child. The same is not true if you've already had two or more C-sections. In this situation, an elective cesarean delivery carries the risk of more complications than a vaginal birth does. Here are several benefits and risks of the procedure to consider.

Maternal benefits Some of the suggested benefits that could come with an elective C-section include:

Protection against urinary incontinence Some women fear that the effort involved in pushing a baby through the birth canal may cause fecal or urinary incontinence, damage pelvic muscles, or injure pelvic nerves. Medical evidence has shown that women who have a cesarean delivery may have a decreased risk of urinary incontinence in the months shortly after delivery. However, that benefit doesn't appear to remain two to five years later. Some women are also concerned that a vaginal delivery may lead to pelvic organ prolapse, a condition where organs such as the bladder and uterus protrude into the vaginal canal. In current evidence, the relationship between elective cesarean birth and decreased pelvic organ prolapse isn't completely clear. But having an elective C-section doesn't guarantee that problems with incontinence or prolapse won't occur. The weight of the baby during pregnancy, pregnancy hormones and genetic factors may weaken pelvic muscles, leading to symptoms of incontinence or prolapse. Even women who've never had babies can develop these problems.

Avoidance of an emergency C-section An emergency C-section, which is usually performed during a difficult labor, has higher risks than both an elective C-section or a vaginal birth. Risks associated with an emergency C-section include infection, a greater chance of injury to organs in the abdomen and pelvis, and bleeding complications.

Avoidance of difficult labor Sometimes, a difficult labor may lead to a forceps or vacuum-assisted delivery. These methods usually don't pose a problem. As with cesarean births, their safety is dependent on the skill of the individual performing the procedure.

Fewer childbirth problems Theoretically, a planned cesarean birth may reduce rare childbirth problems. It might reduce labor-related infant death, shoulder dystocia, birth injury — which is a particular concern for high-risk women who have large babies — and breathing in of meconium, which occurs when a baby has a bowel movement prior to delivery and inhales fecal material. The events of labor also carry a very small risk of cerebral palsy. It's important to remember that the risk of these complications is low with a vaginal delivery, and having an elective cesarean birth is not a guarantee that these problems won't occur.

Decreased postpartum hemorrhage In elective cesarean births, the risk of postpartum hemorrhaging is lower than the combined risk in planned vaginal births and emergency C-sections. The risk of transfusion also appears to be lower.

Reduced risk of transmitting infectious disease Elective C-sections may be associated with a reduction in mother-to-child transmission of infectious diseases such as AIDS, hepatitis B, hepatitis C, herpes and human papillomavirus.

Scheduling of the birth Knowing when you're going to have your baby may allow you to feel better prepared for childbirth.

Maternal risks, short term There are risks and disadvantages associated with an elective cesarean birth. They include longer hospital stays. The average hospital stay after a cesarean birth is three days, compared with two days for a vaginal birth.

Higher infection rate Because surgery is involved, risk of infection after delivery is higher with a C-section than with a vaginal delivery.

Complications of surgery Cesarean birth is major surgery. Thus, it carries associated surgical risks, such as infection, wound complication, bleeding, damage to neighboring organs and formation of blood clots. Anesthetic risks are greater with a cesarean delivery, as well.

Reduced initial infant bonding and breast-feeding Depending on the practices where you deliver, you may not be able to breast-feed or do much with your newborn within the first few hours after a C-section. But this is temporary. You'll have time to feed and bond with your child when you've recovered. Breast-feeding rates are similar at 3 and 24 months for both cesarean and vaginal births.

Insurance coverage An elective cesarean delivery may not be covered by your insurance, and it may be more expensive than a vaginal delivery. Before making your decision, check with your insurance company to see if your insurance covers elective cesarean births.

Maternal risks, long term Long-term risks that can accompany an elective cesarean birth include:

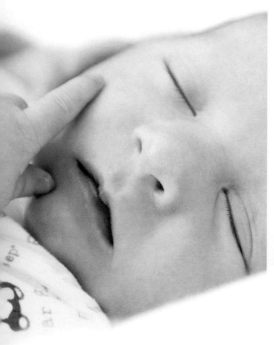

Future complications Multiple cesarean births increase your risk of complications with successive pregnancies. Most women can safely have up to three C-sections. Each repeat C-section is generally more complicated than the last, however. For some women, the risk of surgical complications, such as infection or heavy bleeding, increases only slightly from one C-section to the next. For other women, such as those who have significant internal scarring, the risk of complications increases substantially with each repeat cesarean delivery.

Uterine rupture in subsequent pregnancies A previous cesarean birth may increase your risk of uterine rupture, especially if you decide to try a vaginal birth after a cesarean birth. These risks are small, but should be discussed with your care provider.

Placental problems Women who've had a previous cesarean birth are at an increased risk of placental problems in subsequent pregnancies, such as placenta previa (see page 447). Placenta previa occurs when the placenta covers the opening of the cervix, and often results in preterm delivery. Placenta previa and other placental complications enhanced by cesarean delivery greatly increase the risk of bleeding in the mother.

Increased hysterectomy risk Some placental problems — such as placenta accreta, in which the placenta is attached too deeply to the uterine wall — require the removal of the uterus (hysterectomy) at the time of delivery or shortly after.

Injury to bowel or bladder Inadvertent injury to the bowel or bladder during a cesarean delivery is rare. However, it's much more likely in repeat operations.

Placental complications also can lead to bladder injury.

Fetal risks Some possible risks to baby associated with cesarean birth include:

Respiratory problems One of the more common risks to a baby after a cesarean birth is a mild respiratory condition called transient tachypnea. It occurs when the baby's lungs have difficulty transitioning to breathing air. While your baby is in the uterus, his or her lungs are normally filled with fluid. During a vaginal birth, movement through the birth canal naturally squeezes the baby's chest and pushes the fluid out of the lungs. During a cesarean birth, the squeezing effect isn't present, so your baby's lungs may still contain fluid after birth. This results in rapid breathing and usually requires additional oxygen delivered under pressure to get the fluid out.

Prematurity Even mild prematurity can have significant adverse effects on a newborn. If the timing of baby's due date is not accurate and the C-section is performed too early, the baby may experience prematurity-related complications.

Cuts A baby may be cut during a cesarean delivery, but this is rare. The chance of laceration during a planned C-section is less than during an emergency procedure.

MAKING YOUR DECISION

If your care provider doesn't at least question your request for an elective cesarean delivery, you should ask yourself why. Physicians and surgeons have a duty to avoid unnecessary medical interventions, especially those interventions that carry risk. The lack of scientific evidence to support elective cesarean delivery makes such a procedure unnecessary. While scheduling, efficiency and financial reward favor an elective cesarean from a physician's point of view, a care provider you can trust should at least discuss the topic with serious reservations.

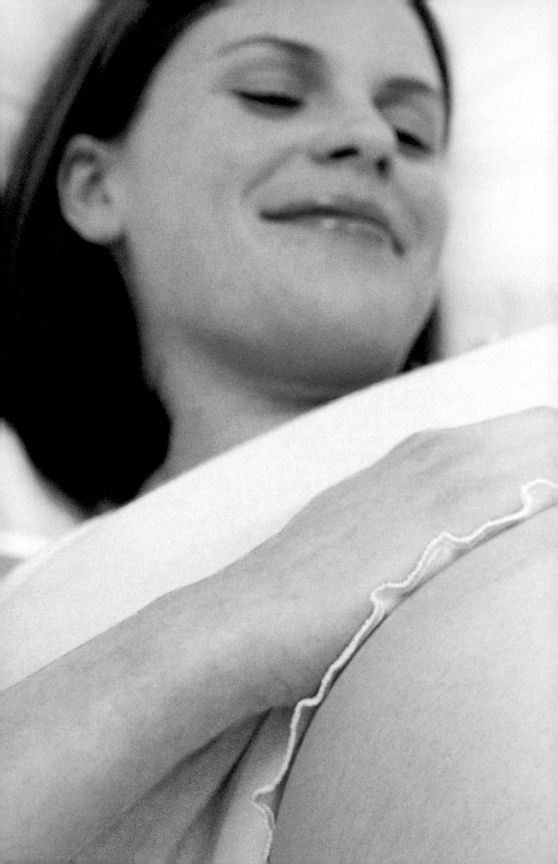

CHAPTER 25

Vaginal birth after a cesarean birth

Your first child was delivered by cesarean birth (C-section), but you would like to experience a vaginal delivery. Now, in another pregnancy, can you have a vaginal birth? The answer is, maybe. It used to be that once you had a C-section, all of your subsequent deliveries would be by cesarean as well. Today, a vaginal birth after cesarean (VBAC) is possible for many women. Attempting a VBAC is also known as trial of labor after cesarean (TOLAC).

Still, a VBAC is not without risk, so several factors must be considered before you and your care provider decide to try it.

Women who choose VBAC go through labor and delivery in the same manner as other women having a vaginal birth. You wait for the first signs of labor and then head to the hospital. If you're attempting a VBAC, it's not recommended that you have a home delivery.

At the hospital, it's important that a doctor and hospital staff closely monitor your active labor. They can be ready to perform a C-section if it's needed. Most women who plan to have a VBAC are able to do so. Sometimes, though, a repeat cesarean birth is necessary.

BENEFITS VS. RISKS

Success rates of VBAC depend on many factors. Consider the following benefits and risks of attempting a vaginal birth.

Benefits of VBAC An advantage to having a vaginal birth is that it's generally safer than a C-section, because it doesn't involve major surgery. Other advantages of a vaginal birth include:

- Lower risk of blood transfusions
- Lower risk of infection
- Shorter hospital stay, generally one to two days instead of three or more
- Lower risk of hemorrhage (compared with a C-section during labor)
- Lower risk of future surgeries and complications such as hysterectomy, bowel or bladder injury, and certain placental problems.

- More energy after childbirth
- A faster return to normal activities

In addition, you may feel more involved in the delivery process during a vaginal birth because of your efforts to push the baby out. Your labor coach and others also may be able to play a greater role in a vaginal delivery.

Risks of VBAC The possible risks of a vaginal birth after cesarean include:

Failure to deliver vaginally A repeat cesarean birth after an unsuccessful attempt at vaginal delivery may increase your risk of complications, which may include the need for a blood transfusion, the formation of blood clots and infection. You may also feel emotionally and physically drained after going through labor and still needing a C-section. Some women feel that they have failed, even though events were beyond their control.

Tearing of the scar from your previous cesarean birth (uterine rupture) The risk of this happening is typically low in women who choose VBAC. However, uterine rupture may be life-threatening to you and your baby. Uterine rupture also increases the chances you'll need a hysterectomy after delivery of your baby. There are several factors that increase the risk of uterine rupture, which you should discuss with your care provider. If you're at high risk of a uterine rupture, your care provider will likely recommend that you have a repeat cesarean delivery.

ISSUES TO CONSIDER

Are you a good candidate for a vaginal birth after a cesarean delivery? It depends mainly on the type of uterine incision used during your initial cesarean birth and the reasons you had a cesarean delivery.

Previous incision During a C-section, your care provider creates an incision in the abdominal wall and in your uterus. The incision in your abdominal wall goes through skin, fat and muscles. From this opening, your surgeon makes an incision in your uterus. The incision in your uterus is different from the incision in your abdomen. The types of uterine incisions are as follows:

A low transverse incision This is the most common type. It's made horizontally across the lower portion of the uterus. It usually bleeds less than an incision made higher on the uterus. It also tends to form a stronger scar and presents less danger of rupture during subsequent labors. If you have had one or even two of these incisions, you may be a candidate for VBAC.

A low vertical incision This incision is made low on the uterus, where the uterine wall is thinner. It may be used to deliver a baby in an awkward position or when the doctor thinks that the incision may need to be extended. At this time, there's no consistent data indicating that this type of incision increases the risk of uterine rupture. Therefore, if you've had this type of incision, you may still be a candidate for VBAC. Unfortunately, not many low vertical incisions are confined to the lower part of the uterus.

A classical incision This type of incision is made higher up on the uterus, on the portion of the uterus that contracts during labor. It was once used for all cesarean births but is now rarely used because a classical incision is associated with the highest risk of bleeding and of subsequent rupture of the uterus. It's generally used only in emergency situations when doctors need to deliver the baby quickly. VBAC is not recommended for women who have had a classical uterine incision.

Unknown type of incision For some women, it's difficult to determine the type of incision used during a previous C-section. Studies haven't shown an increased risk of rupture in this situation because the vast majority of uterine incisions are low transverse uterine incisions. Unless your doctor has concern that your previous incision was a classical one, women with an unknown type of incision may be a candidate for VBAC.

Reason for previous C-section The reasons surrounding your first cesarean birth often influence the type of delivery you have in the next pregnancy:

- If your first cesarean birth was performed for a reason that may not necessarily recur, your chance of having a successful vaginal delivery is almost the same as that of someone who has never had a cesarean birth. Examples include breech presentation, an infection, pregnancy-induced high blood pressure (preeclampsia), placental problems and fetal distress.
- If you've had at least one vaginal delivery either before or after your cesarean birth, you're more likely to have a successful VBAC than is someone who hasn't delivered vaginally.
- If you previously had a difficult labor because of the size of your child or the small size of your pelvis, you may still have a successful VBAC. However, the chances are somewhat lower than if you had a cesarean birth for a nonrecurring condition.
- If you have a chronic medical condition, such as a specific heart condition,

where problems may arise again during labor and delivery, you and your care provider may decide on a repeat cesarean birth.

Who might not be a candidate In some cases, a repeat cesarean birth is a better option than VBAC, because an unsuccessful trial of labor would carry higher risks for both you and baby. If you're interested in VBAC, your care provider will talk with you about your individual potential risks and benefits and whether you may be a good candidate.

According to the American College of Obstetricians and Gynecologists, labor

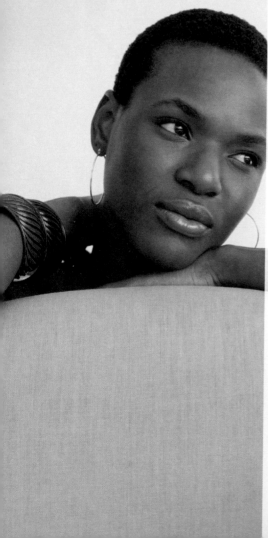

should not be attempted in the following situations:

▶ You have a prior classical or T-shaped incision or another similar type of uterine surgery
▶ You've had a previous uterine rupture
▶ You have a medical or obstetric problem that precludes vaginal delivery
▶ You're at a facility that can't perform emergency cesarean birth

TIPS FOR PLANNING A VBAC

Most women who've undergone a cesarean delivery are candidates for a vaginal birth in their subsequent pregnancies. Yet most choose not to have a vaginal delivery following a previous cesarean. Why don't more women choose VBAC? Part of the reason may be the fear of a possible long (protracted) labor that ends in surgery. Another possible reason is that not all women have access to facilities that are prepared to handle VBACs.

If you and your care provider think that VBAC is right for you, don't be afraid to try it. Although it's impossible to guarantee that a VBAC will be successful, you can increase your chances of a positive experience. Try these suggestions:

▶ *Discuss your fears and expectations.* Your care provider can help you better understand the process and how you may be affected. If you have a new care provider, make sure he or she has your complete medical history, including records of your initial C-section.
▶ *Take a class on VBAC with your labor coach.* These classes often help you work through concerns you may have about VBAC.
▶ *Have your VBAC at a well-equipped hospital.* Look for a hospital that has continuous fetal monitoring, a surgi-

cal team that can be assembled quickly, and the ability to administer anesthetics and blood transfusions 24 hours a day.

- *Discuss use of medications.* Your care provider will avoid certain medications for induction of labor because they may increase the risk of uterine rupture.
- *Make sure a qualified care provider is available.* Constant monitoring by your labor and delivery team can decrease the risk of complications. Make sure your labor and delivery team is aware of your obstetrical history.
- *Think of yourself as an athlete preparing for an event.* Thinking positively, eating a healthy diet, exercising regularly and getting plenty of rest will give you the best chance of a vaginal labor and delivery.
- *Keep your ultimate goal in mind.* You want both you and baby to have a healthy outcome, regardless of how you get there.

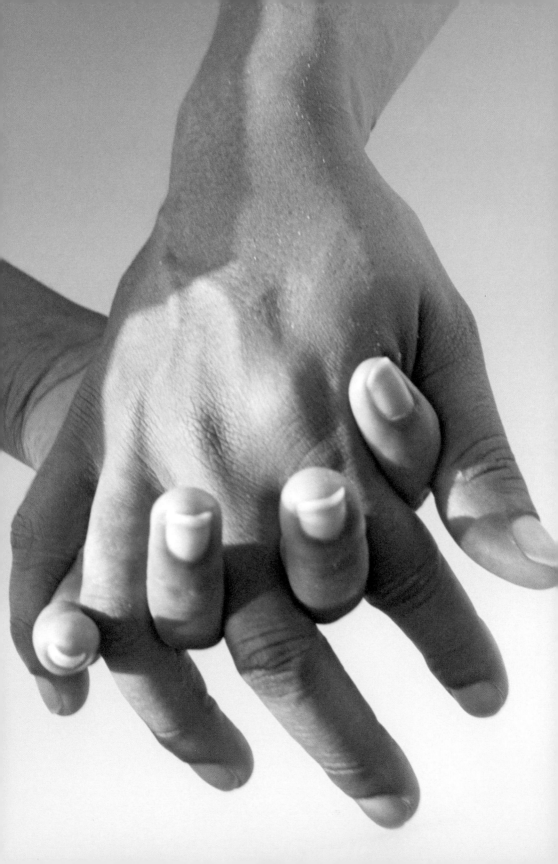

CHAPTER 26

Contraception after delivery

In the blur of sleepless nights and diaper changes, it's easy to forget about birth control. But the fact is, even before you experience your first menstrual period after childbirth, there may be a chance that you could become pregnant again if you have unprotected sex. Conceiving again within 18 months of your delivery may carry certain health risks for you and your baby. These include an increased risk of autism, which may be related to a lasting depletion of nutrients in your body. Not to mention, conceiving again soon would also mean being pregnant while caring for an infant. For these reasons, it's important to consider your birth control options.

There are many different methods of birth control available:

▶ *Hormonal methods.* Examples include birth control pills, as well as the contraceptive patch (Xulane), vaginal ring (NuvaRing), contraceptive implant (Nexplanon) and contraceptive injection (Depo-Provera).
▶ *Barrier methods.* Examples include male and female condoms, as well as the diaphragm, cervical cap, and contraceptive sponge and spermicide.
▶ *Intrauterine devices.* Examples include a copper IUD (ParaGard) and a hormonal IUD (Mirena, Skyla, others).
▶ *Permanent methods.* Examples include tubal ligation and hysteroscopic sterilization (Essure) for women and vasectomy for men.
▶ *Natural family planning.* Examples include the rhythm method and the basal body temperature and cervical mucus methods.

ISSUES TO CONSIDER

Some forms of contraception may be a better fit for you than others. Here are some questions to ask yourself as you consider your options:

How effective is it? To be effective, any method of contraception must be used consistently and correctly. But some methods tend to be more effective than others. For example, IUDs and implants are more effective than contraceptive pills, patches and rings, and injections. It's up to you to determine the level of effectiveness you need.

When do you hope to become pregnant again? If you're planning another pregnancy in the near future, you may want a birth control method that's easy to stop using and quickly reversible, such as a hormonal method or a barrier method. If you'd like to become pregnant again — but not for at least a year or two — you may also consider an IUD, which provides continuous contraception for as long as it's in place. If you're certain that you don't ever want to have more children, you may prefer a permanent method.

Is it convenient? For some people, convenience suggests ease of use, no bothersome side effects or no disruption of the sexual experience. For others, convenience means no prescription is required. When choosing a method of contraception, consider how willing you are to plan ahead or, if necessary, adhere to a rigid schedule. It's important to choose a type of birth control that suits your lifestyle.

Will it impact your milk supply? If you're breast-feeding, you're more limited in your contraception options at first. See the next section to learn more.

What are the side effects? Some methods, particularly those that contain hormones, may have more side effects than others, such as barrier methods and natural family planning methods. Talk to your care provider about your medical history and how it might affect your choice of birth control.

Does the method offer any additional benefits? Besides preventing pregnancy, some contraceptives provide additional benefits — such as more predictable and lighter menstrual cycles, a decreased risk of sexually transmitted infections, or a reduced risk of some cancers.

Will it protect you from sexually transmitted infections? Male and female condoms are the only methods of birth control that offer reliable protection from sexually transmitted infections (STIs). Other birth control options don't protect against STIs.

Is the method acceptable to your sexual partner? Your partner may have birth control preferences that are similar to or different from your own. Discuss birth control options with your partner to help determine which method is acceptable to both of you.

Is the method compatible with your beliefs or practices? Some forms of birth control are considered a violation of certain religious laws or cultural traditions. When deciding on which type of birth control to use, weigh the risks and benefits of a particular method against your personal convictions.

BREAST-FEEDING AND CONTRACEPTION

Contraception after childbirth may require extra consideration if you're breast-feeding. That's because breast-feeding affects fertility and birth control options in a couple of different ways.

Fertility The myth is that you can't get pregnant if you're breast-feeding. And there is some truth behind it: Breast-feeding reduces fertility. In fact, breast-feeding can be as effective as condom use for contraception, for up to six months — but only if *all* of the following are true:

▸ You're exclusively breast-feeding your baby, with no formula supplements or even bottles of breast milk.

▸ You're breast-feeding on demand, feeding at least every four hours during the day and every six hours overnight.

▸ You're not using a breast pump. Pumping doesn't provide the same stimulation for pregnancy prevention as breast-feeding your baby.

▸ You haven't yet gotten a period since giving birth.

For many new moms, juggling feedings and work schedules with a partner can make these conditions unrealistic. Fertility will be reduced, but not reliably. That's why most new parents could still get pregnant while breast-feeding.

Knowing that fertility is reduced, some women choose natural family planning as their form of contraception while breast-feeding. If this is your choice, keep in mind a couple of caveats:

▸ *You may experience your first ovulation before your first period.* That means you can't use your first period as an indicator that you need to take precautions against pregnancy. You could become pregnant again without ever experiencing a period.

▸ *While breast-feeding, your period may not follow a consistent pattern.* This makes natural family planning more difficult than normal.

Hormones and breast milk Birth control methods containing estrogen and progestin (combination hormonal contraceptives) include most pills, the patch and the ring. These traditionally haven't been recommended for women who are breast-feeding. There's a small chance the hormones involved could affect your early milk production, and in the past, there's also been concern that the estrogen in combined hormonal contraceptives could decrease the nutrients in breast milk. However, in well-nourished mothers, this possibility generally isn't a problem. There's also no conclusive evidence that hormonal contraceptives affect baby's development through breast milk.

Here are some things you need to remember if you're considering birth control pills or other hormonal contraceptives while breast-feeding.

▸ *It's best to wait at least 30 days before using a combined hormonal contraceptive.* This is to allow your breast-feeding pattern to become established. Any potential effect on breast milk production is more of a concern before your milk supply is well-established.

▸ *Contraceptives containing estrogen increase the risk of blood clots (deep vein thrombosis, or DVT).* Because postpartum women are already at risk of DVT, they should generally wait at least 30 days after delivery before starting contraceptives containing estrogen, and women with additional risk factors for DVT should wait at least six weeks. Risk factors include older age (age 35 or above), cesarean delivery, previous DVT and a BMI of 30 or more.

▶ *Contraceptives containing only progestin don't affect milk production.* According to the Centers for Disease Control and Protection (CDC) and the American College of Obstetricians and Gynecologists (ACOG), progestin-only methods are safe to use during breast-feeding with no waiting period after delivery. These include some pills (the minipill), hormonal IUDs, contraceptive implants and the contraceptive injection.

▶ *The minipill requires a very consistent dose to be effective.* It has to be taken exactly as prescribed to offer maximum protection. Taking a pill two hours late or more will significantly impact your level of protection over the next several days.

Vaginal dryness Breast-feeding can also cause vaginal dryness. If you're planning to use condoms as contraception while you're breast-feeding, be aware that vaginal dryness may make condom use a bit uncomfortable. However, lubricants can help with this.

OPTIONS

Following is a description of the contraceptives currently available to prevent pregnancy. Keep in mind that correct use is needed for full effectiveness. Talk with your care provider about which choice may be best for you.

Hormonal methods These methods prevent pregnancy by suppressing the release of certain hormones, in turn preventing the release of eggs from your ovaries.

Combination birth control pills Combination birth control pills, commonly referred to as "the pill," are oral contraceptives that contain the hormones estrogen and progestin. Combination birth control pills suppress ovulation — keeping your ovaries from releasing an egg. They also thicken cervical mucus and thin the lining of the uterus (endometrium) to keep sperm from reaching the egg and prevent implantation.

Different types of combination birth control pills contain different doses of estrogen and progestin. Other types of combination birth control pills allow you to reduce the number of periods you have each year. For maximum effectiveness, you must take combination birth control pills at the same time every day.

Types. Combined oral contraceptives come in different quantities of active and inactive pills, including:

▶ *Conventional pack.* The most common type of combination birth control pills contains 21 active pills and seven inactive pills. Formulations containing 24 active pills and four inactive pills, known as a shortened pill-free interval, also are available. Bleeding occurs the week you take the inactive pills.

▶ *Continuous dosing or extended cycle.* These combinations typically contain 84 active pills and seven inactive pills. Bleeding generally occurs only four times a year, during the days when you take the inactive pills.

Combination birth control pills also come in different formulations:

▶ *Monophasic.* With this type of combination birth control pill, each active pill contains the same amount of estrogen and progestin.

▸ *Multiphasic.* With this type of combination birth control pill, the combinations and amounts of hormones in active pills vary. In some types, the progestin content increases through the cycle, while in others the progestin dose remains steady and the estrogen content increases.

Combination birth control pills now typically contain up to 35 micrograms of ethinyl estradiol, a type of estrogen, and are known as low-dose pills. Women who are sensitive to hormones may want to inquire about even lower doses. However, lower dose pills may result in more breakthrough bleeding than other pills.

Effectiveness. An estimated 9 out of 100 women who use combination birth control pills for one year will get pregnant. With perfect use, the pill is even more effective.

Benefits and risks. Combination birth control pills are an easily reversible method of contraception. Your fertility may return to normal two weeks after you stop taking combination birth control pills. Other benefits may include:

▸ A decreased risk of ovarian, endometrial and colorectal cancers, uterine fibroids, benign breast cysts, and iron deficiency anemia
▸ Reduced pain for women who regularly experience severe menstrual cramps (dysmenorrhea)
▸ Relief from premenstrual syndrome (PMS)
▸ Shorter, lighter and more predictable periods or, for some types of combination pills, fewer periods each year
▸ An improvement in acne

Possible side effects of combination birth control pills include:

▸ An increased risk of blood clots in the legs or lungs, heart attack, and stroke, although the overall risk is low
▸ An increased risk of cervical cancer and, possibly, breast cancer
▸ Elevated blood pressure
▸ Nausea
▸ Bloating
▸ Breast tenderness
▸ Headaches

Combination birth control pills may not be the best choice if you are older than age 35 and smoke, have poorly controlled high blood pressure, or have a history of blood clots, stroke, or breast or liver cancer. The risk of complications is higher in these situations.

Minipill The minipill, also known as the progestin-only birth control pill, is an oral contraceptive that contains only the hormone progestin. It does not contain estrogen.

The minipill thickens cervical mucus, preventing sperm from reaching the egg, and it thins the lining of the uterus (endometrium), preventing implantation. The minipill may also suppress ovulation.

Effectiveness. The minipill is estimated to be as effective as combined hormonal pills.

Benefits and risks. The minipill is an easily reversible method of contraception. Your fertility may return to normal immediately after you stop taking the minipill.

Your care provider may recommend the minipill if:

▸ You're breast-feeding. Because there's no estrogen in the pill, you don't have to worry about it interfering with your milk supply.
▸ You have certain health problems, such as a high risk of heart disease, high blood pressure or migraines.

▶ You're older than age 35 and a smoker.

Your care provider may discourage use of the minipill if you have breast cancer or if you're taking medications that contain anticonvulsants or anti-tuberculous agents.

Possible side effects of the minipill include:
▶ Irregular menstrual bleeding
▶ Ovarian cysts
▶ Acne flare

Contraceptive patch The contraceptive patch contains the hormones estrogen and progestin. You apply the small patch to your skin once a week for three weeks. On the fourth week, you don't use a patch, which allows menstruation to occur.

Similar to combination birth control pills, the patch prevents pregnancy by releasing the hormones estrogen and progestin into your bloodstream. The hormones suppress ovulation, keeping your ovaries from releasing an egg. The patch also thickens cervical mucus to keep sperm from reaching the egg.

Effectiveness. An estimated 9 out of 100 women who use the patch for one year will get pregnant. As with the pill, it may be more effective with perfect use according to instructions.

Benefits and risks. The benefits and risks are similar to those of combination birth control pills. However, studies indicate that the patch causes a higher level of estrogen to circulate in the body than combination birth control pills do. As a result, there may be a slightly increased risk of blood clots when using the patch compared with the pill. With either, the overall risk of blood clots is still very low.

Vaginal ring NuvaRing is a flexible, transparent plastic ring that contains the hormones estrogen and progestin. It's inserted deep into the vagina and worn for three weeks. You remove NuvaRing for one week — allowing menstruation to occur — then insert a new ring.

Similar to combination birth control pills, NuvaRing prevents pregnancy by releasing hormones into your body that suppress ovulation — keeping your ovaries from releasing an egg. NuvaRing also thickens cervical mucus to keep sperm from reaching the egg.

Effectiveness. As with other combined hormonal contraceptives, an estimated 9 out of 100 women who use NuvaRing for one year will get pregnant. The ring is over 99 percent effective with perfect use.

Benefits and risks. NuvaRing doesn't require a personalized fitting. It can be removed at any time, followed by a quick return to fertility. It isn't appropriate for everyone, however. You must be comfortable with inserting and removing the device. Your care provider may discourage use of NuvaRing if:
▶ You are older than age 35 and smoke
▶ You're breast-feeding
▶ You recently gave birth or had a second trimester miscarriage or abortion
▶ You have a history of heart attack or stroke
▶ You have a history of breast, uterine or liver cancer
▶ You have a history of blood clots in your legs, lungs or eyes
▶ You have severe high blood pressure

Possible side effects of NuvaRing are similar to combination birth control pills and include an increased risk of blood-clotting problems, heart attack, stroke, liver cancer and high blood pressure. Other possible side effects include breakthrough bleeding or spotting, vaginal infection or irritation, and headache.

Contraceptive implant Nexplanon is a contraceptive implant for women that's placed under the skin of the upper arm. Nexplanon releases a low, steady dose of the hormone progestin to thicken cervical mucus and thin the lining of the uterus (endometrium) — preventing sperm from reaching the egg and implanting. The implant typically suppresses ovulation as well. It prevents pregnancy for up to three years after insertion.

Effectiveness. Fewer than 1 percent of women who use Nexplanon for one year will get pregnant.

Benefits and risks. Nexplanon doesn't require a personalized fitting or regular attention. And it can be removed at any time, followed by a quick return to fertility.

Your care provider may discourage use of Nexplanon if you:

- Have had serious blood clots, a heart attack or stroke
- Have hepatic tumors or liver disease
- Have unexplained vaginal bleeding
- Have known or suspected breast cancer or a history of breast cancer

If you do conceive while using Nexplanon, there's a higher chance the pregnancy will be ectopic, when the fertilized egg implants outside the uterus, usually in a fallopian tube. Other risks associated with the contraceptive implant include:

- Changes in vaginal bleeding patterns, including the absence of menstruation (amenorrhea); irregular bleeding may resolve within three to nine months
- Mood swings
- Depression
- Weight gain
- Acne
- Headaches
- Slight risk of developing ovarian cysts and blood clots

Contraceptive injection Depo-Provera is a contraceptive that's given in the form of a shot. You visit your care provider for an injection once every three months. Depo-Provera suppresses ovulation, keeping your ovaries from releasing an egg. It also thickens cervical mucus to keep sperm from reaching the egg. It may take 10 months or more for fertility to return after stopping contraceptive injections.

Types. Two injectables — Depo-Provera and Depo-subQ Provera 104 — are currently available. Both contain the hormone progestin, but Depo-subQ Provera 104 contains a lower dose.

Effectiveness. An estimated 6 out of 100 women who use Depo-Provera for one year will get pregnant.

Benefits and risks. Among various benefits, the contraceptive injection:
- Doesn't require a personalized fitting or daily attention
- Decreases the risk of endometrial cancer, pelvic inflammatory disease and uterine fibroids
- Can be used while breast-feeding
Your care provider may discourage its use if you have unexplained vaginal bleeding, breast cancer, liver disease or a history of blood-clotting problems. Side effects of the contraceptive may include:
- A temporary loss of bone mineral density (The loss increases the longer Depo-Provera is used and may not be completely reversible.)
- Irregular periods and breakthrough bleeding
- Weight gain
- Breast soreness
- Headaches

Barrier methods These methods prevent pregnancy by creating a "barrier" to prevent male sperm from reaching female eggs.

Male and female condoms Condoms are a very effective way to prevent pregnancy and protect yourself and your partner from sexually transmitted infections (STIs). Condoms are simple to use, inexpensive and widely available. They're sold with or without a lubricant in a variety of lengths, shapes, widths and thicknesses, and they come in different colors and textures.

Types. A male condom is a thin sheath that's placed over the erect penis just before sexual intercourse. The female condom is a soft, loosefitting pouch with a ring on each end. Before sex, one ring is inserted into the vagina to hold the female condom in place. The ring at the open end of the condom remains outside the vagina. While the male condom is fairly easy to use, some women find the female condom difficult to insert.

Effectiveness. Condoms are an effective form of birth control — when they're used properly. With perfect use, about 2 in 100 couples who use male condoms will get pregnant in a year. If you consider more typical use, the statistics are 18 in 100. Chances of pregnancy increase if condoms are used incorrectly or sporadically — a condom isn't effective at all if it lies unopened in a drawer.

An estimated 21 out of 100 women who use the female condom for one year will get pregnant — usually because they don't use condoms every time they have sex. When female condoms are used correctly and all of the time, pregnancy results about 5 percent of the time.

Benefits and risks. Condoms don't have the side effects of some forms of female contraception, such as birth control pills or shots, or potential complications of an intrauterine device (IUD). They are also available without a prescription and are easy to obtain.

Some people are allergic to latex, and if either partner is allergic, he or she may react to contact with a latex condom. The female condom also may cause discomfort, including burning, itching or a rash.

Diaphragm The diaphragm prevents sperm from entering the uterus. It's a small, reusable rubber or silicone cup with a flexible rim that covers the cervix. Before sex, the diaphragm is inserted deep into the vagina so that part of the rim fits snugly behind the pubic bone. The device is held in place by the vaginal muscles. You'll need your care provider to prescribe the right size diaphragm for you.

Effectiveness. An estimated 12 out of 100 women who use the diaphragm for one year will get pregnant. The device is effective at preventing pregnancy only when used with spermicide, which blocks or kills sperm.

Benefits and risks. The diaphragm can be used as a backup method of birth control, and it doesn't pose a risk of side effects. However, your care provider may discourage use of the diaphragm if you just gave birth, or if you:

▶ Have an allergy to silicone, latex or spermicide
▶ Have vaginal abnormalities that interfere with the fit, placement or retention of the diaphragm
▶ Have an infection in your vagina or pelvic area
▶ Have frequent urinary tract infections

Cervical cap The cervical cap is a contraceptive device that prevents sperm from entering the uterus. This reusable, deep cup fits over the cervix and is used with spermicide. Before sex, the device is inserted into the vagina and held in place by suction.

Presently, only one cervical cap — FemCap — has Food and Drug Administration (FDA) approval. FemCap is made of silicone rubber. It must be fitted and prescribed by a doctor.

Effectiveness. An estimated 13 to 16 out of 100 women who've never had a vaginal birth and use the cervical cap for one year will get pregnant. Of women who have given birth vaginally, an estimated 23 to 32 out of 100 will get pregnant while using the cervical cap for one year. This decrease in effectiveness is due to changes in the shape of the cervix after childbirth, making it more difficult for the cap to fit well.

Benefits and risks. The cervical cap can be used as a backup method of birth control and doesn't pose a risk of side effects. It may not be the best choice if you just gave birth, or if you:

▶ Have an allergy to spermicide or silicone
▶ Are experiencing vaginal bleeding or you have an infection in your vagina, cervix or pelvic area
▶ Have vaginal abnormalities that interfere with the fit, placement or retention of the cervical cap
▶ Have a history of pelvic inflammatory disease, toxic shock syndrome, cervical cancer, third-degree uterine prolapse, uterine tract infections, or vaginal or cervical tissue tears

Some women find the cervical cap difficult to insert.

Contraceptive sponge and spermicide The contraceptive sponge is a soft, disk-shaped device made of polyurethane foam that covers the cervix. The device is sold over-the-counter. Before sex, the sponge is moistened with water and inserted deep into the vagina, where it's held in place by vaginal muscles. It has a loop to assist with removal. The contraceptive sponge contains spermicide, which immobilizes or kills sperm before they enter the uterus.

Effectiveness. An estimated 12 out of 100 women who've never given birth and use the contraceptive sponge for one year will get pregnant. That number is estimated at 24 out of 100 for women who've given birth.

Benefits and risks. The contraceptive sponge doesn't require a prescription or fitting, can be inserted hours before sex, and provides protection from pregnancy for 24 hours. However, it may not be appropriate if you just gave birth, or if you:

▶ Are sensitive or allergic to spermicide or polyurethane
▶ Have vaginal abnormalities that interfere with the fit, placement or retention of the contraceptive sponge
▶ Have frequent urinary tract infections
  Spermicide may increase your risk of urinary tract infections and cause vaginal irritation.

Intrauterine devices Intrauterine devices (IUDs) affect the way sperm move, preventing them from joining with an egg. An IUD is a small, flexible, plastic T-shaped device, which is placed in the uterus by a care provider.

Types. There are two types of IUDs, the copper IUD (ParaGard) and the hormonal IUD (Mirena, Skyla, others).

ParaGard continuously releases copper, preventing sperm from entering the fallopian tubes. If fertilization occurs, ParaGard keeps the fertilized egg from implanting in the lining of the uterus.

With the hormonal IUD, the hormone progestin is released from the device. This thickens the cervical mucus and thins the lining of the uterus (endometrium) — preventing sperm from entering the fallopian tubes.

Effectiveness. An estimated 1 out of 100 women who use either type of IUD for one year will get pregnant.

Benefits and risks. An IUD provides continuous contraception as long as it's in place. It stays in your uterus for as long as you want to avoid pregnancy — up to three to five years for hormonal IUDs, and 10 years for ParaGard.

There may be some discomfort with placement of an IUD, and there's a small risk of uterine infection after placement. ParaGard generally tends to cause longer, heavier and more painful menstrual periods. Hormonal IUDs may cause irregular bleeding for the first three to six months after insertion, but after this time, periods tend to be lighter. In fact, some women using them experience an absence of periods. Side effects associated with hormonal IUDs include headache, acne, breast tenderness and mood changes.

In addition, IUDs can dislodge from the uterus, and you may not know it's happened. Expulsion occurs most often during your first period after the device is inserted. If you're worried about expulsion, you may want to see your care provider to make sure the IUD is still in place.

The overall risk of ectopic pregnancy with an IUD is less than the risk in women who don't use contraception. However, if pregnancy does occur with an IUD in place, the risk of ectopic pregnancy is higher. If you have an IUD in place and you're concerned that you might be pregnant, contact your care provider right away so that he or she can determine that it's not an ectopic pregnancy.

Permanent methods Sterilization is generally irreversible. Before undergoing these procedures, you need to be certain that you don't wish to have any more children.

Tubal ligation A tubal ligation — also known as having your tubes tied — is a form of permanent birth control. During a tubal ligation, the fallopian tubes are cut or blocked, disrupting the movement of the egg to the uterus for fertilization and preventing sperm from traveling up the fallopian tubes to the egg.

Tubal ligation is usually done under short-acting general or regional anesthesia. It can be done while you're recovering from vaginal childbirth or during a cesarean delivery. It can also be done as an outpatient procedure at a later time. Postpartum tubal ligation may be more difficult in certain women, such as those with a significantly high BMI. In this situation, your physician may discuss other options with you.

It's possible to reverse a tubal ligation — but reversal requires major surgery and isn't always effective.

Effectiveness. In the first year after a tubal ligation, an estimated 1 out of 100 women will get pregnant. If you do conceive after having a tubal ligation, there's a higher chance that the pregnancy will be ectopic — when the fertilized egg implants outside the uterus, usually in a fallopian tube.

Benefits and risks. A tubal ligation permanently prevents pregnancy, ending the need for any type of contraception. Because it does involve surgery, it carries some risks, which include damage to the bowel, bladder or major blood vessels, adverse reaction to anesthesia, and wound infection.

Hysteroscopic sterilization Hysteroscopic sterilization is the "plugging up" of the fallopian tubes to prevent fertilization. This is done by way of nonsurgical methods performed in a doctor's office or an outpatient surgery setting.

▶ *Essure system.* This method consists of placing a small, coil-shaped metallic device within each fallopian tube. The devices cause scar tissue to form, effectively blocking the fallopian tube and preventing fertilization of the egg. Your doctor inserts the device into each of your fallopian tubes by threading a thin, flexible tube through the vagina into the uterus and on into the fallopian tube. For the following three months, you must use an alternate form of birth control. After this time, you undergo an X-ray to ensure that scar tissue has developed. If the X-ray shows that both tubes are fully blocked, you can discontinue other forms of birth control.

Effectiveness. In the first year after implantation of the Essure system, an estimated 1 out of 100 women will get pregnant. If you do conceive after having this system implanted, there's a higher chance that the pregnancy will be ectopic.

Benefits and risks. Benefits of hysteroscopic sterilization include permanent sterilization and no significant long-term side effects. Your doctor may not recommend these forms of sterilization if you recently gave birth, you're not certain that you don't want to have more children, you're sensitive to nickel or allergic to the contrast agent used to confirm tubal blockage, or you have a condition that prevents access to one or both tubal openings.

Vasectomy Vasectomy is a simple surgery that provides birth control for men. A vasectomy may be done in a doctor's office with a local anesthetic. In this procedure, the vasa deferentia — the ducts through which the sperm travel — are cut and sealed.

Effectiveness. Vasectomy is nearly 100 percent effective in protecting against pregnancy. However, vasectomy doesn't provide immediate protection. Most men become free of sperm after eight to 10 ejaculations. Until your doctor determines that the ejaculate doesn't contain sperm, another form of birth control needs to be used.

Benefits and risks. Vasectomy is a minor outpatient surgery with a low risk of complications or side effects. The cost of a vasectomy is far less than the cost of female sterilization (tubal ligation). Serious side effects or complications are rare. Minor side effects may include swelling, bruising of the scrotum and blood in the semen.

Natural family planning methods Natural family planning methods, also called rhythm methods, involve determining the days during your monthly cycle that you're fertile (ovulating) and avoiding intercourse on those days. No devices or medications are required.

Types. Methods that can be used to assess when you're most fertile include:

▶ *Calendar method.* Using certain calculations, you determine the first and last days during which you can become pregnant in your cycle.
▶ *Cervical position and dilation.* Your cervix opens and changes position at the time of ovulation. With this method, you check your cervical position using your finger. During ovulation, your cervix is slightly higher, softer and more open than it is at other times of the month.
▶ *Mucus inspection method.* This involves tracking changes in your cervical mucus to determine when you're ovulating.
▶ *Temperature method.* Most women have a slight change in basal body temperature related to ovulation. Their temperature drops during ovulation and then rises slightly after ovulation.
▶ *Mucothermal method.* This is a combination of the temperature and mucus inspection methods.
▶ *Symptothermal method.* This is a combination of four different methods — calendar, cervical position and dilation, mucus inspection, and temperature. Using more than one method provides a more accurate estimate of your fertile phase.

If you plan to use a rhythm method, it's best to take a class or receive training from a qualified teacher.

Effectiveness. The effectiveness of natural family planning methods depends on your diligence. Used perfectly, effectiveness ratings can reach more than 90 percent, which means that fewer than 10 out of 100 women who use natural family planning as birth control for a year would become pregnant. However, few couples use these methods perfectly. With typical use, an estimated 24 out of 100 women who use natural family planning methods for one year will become pregnant.

It's easier to be successful with natural family planning if your periods are very regular. Plus, you must carefully chart your cycles and observe signs of ovulation.

Natural family planning is particularly challenging if you're breast-feeding, because you may not have periods or they may be irregular. Mucus inspection and cervical position and dilation become particularly important because ovulation may precede vaginal bleeding.

Benefits and risks. Some women choose natural family planning for religious reasons. It doesn't cause side effects, and it doesn't pose any risks. However, it's less effective than other options.

Emergency methods Emergency contraception isn't meant to be used in place of routine birth control, but it's an option if you've had unprotected sex, your method of birth control failed or you missed a birth control pill.

You may be able to choose from several different types of emergency contraception. Many women opt for the morning-after pill (Plan B One-Step, others), which is sold over-the-counter in most pharmacies. Another formulation of the morning-after pill, ulipristal (Ella), may be even more effective but requires a prescription. It's also possible to use combination birth control pills or ParaGard — an intrauterine device — for emergency contraception.

Depending on where you are in your menstrual cycle, emergency contraception can prevent or delay ovulation, block fertilization, or keep a fertilized egg from implanting in the uterus.

To be effective, emergency contraception must be used as soon as possible after unprotected sex. Emergency contraceptive pills are most effective when taken within 72 hours of intercourse. Ulipristal is designed to prevent pregnancy if taken within five days after unprotected sex. Emergency IUDs may be placed within seven days of intercourse.

Emergency contraceptives are generally very safe and have few side effects, but they are not intended for frequent use and aren't recommended as a routine form of birth control. Common side effects are nausea and vomiting, although they may occur more frequently with combination regimens. If you're breast-feeding, your care provider may recommend a progestin-only regimen. After use of emergency contraceptive pills, your first period may be irregular.

MAKING YOUR DECISION

When you choose a contraceptive method, many factors come into play, including your age, health, emotional maturity, marital status, religious convictions and whether you're breast-feeding. Knowing your options is part of the decision process — but an honest assessment of yourself, your partner and your relationship is just as important. Most people have to make some trade-offs. You might, for instance, prefer to deal with the mild side effects of a hormonal contraceptive in exchange for effectiveness, or forgo the convenience of an IUD for the low cost of a barrier method. Ideally, you and your partner will discuss the options and reach a mutually satisfying decision.

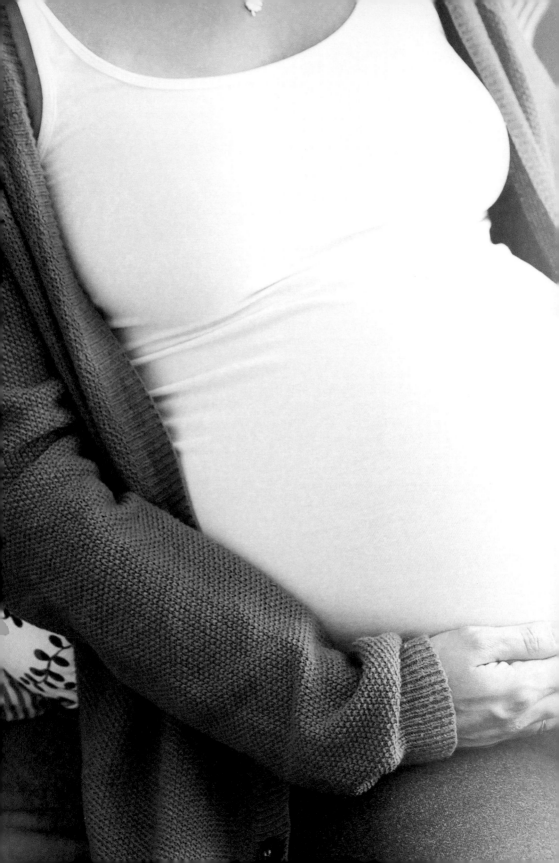

PART 5

Symptoms guide

Pregnancy can bring with it a host of concerns, including acne, morning sickness, fatigue and heartburn. This guide offers tips and insights to help you get through many of the signs and symptoms of pregnancy that may be uncomfortable or worrisome.

ABDOMINAL DISCOMFORT

Pain in the lower abdomen during the first and second trimesters often stems from normal pregnancy changes. As the uterus expands, the ligaments and muscles that support it stretch. This stretching may cause twinges, cramps or pulling sensations on one or both sides of your abdomen. You may notice the pain more when you cough, sneeze or change position.

An example of abdominal or groin discomfort in midpregnancy is stretching of the round ligament, a cord-like muscle that supports the uterus. The discomfort usually lasts for several minutes and then goes away. (See Round Ligament Pain, page 417.)

If you've had abdominal surgery, you may have pain from stretching or pulling of adhesions, the bands of scar tissue that adhere to the walls of the abdomen or other structures. The increasing size of your abdomen can cause these bands of tissue to stretch or even pull apart, which can be painful.

Lower abdominal discomfort that's relatively minor and comes and goes irregularly is probably nothing to worry about. If it's regular and predictable, consider whether you might be entering labor, even if you are still far from your due date.

Prevention and self-care It may help to sit or lie down if abdominal pain is bothering you. You may also find relief by soaking in a warm bath or doing relaxation exercises.

When to seek medical help Pain that's severe and unrelenting may be a sign of a problem, such as an ectopic pregnancy or, later in pregnancy, early labor or a placental abruption (see page 446). With an ectopic pregnancy, which generally causes problems in the first trimester, the pain is often sharp and stabbing (see page 484). Your abdomen may feel tender. You may also have bleeding, nausea and low back pain.

In midpregnancy and beyond, abdominal pain accompanied by continuous low back pain may signal a problem. No matter what the cause, call your care provider right away if:

▶ The pain is severe, persistent or accompanied by a fever
▶ You experience vaginal bleeding, vaginal discharge, burning with urination, gastrointestinal symptoms, dizziness or lightheadedness
▶ You have contractions, which may feel like a tightening in the abdomen and a sensation similar to menstrual cramps

ABDOMINAL PRESSURE

A feeling of pressure in the lower abdomen and pelvis is probably nothing to worry about, if it's not accompanied by other symptoms. In the first trimester, this sensation is common. Most likely, you're feeling your uterus starting to grow. You may also be feeling increased blood flow. In the second or third trimester, the pressure likely has to do with the weight of your baby. Compression of the bladder and rectum and stretching of the pelvic floor muscles also provoke feelings of pressure.

When to seek medical help If the pressure is accompanied by pain, cramping or bleeding early in your pregnancy, contact your care provider. These might

be signs and symptoms of miscarriage or an ectopic pregnancy. An ectopic pregnancy occurs when the embryo implants outside the uterus, usually in a fallopian tube (see page 484).

Later in your pregnancy, pressure in the lower abdomen might indicate preterm labor.

Contact your care provider if the pressure lasts for four to six hours or longer or is accompanied by any of the following:

▶ Pain
▶ Vaginal bleeding
▶ A low, dull backache that lasts four hours or longer
▶ Abdominal cramps
▶ Regular contractions or uterine tightening
▶ Watery vaginal discharge

ABDOMINAL TENDERNESS

During pregnancy, your growing uterus stretches the muscles in your abdomen. This may cause the two large parallel bands of muscles that meet in the middle of the abdomen to separate. This separation, called diastasis, can also cause a bulge where the two muscles separate.

For most women, the condition is painless. Other women may experience some

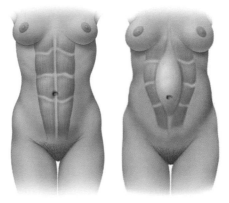

tenderness around the bellybutton. Diastasis can also contribute to back pain.

The condition may first appear during the second trimester, and it may become more noticeable in the third trimester. The problem generally goes away after delivery, but some degree of separation may remain permanently In subsequent pregnancies, it's likely to be worse.

Medical care Usually no medical care is needed for abdominal muscle separation. Your care provider can evaluate whether the amount of muscle separation is more than usual. He or she may suggest ways to remedy the separation after your baby is born.

ACNE

Because pregnancy hormones increase secretion of oil from your skin glands, you may develop acne early in your pregnancy. The change is usually temporary and disappears after you give birth.

Prevention and self-care Most acne can be prevented or controlled with good basic skin care. Try the following:
- *Wash your face as you normally would.* Avoid facial scrubs, astringents and masks because they tend to irritate skin and can make acne worse. Excessive washing and scrubbing also can irritate skin.
- *Avoid irritants such as oily cosmetics or hair-styling products.* Use products labeled water-based or noncomedogenic, which are less likely to clog pores or irritate your skin. Protect your skin from direct sunlight with a noncomedogenic sunscreen.
- *Watch what touches your face.* Keep your hair clean and off your face.

Avoid resting your hands or objects on your face. Tight clothing or hats also can pose a problem, especially if you're sweating. Sweat, dirt and oils contribute to acne.

Medical care It's important to exercise caution during pregnancy — even with over-the-counter products. There's little research on the safety of nonprescription products containing benzoyl peroxide during pregnancy, although problems haven't been reported. Erythromycin (Erygel) is often the drug of choice for pregnancy acne. Azelaic acid (Azelex, Finacea) may be another option. Both are typically applied to the skin as a lotion or gel and are available by prescription.

ALLERGIES

A stuffy nose in pregnancy is common because pregnancy provokes swelling of the tissues lining the nose. Still, many women experience allergies, either seasonal or year round, before getting pregnant. Others develop allergy-related symptoms during pregnancy, even if they haven't had the problem before. In addition to a runny or stuffy nose, you may experience sneezing and itchy, watery eyes.

Many of the usual remedies for these common signs and symptoms — including some antihistamines and decongestants — have not been proved safe to use during pregnancy. For information on how best to treat allergies during pregnancy, see page 62.

When to seek medical help If your signs and symptoms are severe or don't improve with self-care techniques, talk to your care provider.

BABY'S HICCUPS

Starting about midway through your pregnancy, you may occasionally notice a slight twitching or little spasms in your abdomen. What you may be feeling is your baby's hiccups. Fetal hiccups develop as early as the 15th week of pregnancy. Some fetuses experience hiccups several times a day, and others never get them. After they're born, most babies have frequent bouts of hiccups. Hiccups are common after a feeding, particularly after burping. No one knows exactly why they occur — in babies or adults — or why babies have them so often.

BABY'S KICKS

The first movements or kicks you feel from the fetus is called quickening. In first pregnancies, this exciting development typically occurs by about 20 weeks' gestation, although some women experience them a few weeks earlier or later. The movements might feel like a light tapping or the fluttering of a butterfly. At first you might attribute the sensation to gas or hunger pangs.

It's normal during the second trimester for fetal movements to be somewhat erratic. Later, the kicks and movements usually become stronger and more regular, and you'll be able to feel them by placing a hand on your lower abdomen. Some women may feel discomfort or have difficulty sleeping due to particularly active babies. This is normal and, while sometimes uncomfortable, is a reassuring sign of a happy baby.

As your pregnancy progresses, you'll probably become aware of your baby's typical movement patterns. Each fetus has its own pattern of activity and devel-

opment. The most active time is between 27 and 32 weeks. Activity tends to slow down in the last weeks of pregnancy. If you notice any major changes in your baby's activity level after 22 weeks — such as an absence or slowdown of movement for more than 24 hours — contact your care provider.

BACKACHE

Pregnant women are prone to backaches and back pain for a number of reasons. During pregnancy, the joints and ligaments in your pelvic region begin to soften and loosen in preparation for the baby to pass through your pelvis. As your uterus grows, your abdominal organs shift and your body weight is redistributed, changing your center of gravity. In response, you begin to adjust your posture and the ways you move. These compensations often lead to backaches and back pain.

Prevention and self-care To help you feel more comfortable:

- Practice good posture. Tuck your buttocks under, pull your shoulders back and downward, and stand straight and tall. Be aware of how you stand, sit and move.
- Change position often, and avoid standing for long periods of time.
- Avoid lifting heavy objects or children.
- Lift correctly. Don't bend over at the waist. Instead, squat down, bend your knees, and lift with your legs rather than your back (see page 55).
- Place one foot on a low stool when you have to stand for a long time.
- Wear supportive low-heeled or flat shoes.

- Exercise (swim, walk or stretch) at least three times a week. Consider joining a prenatal exercise or yoga class.
- Try to avoid sudden reaching movements or stretching your arms high over your head.
- Sit with your feet slightly elevated.
- Sleep on your side with one knee or both knees bent. Place a pillow between your knees and another one under your abdomen. You may also find relief by placing a regular pillow or a specially shaped body pillow under your abdomen.
- Apply heat to your back. Try warm bath soaks, warm wet towels, a hot water bottle or a heating pad. Some women find relief by alternating ice packs with heat.
- Have a back massage or practice relaxation techniques.
- Wear maternity pants with a low, supportive waistband. Or consider using a maternity support belt.
- Do low back stretches. Rest comfortably on your hands and knees with your head in line with your back (see page 167). Pull in your stomach, arching your back upward. Hold the position for several seconds, then relax. Repeat five times, gradually working up to 10 repetitions.

When to seek medical help If your back pain is severe, tell this to your care provider. He or she may suggest a variety of approaches, such as special stretching exercises, to alleviate the pain. Also contact your care provider if your back pain lasts four to six hours or longer or if you're also experiencing any of the following signs or symptoms:
- Vaginal bleeding
- Blood in your urine or burning when you urinate
- Cramping or abdominal pain
- Passing of tissue from the vagina
- Fever
- Regular uterine contractions (every 10 minutes or more often), which may feel like a tightening in your abdomen
- A feeling of heaviness or pressure in the pelvis or lower abdomen
- Watery discharge (clear, pink or brownish fluid) leaking from your vagina
- Menstrual-like cramps, which may come and go and may be accompanied by diarrhea

BLURRY VISION

Eye changes during pregnancy can cause slightly blurred vision. Because your body retains extra fluid, the outer layer of your eye (cornea) becomes slightly thicker.

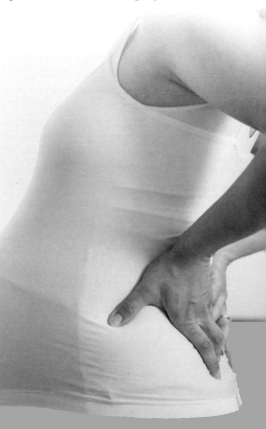

This change may become apparent by the 10th week of pregnancy and persist until about six weeks after the baby is born. In addition, the pressure of fluid within your eyeball (intraocular pressure) decreases during pregnancy. In combination, these changes can cause blurry vision. If you wear contact lenses, particularly hard lenses, you may find them uncomfortable because of these changes.

Prevention and self-care If your contact lenses are uncomfortable, you may want to wear your glasses more often. It's not necessary to change your glasses prescription during pregnancy because your vision will typically return to normal after you give birth.

When to seek medical help If you experience a sudden onset of blurry vision, or you develop additional symptoms such as headaches with the onset of blurry vision, contact your care provider. This is especially critical if you have diabetes. Talk to your care provider about establishing good control of your diabetes and monitoring your blood sugar, and about any vision problems you experience.

Blurry vision may also be related to preeclampsia, a disease that produces an increase in blood pressure. Talk to your care provider if you notice a sudden change in your vision, if your vision is very blurry or if you're seeing spots in front of your eyes.

BREAST DISCHARGE

In the final weeks of pregnancy, you may notice a thin, yellowish or clear substance leaking from one or both nipples. This discharge is colostrum, the yellowish fluid produced by your breasts before your milk comes in several days after giving birth.

Colostrum can range in color and consistency, and variations are normal. It may be sticky and yellow at first and become more watery as you approach your due date. The older you are and the more pregnancies you've had, the more likely it is you'll have some breast discharge. But it's no cause for concern if you don't leak colostrum — it doesn't mean you won't be able to produce breast milk.

If you're breast-feeding, you'll produce colostrum for the first few days after your baby is born.

Prevention and self-care If you're leaking colostrum, you can wear disposable or washable breast pads. It may also be helpful to allow your breasts to air-dry a few times a day and after showers.

When to seek medical help Call your care provider if your nipple discharge is bloody or contains pus or is accompanied by pain. This could indicate a breast abscess or other problem.

BREAST ENLARGEMENT

One of the first signs of pregnancy is an increase in breast size. As early as two weeks after conception, your breasts start to grow and change in preparation for producing milk. Stimulated by the hormones estrogen and progesterone, the milk-producing glands inside your breasts get bigger and fatty tissue increases slightly.

By the end of your first trimester, your breasts and nipples will be noticeably larger, and they may keep growing throughout your pregnancy. Breast enlargement accounts for at least a pound of the weight you gain while pregnant. Your breasts may remain enlarged for a while after your baby's birth.

Prevention and self-care As your breasts grow, wear a bra that fits well and provides good support to ease the strain on your breasts and back muscles. If your breasts make you uncomfortable at night, try sleeping in a cotton bra. Over the course of your pregnancy, you may need to replace your bras several times as your breasts change in size.

BREAST TENDERNESS

Often the first hint of pregnancy is a change in the way your breasts feel. A few weeks after conception, you may notice tingling sensations in your breasts, and they may feel heavy, tender and sore. Your nipples may be more sensitive.

As with breast enlargement, the primary reason for these changes is an increased production of the hormones estrogen and progesterone. Breast tenderness normally decreases after the first trimester.

Prevention and self-care A good support bra that fits well can help alleviate breast tenderness. Try a maternity bra or an athletic bra — these tend to be breathable and comfortable. At night you may feel more comfortable sleeping in a cotton bra.

BUTTOCK AND LEG PAIN

Pain, tingling or numbness running down your buttock, back or thigh is called sciatica because it follows the course of the sciatic nerve, a major nerve that runs from your lower back down the back of your legs to your feet. Sciatica is caused by pressure on the sciatic nerve from your growing uterus or baby or by relaxed pelvic joints. Lifting, bending and even walking may aggravate sciatica.

Although sciatica is no fun, it's generally not a cause for concern. When your baby changes position closer to the time of delivery, the pain is likely to ease.

Prevention and self-care Warm baths, a heating pad and switching the side of your body that you sleep on may help with sciatic nerve pain. You may also find relief by changing your position regularly during the day, such as by getting up and moving around once every hour or so.

Swimming is another way to ease the discomfort. Being in the water temporarily takes some of the weight of your uterus off your sciatic nerve.

When to seek medical help Tell your care provider if you're experiencing sciatica. Seek care if the numbness or pain causes you to trip when you walk or if you feel that you can't move your foot with equal strength in all directions. It's fairly common to need physical therapy to help relieve sciatic nerve pain.

CARPAL TUNNEL SYNDROME

Carpal tunnel syndrome is most often caused by repetitive movements of the hand and wrist. You may be surprised to learn that it's also common in pregnant women. That's because hormonal changes, swelling and weight gain can compress the nerve beneath the carpal tunnel ligament in your wrist.

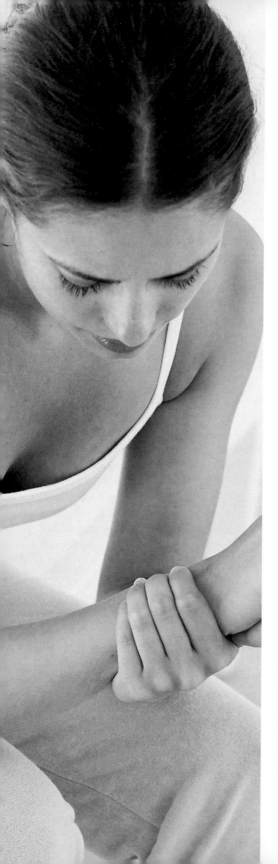

The carpal tunnel ligament is a tough membrane that holds the wrist bones together. A nerve called the median nerve enters the hand through the carpal tunnel, a space between the wrist bones and the carpal tunnel ligament. This passageway is rigid, so any swelling in the area can pinch or compress the median nerve, which supplies sensation to the ball of the thumb, the first two fingers and half of the ring finger.

Symptoms of carpal tunnel syndrome include numbness, tingling, weakness, pain, or a burning sensation in the hands and lower arms. In pregnant women, carpal tunnel syndrome often occurs in both hands.

Prevention and self-care You may be able to relieve the discomfort by rubbing or shaking your hands. The first line of treatment is to wear a wrist splint at night and during activities that make the symptoms worse, such as typing, driving a car or holding a book. Applying cold compresses or heat to your wrists also may help.

Medical care Carpal tunnel syndrome almost always disappears after delivery. In the rare cases when it doesn't, or when the effects are severe, you may be given steroid injections. Sometimes, minor surgery is needed to correct the problem.

CLUMSINESS

During pregnancy, you may find yourself stumbling or tripping, bumping into things, or dropping everything you pick up. You may worry that you're going to fall and hurt your baby.

It's perfectly normal to be clumsier than usual at this time. As your uterus grows, your sense of balance is thrown off. Your usual ways of moving, standing and walking change.

In addition, the hormone relaxin, produced by the placenta, relaxes the binding ligaments that hold the three pelvic bones together. This allows the pelvis to open wider so that the baby's head can move through the pelvis. It can also contribute to the feeling of clumsiness.

Other factors that may make you clumsier include water retention and lack of dexterity due to carpal tunnel syndrome. Late in pregnancy, your large abdomen can block your view of stairs or hazards on the floor. All of these effects are temporary, and you'll be back to your old self again after the baby is born.

If you do fall, know that your baby is well-protected and probably won't be harmed. An injury would normally have to be severe enough to hurt you before it would harm your baby.

Prevention and self-care You can't do much about the physical changes that can make you feel like a bull in a china shop, but you can decrease your chances of falling by taking a few precautions:

▶ Avoid wearing high heels. Instead, wear stable, flat or low-heeled shoes with soles that provide good traction.

▶ Avoid situations that require careful balance, such as perching on ladders and stools.

▶ Take a little extra time with tasks that require many changes of position.

▶ Use extra caution when going up or down stairs and in other situations that put you at risk of tripping or falling, such as walking on an icy stretch of sidewalk.

When to seek medical help If you fall, especially if you strike your abdomen or are worried about the welfare of your baby, contact your care provider for reassurance or treatment, if needed. If you fall on your abdomen late in pregnancy, your care provider will likely monitor the baby to be sure that the placenta's attachment to the uterus wasn't damaged. Also contact your care provider if after a fall or injury you begin to experience contractions or vaginal bleeding, or you feel you've hurt yourself.

CONSTIPATION

Constipation is one of the most common side effects of pregnancy, affecting at least half of all pregnant women at some point. It's usually more troublesome in women who were prone to constipation before pregnancy.

When you're pregnant, an increase in the hormone progesterone causes digestion to slow, so food passes more slowly through the gastrointestinal tract. In the later months, your ever-expanding uterus puts pressure on the lower bowel. In addition, your colon absorbs more water during pregnancy, which tends to make stools harder and bowel movements more difficult.

Other factors that can contribute to the problem include irregular eating habits, stress, changes in environment, and added calcium and iron in your diet. Constipation can give rise to hemorrhoids.

Prevention and self-care The first step in dealing with constipation is to evaluate your diet. Eating fiber-rich foods each day and drinking plenty of fluids, especially water, will help prevent or ease constipation. Follow these suggestions:

▶ Eat high-fiber foods, including fresh fruits, raw and cooked vegetables, bran, beans, and whole-grain foods, such as whole-wheat bread, brown rice and oatmeal. The age-old remedy of prunes (also called dried plums) can help, as can prune juice.

▶ Eat small, frequent meals and chew your food thoroughly.

▶ Drink plenty of fluids, especially water. Aim for eight 8-ounce glasses a day. Drink a glass of water before going to bed.

▶ Get more exercise. Just adding a little time to your daily walks or other physical activities can be effective.

▶ Iron supplements can cause constipation. If your care provider has recommended iron supplements and you have constipation, take the iron pills with prune juice. Or check to see if you could take a smaller dose of iron. Certain antacids and calcium supplements also can cause constipation, especially if you use frequent doses. If you have heartburn that requires multiple antacids per day and you develop constipation, talk to your provider for other recommendations.

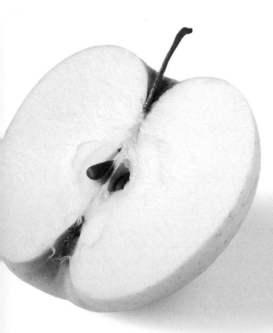

Medical care If self-care measures don't work, your care provider may recommend a mild laxative such as milk of magnesia, a bulking agent such as Metamucil or Citrucel, or a stool softener containing docusate. Stronger measures are sometimes needed, but they should only be used on the advice of your doctor.

Don't take cod liver oil because it can interfere with the absorption of certain vitamins and nutrients.

CONTRACTIONS

When you're about to go into labor, you'll notice an increase in contractions, the tightening and relaxing of the uterine muscles. During labor, the uterus repeatedly contracts, causing the cervix to thin (efface) and open up (dilate) so that you can push your baby out. The contractions gradually dilate the cervix until it's wide enough for the baby to pass through.

During the early phase of labor, contractions can vary greatly from one woman to another. They might last 30 seconds at the beginning and be irregularly spaced, 15 to 30 minutes apart. Or they might start out fast and then slow down. But they will continue to increase in frequency and duration as the cervix dilates.

Contractions may be relatively painless at first but gradually build in intensity. You may feel like your uterus is knotting up. Or the pain may feel like an aching sensation, pressure, fullness, cramping or a backache. For more information about contractions and labor, see Chapter 14.

Most expectant mothers feel occasional contractions in the last weeks of pregnancy, before they're actually in labor. When you put your hands on your abdomen, you may be able to feel your uterus tighten and relax. These mild contractions, also known as Braxton Hicks contractions, are called false labor. Your uterus is warming up, preparing for the big job ahead.

As you approach your due date, false labor contractions become stronger and may be uncomfortable or even painful at times. It can be easy to mistake them for the real thing.

Prevention and self-care If false labor contractions are making you uncomfortable, take a warm bath and drink plenty of fluids. If you're in true labor, and walking feels comfortable, go ahead and walk, stopping to breathe through contractions, if necessary. Walking may help your labor. Some women find that as the pain intensifies, rocking in a rocking chair or taking a warm shower helps with relaxation between their contractions.

When to seek medical help Monitor your contractions closely to see if they:
◗ Last at least 30 seconds
◗ Occur regularly
◗ Occur more than six times in an hour
◗ Don't go away when you move around

If you're in doubt about whether you are in labor, call your care provider. He or she will want to know what other symptoms you're feeling, how far apart your contractions are and whether you can talk during them. Go to the hospital if:
◗ Your water breaks (membranes rupture), even if you're not having contractions.
◗ Your contractions come five minutes apart or closer. Frequent contractions may be a sign of a rapid delivery.

FALSE LABOR VS. TRUE LABOR

Contraction characteristic	False labor (Braxton Hicks contraction)	True labor
Frequency of contractions	• Irregular • Don't become consistently closer together	• Regular pattern • Grow closer together
Length and intensity of contractions	• Vary • Usually weak • Don't become stronger	• At least 30 seconds at onset • Become longer • Become stronger
	• Usually stop if you walk, rest, change positions or drink water	• Won't go away no matter what you do • May grow stronger with activity, such as walking
Location of contractions	• Centered in lower abdomen and groin	• Wrap around from back to abdomen • Radiate throughout lower back and high on abdomen

- You have constant, severe pain.
- You have bleeding that's heavier than spotting.

CRAMPING

Abdominal cramping or pain is not uncommon in pregnancy. However, in early pregnancy, abdominal cramping that's accompanied by bleeding may be associated with a miscarriage or an ectopic pregnancy.

In midpregnancy and beyond, cramping is often associated with uterine contractions (see page 395). Occasionally,

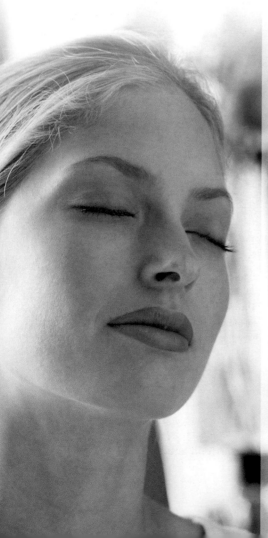

constipation is the cause. Abdominal pain that's sudden and severe may be an indication of placental separation. Abdominal pain combined with a fever and vaginal discharge may signal an infection.

When to seek medical help Contact your care provider if cramping or back pain is severe, persistent or accompanied by a fever, bleeding or vaginal discharge.

DIZZINESS AND FAINTNESS

Feeling a little dizzy? It's common for pregnant women to experience light-headedness, dizziness or faintness. These sensations can result from circulatory changes, such as decreased blood flow to your upper body because of the pressure of your uterus on the blood vessels in your back and pelvis. You're particularly susceptible to this early in the second trimester, when your blood vessels have dilated in response to pregnancy hormones but your blood volume hasn't yet expanded to fill them.

Dizziness or faintness may also occur during hot weather or when you're taking a hot bath or shower. When you're overheated, the blood vessels in your skin dilate, temporarily reducing the amount of blood returning to your heart.

Low blood sugar (hypoglycemia), common in early pregnancy, also can cause dizziness, as can having too few red blood cells (anemia). Stress, fatigue, hunger and, rarely, abnormal heart rhythms can make you feel dizzy or faint as well.

Prevention and self-care To prevent faintness and dizziness:
- Move slowly as you get up from a lying or sitting position.

- Move or walk at a slower pace. Take frequent rest breaks.
- Avoid standing for long periods of time.
- Avoid lying flat on your back. Instead, lie on your side, with a pillow tucked under your hip.
- Avoid getting overheated. Stay away from warm, crowded areas. Dress in layers. Make sure your bath or shower isn't too hot. Leave the door or window open to keep the room from getting too hot.
- Eat several small meals or snacks each day instead of three large meals. Munch on snacks such as dried or fresh fruit, whole-wheat bread, crackers or low-fat yogurt.
- Stay physically active to help with your lower body circulation. Good activities include walking, water aerobics and prenatal yoga.
- Wear compression garments to help with lower body circulation.
- Drink plenty of fluids, particularly early in the day. Water is best. Sports drinks may also be effective.
- Eat foods that are rich in iron, such as beans, red meat, green leafy vegetables and dried fruits. Also take iron supplements or prenatal vitamins as recommended by your care provider.

When to seek medical help It's always a good idea to tell your care provider if you've been feeling faint or dizzy. Early in pregnancy, if faintness or dizziness is severe and occurs with abdominal pain or vaginal bleeding, it may be a sign of the fertilized egg attaching outside the uterus (ectopic pregnancy). Also inform your care provider if you're experiencing headaches, blurred vision, impaired speech, chest pain or palpitations along with dizziness.

DREAMS

You're being grabbed by a gorilla ... flying over tall buildings ... talking to your newborn, who is talking back! Vivid dreams and nightmares are common during pregnancy. Dreams may be the mind's way of processing unconscious information. During this time of emotional and physical changes, your dreams may seem more intense and strange. You may find that you're dreaming more frequently or remembering your dreams more clearly when you wake up.

You may have anxiety dreams or nightmares. Try not to be disturbed about them. They reflect your apprehension and excitement about this major life change.

One way to enjoy your heightened dream world is to record your dreams in a dream journal. Writing about dreams can be a way to reflect on and come to terms with your experiences. If disturbing dreams or nightmares are causing you distress, it might be helpful to talk with a therapist or counselor to help discover what's troubling you.

ENLARGED VEINS

During pregnancy, veins throughout your body become larger to accommodate increased blood flow to your baby. These enlarged vessels often show up as fine bluish or purplish lines under the skin, most often on the legs and ankles. Blood vessels in the skin on your breasts also become more visible and appear as blue or purplish lines. These lines usually disappear after pregnancy.

Some women develop varicose veins — protruding, swollen veins, particularly in the legs (see page 427). The veins may also extend into the vulva, where they

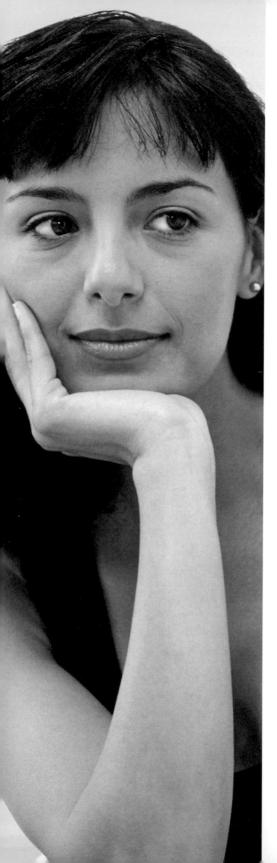

can be quite painful. Varicose veins usually surface late in pregnancy, when the uterus exerts greater pressure on the veins in the legs and lower body. They typically resolve within a few months after delivery. To help minimize the effects of varicose veins, elevate your legs while at rest, avoid prolonged standing or sitting, and wear compression stockings. Contact your provider if your varicose veins become swollen, red, or tender or they begin to bleed.

EXCESSIVE SALIVATION

Along with feeling nauseated, you may be experiencing excessive salivation. This is called ptyalism. It's a somewhat unusual side effect of pregnancy, but it's very real and can be annoying. However, it's not an indication that anything is wrong. It may be that you're not really producing more saliva, but that you're not swallowing as much as usual because of nausea.

Prevention and self-care It may be helpful to cut back on starchy foods. Usually, when your nausea begins to decrease, this problem tends to ease up.

When to seek medical help Excessive salivation by itself doesn't require medical care. However, if you have pain while swallowing or difficulty swallowing, tell your care provider.

EYE CHANGES

Some of the changes your body undergoes during pregnancy can affect your eyes and your vision. During pregnancy, the outer layer (cornea) of the eyes becomes a little thicker, and the pressure of fluid within your eyeballs (intraocular pressure) decreases by about 10 percent. These changes occasionally result in slightly blurred vision (see page 389). In addition to blurry vision, you may experience other changes:

> *Refractive changes.* Changes in hormone levels appear to temporarily alter the strength you need in your eyeglasses or contact lenses.
> *Dry eyes.* Some pregnant women develop dry eyes, which may involve a stinging, burning or scratchy sensation, increased eye irritation or fatigue, and difficulty wearing contact lenses.
> *Puffy eyelids.* Because of water retention during pregnancy, you may have puffiness around the eyes. Puffy eyelids can interfere with your peripheral vision.

Diabetes complications such as diabetic retinopathy — which damages the retina of your eye — can worsen during pregnancy. It's essential to have your eyes examined during pregnancy if you have diabetes. Women with high blood pressure (hypertension) also are susceptible to vision problems. High blood pressure during pregnancy also requires close observation.

Prevention and self-care To lessen the discomfort of dry eyes, use lubricating eyedrops, also referred to as artificial tears. Lubricating eyedrops are safe to use during pregnancy. If your contacts are uncomfortable because of dry, irritated eyes, try cleaning the lenses with an enzymatic cleaner more often. If they remain uncomfortable, don't worry. Your eyes will likely return to normal a few weeks after delivery. Meanwhile, you may need to stop wearing your contact lenses during pregnancy.

When to seek medical help Contact your care provider immediately if you have a new onset of blurred vision or blind spots. If you have diabetes or high blood pressure, work with your care provider to closely monitor your vision.

FACIAL SKIN DARKENING

More than half of all pregnant women develop mild skin darkening on the face. Commonly called the mask of pregnancy, this brownish coloration is also known as chloasma or melasma. It can affect any woman who's pregnant, though women who are dark haired and fair skinned are more susceptible. Melasma usually appears on sun-exposed areas of the face, such as the forehead, temples, cheeks, chin, nose and upper lip. It can occur on both sides of the face (symmetrical), but often develops in just one area.

Melasma is often aggravated or intensified by exposure to sunlight or other sources of ultraviolet (UV) light. The condition usually fades after delivery, although it may not fade completely, and it can return with subsequent pregnancies or sun exposure.

Prevention and self-care Because exposure to sunlight often worsens skin darkening, protect yourself from getting too much sun:

> Always wear sunscreen with a sun protection factor (SPF) of 15 or greater when you're outdoors, whether it's sunny or cloudy. The sun's UV rays can reach your skin even when the sky is overcast.
> Avoid the most intense hours of sunlight, during the middle of the day.
> Wear a wide-brimmed hat that shades your face.

Medical care Avoid creams or other agents that bleach the skin. If your skin darkening is extreme, your care provider or a dermatologist may prescribe a medicated ointment. If melasma persists long after you've delivered your baby, consult a dermatologist. He or she may recommend a medicated cream or ointment or a chemical peel.

FATIGUE

"I'm so tired!" This is one of the most common comments of pregnancy. During the early months, your body is working hard — pumping out hormones, producing more blood to carry nutrients to the fetus, speeding your heart rate to accommodate the increased blood flow, and changing the way you use water, protein, carbohydrates and fat. During the last couple of months of pregnancy, carrying the extra weight of the baby is tiring.

In addition to physical changes, you're probably dealing with a range of emotions and thoughts that may sap your energy and disturb sleep. It's natural to have conflicting feelings about a pregnancy, whether it's planned or unplanned, your first or your fourth. Even if you're overjoyed, you're probably facing added stresses. You may have fears about whether the baby will be healthy, anxiety about how you will adjust to motherhood and concerns about increased expenses. If your job is demanding, you may worry about being able to stay productive throughout your pregnancy. These concerns are normal and natural.

Rarely, fatigue is related to a medical condition. If your fatigue is severe, discuss it with your care provider. He or she

might want to check your bloodwork to make sure you're not developing anemia.

Prevention and self-care Fatigue is a sign from your body that you need extra rest. Don't push yourself. Here are some ways to keep fatigue from getting the best of you:

- *Rest.* Accept the fact that you need extra rest during these ten months, and plan your daily life accordingly. Take naps when you can during the day. If you can't nap during the day, maybe you can after work or before dinner. If you need to go to bed at 7 p.m. to feel rested, do it.
- *Avoid taking on extra responsibilities.* Cut down on volunteer commitments and social events if they're wearing you out.
- *Ask for the support you need.* Get your partner or other children to help out as much as possible.
- *Exercise.* Regular physical activity will help increase your energy level. Even walking for 30 minutes a day can make you feel more energized.
- *Eat well.* Eating a nutritious, balanced diet is more important now than ever. Make sure you're getting enough calories, iron and protein. Fatigue may be worse if your diet is short on these.

Medical care No medications for fatigue are safe or effective during pregnancy. You also want to limit stimulants such as caffeine, which may be harmful in high doses.

FEELING WARM

Overheated? It's not just because you're getting bigger or because the weather is warm. During pregnancy, your metabolism — the rate at which your body expends energy at rest — speeds up. And you're probably perspiring more as a result of needing to lose all the heat your baby is making. This can leave you feeling too warm, even in winter.

Prevention and self-care It's important to avoid getting overheated while pregnant. Follow these tips to keep cool:

- Drink plenty of water and other fluids. Carry a water bottle with you.
- Dress lightly in breathable fabrics such as cotton.
- Avoid exercising outside in the warmest part of the day. Take a walk before breakfast or after dinner, or go to a fitness center.
- Try to stay out of the sun as much as possible.
- Go for a swim, or take a tepid or cool shower or bath.
- When the temperature is over 90 F, stay in air-conditioned environments as much as possible.

FLUID LEAKAGE

When the amniotic sac leaks or breaks, the fluid that has been cushioning the baby comes out in a trickle or gush. This dramatic event is known as the water breaking, or the rupture of membranes. Only about 10 percent of women experience their water breaking before labor. Your membranes are more likely to rupture sometime during labor. When it happens, labor usually starts or becomes more intense.

Contact your care provider if your water breaks. Most care providers want to evaluate you as soon as it happens because there's a risk of infection after the membranes rupture. Generally, unless

the baby is very premature, it's best that the baby is born within about 24 hours. Let your care provider know if the fluid is anything other than clear and odorless. A greenish or foul-smelling fluid could be a sign of a uterine infection.

If you're uncertain whether the leaking fluid is amniotic fluid or urine, have it checked by your care provider. Many pregnant women leak urine during the later stages of pregnancy. In the meantime, don't do anything that could introduce bacteria into your vagina, such as having sex or using tampons.

FOOD AVERSIONS

Early in pregnancy, you may find yourself repulsed by certain foods, such as fried foods or coffee. Just the smell of these foods may send a wave of nausea through your stomach. You may have a mildly metallic taste in your mouth that contributes to the problem. Most food aversions disappear or weaken by the fourth month of pregnancy.

Food aversions, like so many other complaints of pregnancy, can be chalked up to hormonal changes. Most pregnant women find that their food tastes change somewhat, especially in the first trimester, when the hormones are having the strongest impact. Food aversions can be accompanied by a heightened sense of smell and, at times, increased salivation, making your distaste even more acute.

Prevention and self-care As long as you continue to eat a healthy diet and get all the nutrients you need, appetite changes aren't a cause for concern. If your aversion is to coffee or tea, that works in your favor because you'll find it easier to give up these foods. But if your aversion is to healthy foods such as fruits or vegetables, you'll have to find other sources of the nutrients that these foods provide.

FOOD CRAVINGS

You may not have had the classic pickles-and-ice-cream craving, but chances are you've had a strong desire for certain types of food during your pregnancy. Most expectant mothers experience food cravings, which are likely caused by pregnancy hormones.

You may wonder if a food craving is a signal from your body that you need the nutrients in that food; however, a craving for ice cream doesn't mean your body

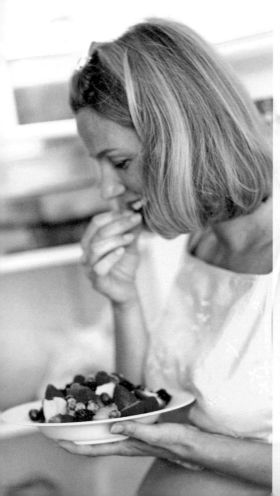

needs the saturated fat. Similarly, if you're not in the mood for citrus fruits, that doesn't mean you don't need vitamin C.

Most food cravings disappear or weaken by the fourth month of pregnancy. Cravings that last longer could be a sign of iron deficiency and the anemia that results. Discuss this with your care provider if strong cravings continue into the second trimester.

Prevention and self-care As long as you're eating a healthy diet and getting the nutrients you need, you don't have to worry about changes in your food tastes. It's OK to indulge occasionally. However, try not to use your cravings as an excuse for overeating. You can respond to cravings without compromising your own or your baby's nutrition.

Try to satisfy your food urges without filling up on empty calories. For example, if you crave chocolate, choose dark chocolate rather than chocolate ice cream. If you crave a burger and fries, try a hot sub sandwich and baked chips instead.

In addition, try diverting your attention by taking a walk, reading a good book or calling a friend to see whether a craving goes away or hunger persists. Even though you're "eating for two," there's usually no need to eat if you don't actually feel hungry.

When to seek medical help Rarely, some pregnant women have a craving for unusual, inedible and possibly harmful substances. These may include items such as clay, laundry starch, dirt, baking soda, ice chips or frost from the freezer, ashes, or road salt. Such uncommon cravings result from a disorder known as pica. It can be dangerous and may be caused by an iron deficiency. If you experience a craving to eat something that isn't food, report it to your care provider.

FORGETFULNESS

You misplace your keys, forget an appointment and can't focus on your work. If you feel like you've turned into a scatterbrain since becoming pregnant, don't worry. During pregnancy, some women become more forgetful or absent-minded or have trouble concentrating. These symptoms, similar to what some women experience premenstrually, are a temporary effect of hormonal changes. Sometimes, forgetfulness can persist for a while after delivery.

Prevention and self-care To help yourself feel more in control:

▶ Accept that being a little absent-minded during pregnancy is normal. Getting uptight about it may make it worse. Now's the time to have a sense of humor.

▶ Reduce the stresses in your life as much as possible.

▶ Keep lists at home and at work to remind you about things you need to do. Use your phone or personal device to help you remember your to-do list, too.

GAS AND BLOATING

Gas, bloating, flatulence — more fun aspects of being pregnant! Under the influence of pregnancy hormones, your digestive system slows down. Food moves more slowly through your gastrointestinal tract. This slowdown serves an important purpose: It allows nutrients more time to be absorbed into your bloodstream and to reach the fetus. Unfortunately, it can also cause bloating and gas. The problem may be aggravated during the first trimester, when many women

have a tendency to swallow air in response to nausea.

Prevention and self-care To minimize the amount of gas and bloating you experience during pregnancy, follow these suggestions:

▶ Keep your bowels moving. Constipation is a common cause of gas and bloating. To avoid it, drink plenty of liquids, eat a variety of high-fiber foods and stay physically active.

▶ Eat small, frequent meals, and don't overfill your stomach.

▶ Eat slowly. When you eat in a hurry, you're more likely to swallow air, which can contribute to gas. Take a few deep breaths before meals to relax.

▶ Avoid gas-producing foods. These vary from one person to another, but some common culprits include beans, cabbage, broccoli, cauliflower, Brussels sprouts, onions, carbonated beverages, fried foods, greasy or high-fat foods, and rich sauces. Some of these foods are good sources of nutrients. Instead of giving them up, try eating them in small amounts.

▶ Don't lie down immediately after eating.

Medical care Some over-the-counter medications for gas and bloating are safe, but talk with your care provider before taking medications. If you're uncomfortable — the problem is more than a social nuisance — your care provider can suggest alternative treatment approaches.

GUM DISEASE AND BLEEDING

Like the rest of your body, your gums receive more blood flow during pregnancy. This can cause them to swell and soften, and they may bleed a little when you brush your teeth.

You're more susceptible to dental problems when you're pregnant, too. The oral changes of pregnancy are linked to an increased amount of plaque that coats your teeth. Hormonal changes also make your gums more susceptible to the damaging effects of plaque. If plaque hardens, it turns into tartar. When plaque and tartar build up around the base of your teeth, they can irritate your gums and create pockets of bacteria between your gums and teeth. This condition is called gingivitis, a form of gum disease. If it occurs, gingivitis usually starts in the second trimester.

Prevention and self-care Because your teeth are more susceptible to the harmful effects of bacteria while you're pregnant, it's important to keep up good dental hygiene. Follow these steps to keep your gums healthy:
- Brush your teeth with fluoride toothpaste at least twice a day, as well as after meals, if possible.
- Rinse your mouth with water or with anti-plaque and fluoride mouthwashes.
- Floss your teeth gently but thoroughly each day. Flossing removes plaque between your teeth and helps massage your gums.
- Even if you're not having problems with your teeth or gums, schedule an appointment to have your teeth checked and cleaned at least once during your 10 months.

Medical care If you have severe gum disease, you'll want to have it treated. Contact your dentist and your care provider if you have signs and symptoms of periodontitis:
- Swollen or recessed gums
- An unpleasant taste in your mouth
- Bad breath
- Loose teeth or a change in your bite
- Drainage of pus around one or more teeth

HEADACHES

Many pregnant women are troubled by headaches. Early in pregnancy, increased blood circulation and hormonal changes can cause headaches. Other possible causes include stress or anxiety, fatigue, nasal congestion, eyestrain, and tension. If you suddenly eliminated or cut down on caffeine when you learned you were pregnant, this withdrawal can cause headaches for a few days.

If you already have problems with migraines, during your pregnancy they may stay the same, improve or worsen. They might be worse in the first trimester, then improve in the second.

Prevention and self-care To prevent headaches, you might try to determine what triggers them and avoid those things. Triggers may include cigarette smoke, stuffy rooms, eyestrain and certain foods. Here are some other suggestions for minimizing headaches:
- Get plenty of sleep each night, and rest during the day when possible.
- Drink plenty of liquids.
- Soothe a sinus headache by applying a warm washcloth to the front and sides of your face, around your nose, eyes and temples. If you feel a tension headache coming on, apply an ice pack or cold compress to your forehead and the back of your neck.
- Take a warm shower or bath.
- Massage your neck, shoulders, face and scalp, or ask your partner or a friend to give you a massage.

- Practice relaxation techniques and exercises, such as relaxed breathing and meditation (see page 353).
- Minimize the stresses in your life. If you're under more stress than you feel you can handle, it might be helpful to talk to your care provider.

When to seek medical help Contact your care provider right away if you're having headaches that are severe, persistent or frequent, or that are accompanied by blurry vision or other vision changes. Also talk to your care provider before taking pain relievers or headache medications. Acetaminophen (Tylenol, others) is safe for most women to use in pregnancy, but if overused, it can cause liver issues or worsening headaches.

If you have migraines, talk to your care provider about how to manage them during pregnancy. He or she may advise you to avoid certain medications.

HEARTBURN

More than half of all pregnant women get heartburn, and for many it's their first experience with it. Heartburn actually has nothing to do with your heart. It's caused by the backward flow of stomach contents passing up into the esophagus (acid reflux). When this happens, stomach acids irritate the lining of the esophagus. The resulting burning sensation at about the level of the heart gives the condition its misleading name.

Heartburn is more common during pregnancy because pregnancy hormones cause your digestive system to slow down. This gives nutrients more time to be absorbed into your bloodstream and to reach the fetus, but it also takes longer for your stomach to empty. The result is often indigestion and heartburn. In addition, during the later months of pregnancy, your growing uterus continually pushes on your stomach, moving it higher and compressing it. This pressure can force stomach acids upward, causing heartburn.

Prevention and self-care Heartburn is unpleasant, but you can take steps to prevent it or treat it:

▶ Eat more-frequent but smaller meals. For example, have five or six small meals a day rather than three large meals.

▶ Some foods are more likely to irritate your stomach and esophagus than are others. Try to determine which foods give you heartburn, and avoid them. Stay away from fatty, greasy or fried foods, coffee and tea, chocolate, peppermint, alcohol, carbonated beverages, very sweet foods, acidic foods such as citrus fruits and juices, tomatoes and red peppers, and highly spiced foods.

▶ Drink plenty of fluids, especially water.

▶ Sit with good posture when eating. Slouching can put extra pressure on your stomach.

▶ Wait an hour or longer after eating before you lie down, and avoid eating for two to three hours before you go to bed. An empty stomach produces less acid.

▶ Avoid movements and positions that seem to aggravate the problem. When picking things up, bend at the knees, not the waist.

▶ When resting or sleeping, prop yourself up on pillows to elevate your head and shoulders, or raise the head of your bed 4 to 6 inches.

When to seek medical help If heartburn becomes a frequent, significant problem, see your care provider. Don't take any antacid or acid blocker without consulting your care provider first. Antacids can be high in salt and can increase fluid buildup in body tissues during pregnancy or worsen constipation. You also want to avoid heartburn medications that contain aspirin, such as Alka-Seltzer.

HEMORRHOIDS

Hemorrhoids during pregnancy are caused by increased blood volume and pressure from the uterus on the veins in your rectum. The veins may enlarge into firm, swollen pouches underneath the mucous membranes inside or outside the rectum. Hemorrhoids may occur for the first time during pregnancy or become more frequent or severe.

Constipation also can contribute to hemorrhoids because straining can enlarge the rectal veins. Constipation is common throughout pregnancy, especially during the later months, when your uterus crowds other organs and may push against your large intestine.

Hemorrhoids can be painful, and they may bleed, itch or sting, especially during or after a bowel movement. Usually, hemorrhoids recede or disappear after you give birth.

Prevention and self-care The best way to deal with hemorrhoids is to avoid constipation. To prevent hemorrhoids or to ease their discomfort, try the following tips:

▶ Eat high-fiber foods, such as fruits and vegetables, and drink plenty of fluids.
▶ Exercise regularly.
▶ Avoid straining during bowel movements. Put your feet on a stool to reduce straining, and avoid sitting on the toilet for long periods of time.
▶ Keep the area around your anus clean. Gently wash the area after each bowel movement. Pads of witch hazel may help relieve pain and itching. You can refrigerate the pads, which may be more soothing when applied cold.
▶ Try warm soaks in a tub or sitz bath. Add an oatmeal bath formula or baking soda to the water to combat itching.
▶ Avoid sitting for long periods, especially on hard chairs.

Medical care Consult your care provider to develop a plan to manage hemorrhoids during pregnancy. If self-care measures don't work, your care provider may prescribe a cream or an ointment that can shrink them.

HIP PAIN

It's not uncommon to feel some soreness or pain in your hips during pregnancy, especially when you're sleeping on your side at night. In preparation for the birth of your baby, the connective tissues in your body soften and loosen up. The ligaments in your hips stretch, and the joints between the pelvic bones relax. The greater flexibility makes it easier for the baby to pass through the pelvis at birth.

In late pregnancy, your heavier uterus might contribute to changes in your posture, adding to your hip soreness. Hip pain is often stronger on one side because the baby tends to lie more heavily to one side. If you have other young children you carry on your hip, this may also contribute to hip pain.

Prevention and self-care Exercises to strengthen your lower back and abdominal muscles may ease hip soreness. Warm baths and back and hip massages also may help. Try elevating your hips above the level of your chest a few minutes at a time.

HUNGER

Feeling hungrier than usual is normal — most women experience an increase in appetite throughout pregnancy. Some women have the opposite problem: a lack of appetite due to nausea. Or you may be hungry for a certain type of food, such as fruit, chocolate, mashed potatoes or cereal. Especially during the first trimester, hormonal changes can cause changes in appetite. The main thing is to eat a variety of nutritious foods (see page 38). If you're frequently hungry, eat small meals throughout the day.

INCREASED HEART RATE

Throughout pregnancy your heart pumps more blood than it does normally. This helps meet the fetus's needs for oxygen and nutrients, which are carried in the blood through the placenta.

As the heart pumps additional blood, your heart rate speeds up as well. Your heart beats progressively faster throughout pregnancy — what may feel like a pounding in your chest. By the third trimester, your heart rate may be 20 percent faster than it was before you were pregnant.

Medical care Because of increases in blood volume, some pregnant women develop heart murmurs. This occurrence is normal because more blood is flowing through your heart valves. Occasionally, however, the murmur may sound different enough that your care provider will investigate the condition further.

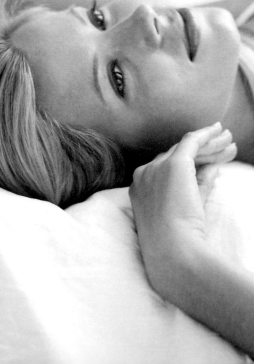

INSOMNIA

You go to bed exhausted, sure that you'll nod off the minute your head hits the pillow. Instead, you find yourself wide awake and watching the minutes tick by. Or you wake up at 4 o'clock in the morning, unable to fall back asleep. Insomnia is very common during pregnancy. There are many reasons why.

Although many women sleep more during the first trimester than before they were pregnant, hormonal changes can make it more difficult for some women to sleep through the night. In addition, as your growing uterus puts pressure on your bladder, the frequent need to urinate also can get you out of bed at night to go to the bathroom.

As the baby gets larger, you may find it harder to find a comfortable position for sleeping. An active baby also can keep you awake. Heartburn, leg cramps and nasal congestion are other common reasons for disturbed sleep in the later months of pregnancy.

Then there's the natural anticipation, excitement and anxiety you're bound to feel about your baby's arrival. You may have worries about the health of the baby and the changes the baby is going to create in your life. These feelings can make it hard to relax your mind and body. If you have frequent and vivid dreams about birth and the baby, these can also contribute to insomnia.

Prevention and self-care If you have difficulty falling or staying asleep, try these suggestions:
- Start winding down before going to bed. Take a bath or do relaxation exercises. Ask your partner for a massage.
- Make sure your bedroom is at a comfortable temperature for sleeping and that it's dark and quiet. Avoid watch-

ing TV or using your smartphone or other personal devices soon before bed. Store your personal devices away from the bed at night.

▶ Cut down on your fluids in the evening before bed.

▶ Avoid beverages containing caffeine.

▶ Exercise regularly, but avoid exercising right before bedtime.

▶ The best position for sleeping in late pregnancy is on your left or right side, with your legs and knees bent. Lying on your side takes pressure off the large vein that carries blood from your legs and feet back to your heart. This position also takes pressure off your lower back. Use one pillow to support your abdomen and place another between your knees to support your upper leg. You can also try placing a bunched-up pillow or rolled-up blanket in the small of your back. This will help relieve pressure on the hip you're lying on.

▶ If you can't sleep, get up and read, listen to relaxing music, work on a hobby or do some other calming activity outside of the bedroom.

▶ Avoid making up for lost sleep by excessive napping, which could make it more difficult to sleep the next night.

Medical care If insomnia is frequent and is causing you problems, talk to your care provider. If disturbing dreams or nightmares are ongoing and are worrying you, it might be helpful to talk with a therapist or counselor.

IRRATIONAL FEARS

Everyone has some fears. You likely are concerned about the health and condition of your baby. You may also have fears about labor — such as not making it to the hospital in time or having an emergency cesarean delivery.

It's normal to feel a moderate amount of worry, but fears that are all-consuming and interfere with your day-to-day functioning may need attention.

Prevention and self-care Sit down and make a list of your fears. Share them with your partner or labor companion. Talking about your fears can lighten an unnecessarily heavy emotional load. You might also want to talk with your care provider and with other expectant mothers, perhaps in a pregnancy class or an online forum. When you voice your fears, they have less power over you.

Childbirth preparation classes offer a unique opportunity to talk with other couples who may have the same worries. The instructor also can help address fears about giving birth.

When to seek medical help If your fears are interfering with your daily functioning, talk with your care provider. Your care provider's reassurance may help you let go of some of your fears so that you can get on with caring for yourself and your baby.

ITCHINESS

Some pregnant women experience itchiness, which usually goes away after birth. The itchiness may be on your abdomen or all over your body, and it may accompany patches of red, flaky rash. (For more information on rashes, see page 415.) Skin stretching over the abdomen probably accounts for some of the itching and flaking, and dry skin can contribute to it as well.

Prevention and self-care Scratching isn't the best way to relieve an itch. Try these measures:

- Moisturize your skin with lotion, creams or oils.
- Wear loose clothing made from natural fibers, such as cotton.
- Use an oatmeal bath formula.
- Avoid getting overheated because you'll itch more if you're too warm.

When to seek medical help If self-care measures don't provide relief for your itches, your care provider may prescribe medication or other treatment techniques that can help.

If severe itching develops late in your pregnancy, or if your itching is primarily in the palms of your hands and soles of your feet, your care provider may order blood tests to check your liver function. Rarely, a liver condition called cholestasis of pregnancy can cause itchiness. Because there are fetal risks associated with cholestasis, let your care provider know if you experience severe itching.

LEG CRAMPS

Cramps in the lower leg muscles are fairly common in the second and third trimesters of pregnancy. They most frequently occur at night, and they may disrupt your sleep. Although the exact cause of leg cramps is unknown, slow blood return associated with the pressure of the baby on your leg veins may be responsible.

Prevention and self-care Here are some tips for relieving the discomfort of leg cramps or calf tenderness:

- Try exercises to stretch your calf muscles, particularly before bed.

- Stretch the affected muscle. Try straightening your knee and gently flexing your foot upward.
- Walk. You may find walking to be uncomfortable at first, but it helps relieve the cramping.
- Wear support hose, especially if you stand a lot during the day.
- Take frequent breaks if you sit or stand for long periods.
- Massage your calves.
- Try resting with your legs up on pillows or the arm of a sofa.
- Wear flats or low-heeled shoes.
- Stay hydrated by drinking plenty of water.

When to seek medical help If leg cramps persist, talk to your care provider. These cramps might be caused by a circulation problem. Contact your care provider right away if you notice redness, swelling or an increase in pain. Also let your provider know if you have a history of blood clots or a blood-clotting disorder.

LINEA NIGRA

Even when you're not pregnant, you have a pale line that runs vertically down your abdomen to your pubic bone. It's often barely noticeable — until pregnancy, when it can darken. Then it's known as the linea nigra, which means "black line." As your pregnancy continues, you may notice this line stretching from the bottom of your sternum to below your navel.

As with so many other changes that occur during pregnancy, this skin darkening is the result of hormones. These hormones cause the body to produce more pigment. You can't prevent this skin darkening, but it will usually fade after delivery.

MOOD SWINGS

One minute you're giddy with happiness. A few minutes later, you feel like crying. Especially in the first trimester, mood swings are common. Your emotions may span from exhilaration and joy to exhaustion, irritation, weepiness or depression. If you've typically experienced premenstrual syndrome, you may have more extreme mood swings when you're pregnant.

What causes this moodiness? Some of it is likely related to changing hormones and changes in your metabolism. Just as fluctuations in progesterone, estrogen and other hormones are linked to the blues many women feel before their periods or after giving birth, these hormonal changes may play a role in the mood changes of pregnancy.

Mood changes also may be linked to pregnancy-related discomforts such as nausea, frequent urination, swelling and backache, all of which can interfere with sleep. Fatigue, changing sleep patterns and new bodily sensations can all influence how you feel. You may also be adjusting to a new body image.

In addition, pregnancy can bring a number of new stresses to your life.

Prevention and self-care Knowing more about why you're feeling moody, and realizing these mood swings are temporary, can help you weather your moody storms. These tips may help you prevent mood swings altogether:

▸ *Keep healthy and fit by eating nutritious foods, getting plenty of sleep and exercising regularly.* Exercise is a natural stress reducer and can help prevent backache, fatigue and constipation.
▸ *Boost your support network.* This may include your partner, family, friends and a support group. A good support network can provide emotional support as well as practical support, helping with tasks as needed.
▸ *Find time to relax each day.* You might try techniques such as meditation, guided imagery and progressive muscle relaxation. These kinds of relaxation exercises are often taught in childbirth classes.
▸ *Accept that you may not be able to do everything you did before getting pregnant.* Cut back on unnecessary activities that may be contributing to stress or discomfort.

When to seek medical help Exaggerated mood swings that last more than two weeks could be a sign of depression. Mild depression is quite common in pregnant women. You may be experiencing depression if you're consistently feeling sad, weepy or worthless, your appetite

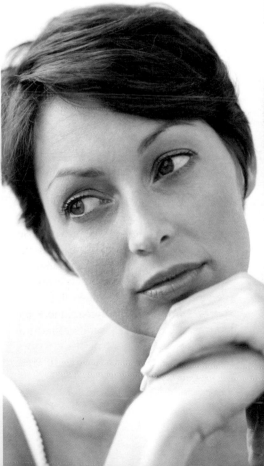

and sleeping habits have changed, you're having difficulty getting your work done, and you take less pleasure in things you normally enjoy.

If your mood swings seem to be more than you can handle or if these feelings get in the way of your daily life, talk to your care provider. Depression is treatable.

MORNING SICKNESS

Morning sickness is one of the classic signs of pregnancy. It refers to nausea and vomiting that often accompany pregnancy, especially in its early stages. For more information on morning sickness and how to cope with this common problem, see page 102.

MUCOUS DISCHARGE

As you approach your delivery date, you may notice an increase in mucous discharge from your vagina. During pregnancy, the opening of the cervix becomes blocked with a thick plug of mucus that helps keep bacteria and other germs from entering the uterus. When you get closer to labor, your cervix begins to thin and relax, and the mucous plug may loosen, causing discharge to increase and thicken. The plug is sometimes dislodged as thick, stringy or blood-tinged mucus.

Prevention and self-care Mucous discharge is normal toward the end of pregnancy. If you need something to absorb the flow, use sanitary napkins. Keep your genital area clean, and wear cotton underwear. Avoid tight or nylon pants, and don't use perfume or deodorant soap in the genital area.

When to seek medical help Call your care provider if your discharge is foul smelling, yellow or green or causes itching or burning. These could be signs or symptoms of an infection. Mucous discharge before 35 weeks could be a sign of preterm labor. Vaginal discharge that's watery and profuse enough to soak through a pad or your underwear should also be evaluated, so report it to your care provider.

NAVEL SORENESS

Along with the other aches and pains associated with your expanding uterus, your bellybutton (navel, or umbilicus) may feel tender or sore. This tenderness might be most noticeable around the 20th week of pregnancy. You may feel most uncomfortable when sitting upright. In some cases, as the skin around the navel continues to stretch, it may become increasingly tender and irritated by clothing and contact. The stretching and separation of the two large bands of muscles that run along your abdomen also can cause some soreness around your navel.

Prevention and self-care To relieve tenderness around your navel, use the pads of your fingers to massage your abdomen in a circular pattern, or ask your partner to do this for you. Apply a cold or warm compress to your bellybutton to soothe it. Sometimes, placing a large bandage over your naval can relieve irritation from clothing and other contact.

NESTING

As your due date nears, you may find yourself cleaning cupboards, washing walls, organizing your closets, cleaning out the garage, sorting the baby's clothes or decorating the nursery. The powerful urge to clean, organize and decorate before the baby arrives is called the nesting instinct. It's usually strongest just before delivery.

Nesting gives you a sense of accomplishment before birth and allows you to come home afterward to a clean house. This desire to prepare your home can be useful because it'll give you more time later to recover and spend time with your baby. But don't overdo it and wear yourself out. You'll need your energy for the hard work of labor.

NIPPLE DARKENING

Like other areas of your skin, the skin on or around your nipples may darken during pregnancy. Skin darkening is the result of pregnancy hormones, which cause your body to produce more pigment. The increased pigment isn't distributed evenly like a smooth tan, but often appears as splotches of color.

Darkening of the nipples and other areas of skin typically fades after delivery. In the meantime, avoid using agents that bleach the skin.

NOSEBLEEDS

Some women experience nosebleeds during pregnancy, even though they never or rarely did before. With the extra blood flowing throughout your body, the tiny blood vessels lining the nasal passages are more fragile and likely to rupture.

Prevention and self-care To prevent nosebleeds, take the following steps:

▶ Be gentle when blowing your nose, and don't pack your nose with gauze.
▶ Dry air may make you more susceptible to nosebleeds. Use a humidifier during the winter months.

If you do get a nosebleed, try this sequence to stop it:

▶ Sit up and keep your head above your heart.
▶ Lean forward to avoid swallowing the blood, and breathe through your mouth.
▶ Pinch the soft parts of your nose together between your thumb and index finger. Press firmly but gently, compressing the pinched parts of the nose toward the face.
▶ Hold this position for five minutes.

When to seek medical help Call your care provider if the nosebleed persists, if you have high blood pressure or if the nosebleed occurs after a head injury.

PELVIC PRESSURE

In the last weeks of pregnancy, you may feel a sense of pressure, heaviness, soreness or tenderness in your pelvic area. This is caused by the baby pushing into the pelvis and compressing the bladder and rectum. In addition, the baby is likely to compress some veins and cause blood to pool. Finally, the bones of the pelvis are being pushed outward a bit, causing further discomfort.

A feeling of pelvic pressure before the 37th week of pregnancy could be the start of preterm labor, particularly if the pressure seems to radiate toward your thighs, or you feel as if the baby is pushing down.

Prevention and self-care If you experience pelvic pressure in the last weeks of pregnancy, you may find some relief by resting with your feet up. Kegel exercises also may help with pelvic soreness: Squeeze the muscles around your vagina tightly, as if you were stopping the flow of urine for a few seconds, then relax. Repeat 10 times.

When to seek medical help Call your care provider or go to the hospital if you think you're experiencing preterm labor. In addition to pelvic pressure, other signs and symptoms of preterm labor may include:

▶ Cramping in the lower abdomen. The cramps may be similar to menstrual cramps and may be continuous or come and go.
▶ A low, dull backache that radiates to the side or front of your body and isn't relieved by any change in position.

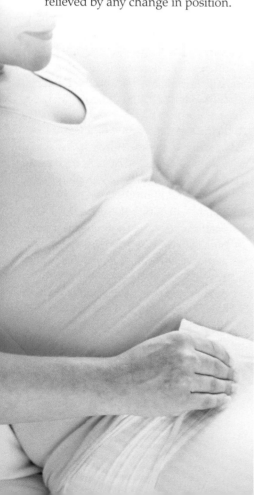

▶ Contractions every 10 minutes or more often.
▶ Clear, pink or brownish fluid leaking from your vagina or vaginal bleeding.

When you call, your care provider may ask you to come into the office or go to the hospital, or you may be advised to rest on your left side for an hour to see if the symptoms lessen or go away.

PERINEAL ACHING

During the last month of pregnancy, after the baby has dropped into the pelvis, you may feel a sensation of increased pressure or aching in the perineal area — the area between the vulva and the anus. This dropping, referred to as lightening, indicates that the presenting part of the baby, usually the head, is engaged in the upper portion of the pelvis. If this is your first pregnancy, baby may drop down into the birth canal several weeks before labor. If you've had a child before, lightening usually occurs just before labor.

In addition to aching or pressure in the perineal area, you may feel sharp twinges when the fetal head presses on the pelvic floor.

Prevention and self-care Kegel exercises can help strengthen your perineal muscles, and they may help with the aching. To do Kegels, squeeze the muscles around your vagina tightly, as if you were stopping the flow of urine for a few seconds, then relax. Repeat 10 times. For more on Kegels, see page 183.

When to seek medical help If perineal aching or pressure grows stronger and is accompanied by a feeling of tightening or contractions, you may be in labor. Contact your care provider.

PERSPIRATION

The effects of pregnancy hormones on your sweat glands, along with your need to get rid of all the heat the baby produces, may leave you feeling a little damp. Increased perspiration during pregnancy makes heat rashes more common. Hot summer weather also can be quite trying in late pregnancy.

Prevention and self-care To relieve excessive perspiration and avoid overheating, rest, drink cold liquids and take cool showers.

PUBIC BONE PAIN

Some pregnant women are troubled by pain in the pubic bone. The sensation may be mild or sharp and feel like an ache or a bruise. The pain is caused by softening and loosening of your tissues and joints. As the cartilage that connects the two pubic bones in the center of your pelvis softens, your pubic bone may feel very sore when you're moving or walking. Some pregnant women feel this more than others, and some have it only later in their pregnancies. Pubic bone pain should disappear within a few weeks after you give birth.

Prevention and self-care To ease the discomfort of pubic bone pain, you might try wearing support pantyhose. It may also help to take a warm bath. Alternating heat and cold may provide pain relief.

When to seek medical help Very rarely, pubic bone pain may result from joint inflammation. In this situation, the pain is constant, gets worse and may be accompanied by fever. If these signs and symptoms develop, contact your care provider.

RASHES

Red, itchy skin is probably not the pregnancy glow you had in mind. But some women develop rashes during pregnancy. Heat rashes, sometimes called prickly heat, are most common. They're caused by the increased perspiration and dampness triggered by pregnancy hormones. Other types of rashes also may appear during pregnancy.

- ▶ *Intertrigo.* This rash may result from inflammation due to skin rubbing, a bacterial infection or a fungal infection in the skin folds. It's typically found in the sweaty skin folds under the breasts or in the groin area — warm, moist areas where fungi can thrive. Intertrigo should be treated as early as possible because the longer it continues, the more difficult it may be to treat.
- ▶ *PUPPP.* About 1 in every 160 pregnant women develops a severe rash with the tongue-twisting name pruritic urticarial papules and plaques of pregnancy (PUPPP). This condition is characterized by itchy, reddish, raised patches on the skin. These itchy bumps are called papules, and the larger raised areas are called plaques. They usually show up first on the abdomen and often spread to the arms, legs and buttocks. In some women, the itching can be extreme. Although PUPPP can be miserable for you, it doesn't pose risks to the baby. The rash should go away after you deliver. Although it's not known for certain what causes PUPPP, a genetic factor

appears to be involved because the condition tends to run in families. PUPPP is more common in women who are pregnant for the first time, and it rarely recurs in later pregnancies.

Prevention and self-care Most common rashes will improve with gentle skin care. Avoid scrubbing the skin, and use gentle cleansers. Minimize the use of soap. Oatmeal baths or baking soda baths can help relieve itchiness. Heat rash can be soothed by applying cornstarch after bathing, avoiding very hot baths or showers, and keeping the skin cool and dry.

To help prevent intertrigo, wear loose-fitting cotton clothing, and wash and dry the affected areas frequently. Use a gentle cleanser or unscented soap. Apply baking soda or zinc oxide powder to the affected areas to help keep them dry. You can also try blowing a fan or hair dryer on a cool setting across moist areas.

Medical care If self-care measures are ineffective or if your rash persists, worsens or is accompanied by other symptoms, let your care provider know. In some cases, treatment with a medicated ointment or an oral drug may be necessary.

RECTAL BLEEDING

Rectal bleeding always requires evaluation. Most often rectal bleeding is caused by hemorrhoids, which are fairly common during the last trimester and in the weeks after delivery. Another possible cause of rectal bleeding is a tiny crack or cracks in the anus (anal fissure). Fissures are usually caused by constipation, another common problem during pregnancy. Anal fissures are usually quite painful, especially during passage of hard stool. Only rarely is rectal bleeding related to a serious colorectal disorder.

Prevention and self-care To prevent hemorrhoids and fissures, your best strategy is to keep your stools regular. Stay well-hydrated, eat foods that are high in fiber and exercise frequently. For more tips on avoiding constipation, see page 393.

When to seek medical help Always report rectal bleeding to your care provider. He or she will want to determine the cause of the bleeding. If you have bleeding accompanied by diarrhea with mucus and abdominal pain, that may indicate the possibility of an inflammatory bowel disorder.

RED PALMS AND SOLES

Many pregnant women find that during pregnancy their palms and the soles of their feet become red. This skin change occurs in one-third to two-thirds of women and is most common in white women. The redness can appear as early as the first trimester and is generally the result of increased blood flow to the hands and feet. In addition to being red, these areas may itch. Like most skin changes of pregnancy, the redness fades after delivery.

Prevention and self-care As with other pregnancy skin changes, there's no specific treatment or prevention. But if your hands and feet itch, moisturizing creams may help.

When to seek medical help If the redness doesn't fade after delivery, or if you have itching on your palms and soles without redness, talk to your care provider.

RIB TENDERNESS

In the later months of pregnancy, the fetus has less room to stretch and may find it handy to rest his or her feet between your ribs. It may be surprising how much those little toes and feet jamming into your rib cage can hurt.

In addition to the pressure the baby is exerting, the shape of your chest is being altered to maintain room for your lungs while the diaphragm is pushed upward by the uterus. This reshaping pushes your ribs outward and can lead to pain between the ribs and the cartilage that attaches them to your breastbone.

If baby's position is causing pain on your ribs, gently pushing the baby's feet or bottom away from the painful side is quite safe. You can also try this stretch (see page 167): Get down on your hands and knees, with your back relaxed but not sagging. Keeping your head straight and your neck aligned with your spine, round your back upward toward the ceiling. Allow your head to drop all the way down. Gradually release your back and raise your head to the original position. Repeat several times.

Rib tenderness may disappear after the baby drops into your pelvis, which usually happens two to three weeks before delivery in first pregnancies — but usually not until labor begins in subsequent ones.

ROUND LIGAMENT PAIN

The round ligaments are among several ligaments that hold your uterus in place within your abdomen. A round ligament attaches on each side of the uterus, connecting it to the groin. As the ligaments stretch, they can cause pain in the abdomen, pelvis or groin, typically during the second and third trimesters.

These cordlike structures are less than a quarter of an inch thick before pregnancy. At that time, your uterus is about the size of a pear. But as the uterus grows in size and weight, the ligaments supporting it become longer, thicker and more taut, stretching and tensing like rubber bands. If you move or reach suddenly, the round ligament can stretch, causing a pulling or stabbing pang in your lower pelvic area or groin or a sharp cramp down your side.

Round ligament pain can be severe, but the discomfort usually goes away after several minutes. You may wake up at night with this type of pain after rolling over in your sleep. The pain may also be triggered by exercise. Round ligament pain may ease as your pregnancy progresses. It should go away after you have your baby.

Prevention and self-care Although round ligament pain is uncomfortable, it's normal with pregnancy and isn't generally a sign of anything to worry about. Try the following suggestions to relieve the pain:

- Change the way you move. Sit down and get up more slowly, and avoid sudden movements.
- Sit or lie down when abdominal pain becomes bothersome.
- Apply heat by soaking in a warm bath or using a heating pad on a low setting.

When to seek medical help If you're not sure of the cause of your abdominal pain, and the pain is persistent and severe, call your care provider. Contact your care provider right away or go to a hospital emergency department if abdominal pain is accompanied by fever, chills, pain when urinating or vaginal bleeding.

SENSITIVITY TO SMELLS

You normally love the smell of bacon cooking and coffee brewing, but now that you're pregnant these odors make you gag. Your co-worker's perfume makes you feel sick, and you have to fight off nausea when you fill up the gas tank. Research confirms that pregnant women have a sharper sense of smell — they notice odors that they don't normally notice, and previously acceptable smells become repugnant. This heightened sense of smell is also connected to the nausea and vomiting that many pregnant women experience. A variety of odors, such as foods cooking, coffee, perfume, cigarette smoke or particular foods, can trigger nausea.

A sensitive sense of smell may be due in part to the increase in estrogen during pregnancy. Like nausea, this symptom may indicate a rapidly growing placenta and embryo, and that's a good sign. Most women find this symptom to tightly parallel nausea in pregnancy, so it usually improves by 13 to 14 weeks.

Prevention and self-care To keep your overactive olfactory cells from getting the best of you, be aware of the odors that trigger or aggravate your nausea, and avoid them whenever possible. You might have to eat lunch at your desk instead of the cafeteria, or you may want to ask a co-worker not to wear a particular perfume or cologne until your nausea subsides. It shouldn't be too long before it improves.

SHORTNESS OF BREATH

Having trouble catching your breath? Many pregnant women experience mild breathlessness beginning in the second trimester. This is because your expanding uterus is pushing against your diaphragm — the broad, flat muscle that lies under your lungs. The diaphragm rises about $1^1/_2$ inches from its usual position during pregnancy. That may seem like a small amount, but it's enough to crowd your lungs and alter the amount of air your lungs are able to take in.

At the same time, your respiratory system makes some adaptations to allow your blood to carry large quantities of oxygen to the placenta and to remove more carbon dioxide than normal. Stimulated by the hormone progesterone, the respiratory center in the brain causes you to breathe more deeply and more frequently. Your lungs will inhale and exhale

30 to 40 percent more air with each breath than they did before. These changes may give you the feeling that you're breathing hard or short of breath.

The larger your uterus becomes, the harder you may find it to take a deep breath because your diaphragm is pushing against the baby. A few weeks before you give birth, the baby's head may move down in the uterus (drop), taking the pressure off the diaphragm. When the baby drops, you'll find it easier to breathe. But this may not happen until the start of labor, especially if you've had a baby before.

Despite the discomfort of feeling short of breath, you don't have to worry that your baby isn't getting enough oxygen. Thanks to your expanded respiratory and circulatory systems, the oxygen level in your blood increases during pregnancy, ensuring that your growing baby is getting plenty of oxygen.

Prevention and self-care If you're short of breath, try these tips:
▶ *Practice good posture.* It will help you to breathe better, both during pregnancy and afterward. Sit and stand with your back straight and shoulders back, relaxed and down.
▶ *Do aerobic exercise.* It will improve your breathing and lower your heart rate. But take care not to overexert yourself. Talk to your care provider about how to safely stay active throughout your pregnancy.
▶ *Sleep on your side to help lessen the pressure on your diaphragm.* Prop yourself up with pillows that support your abdomen and your back, or use a body pillow.

When to seek medical help Mild shortness of breath is common in pregnancy, but severe shortness of breath, es-

pecially if it's accompanied by chest pain, may indicate a more serious problem, such as a blood clot in a lung.

Call your care provider immediately or go to an emergency room if you have:
▶ Severe shortness of breath along with chest pain
▶ Discomfort while taking a deep breath
▶ Rapid pulse or rapid breathing
▶ Bluish-colored lips or fingertips

SKIN TAGS

During pregnancy, you may discover a few new skin growths under your arms, on your neck or shoulders, or elsewhere on your body. These tiny, loose protrusions of skin, called skin tags, are usually painless and harmless. They typically don't grow or change. No one knows what causes them. They often disappear after you give birth. But they're common after midlife.

Generally, skin tags aren't bothersome and don't require treatment. If the growths are irritating or cosmetically displeasing, they can easily be removed. Let your care provider know if a skin growth changes in appearance.

SNORING

Pregnant women are more likely to snore because the upper airway is narrower, due to increased swelling in the nasal passages and nasal congestion during pregnancy.

Although snoring is often the subject of jokes, it can have some serious consequences. Snoring can be related to high blood pressure (hypertension). It may also be a sign of sleep apnea, a sleep disorder in which you stop breathing for short periods during sleep. The lack of oxygen disrupts the mother's sleep and may stress the fetus.

Overweight women may be at particularly high risk of snoring-related problems. In one study, women who reported regular snoring during pregnancy were heavier before becoming pregnant and gained more weight during pregnancy.

Prevention and self-care To minimize your chance of snoring:
▶ Sleep on your side rather than your back. Sleeping on your back can cause your tongue and soft palate to rest against the back of your throat and block your airway.
▶ Nasal strips may help increase the area of your nasal passages and airway.
▶ Keep your weight gain in check. Avoid gaining more than recommended based on your weight before becoming pregnant.

When to seek medical help Contact your care provider if your partner thinks your snoring is interrupted by periods of stopped breathing, and you find yourself excessively sleepy during the day. These signs may indicate obstructive sleep apnea.

STRETCH MARKS

Get a group of new or expecting moms together, and you're likely to hear something about stretch marks. Stretch marks are pink or purplish streaks that typically appear on the abdomen, breasts, upper arms, buttocks and thighs. More than half of pregnant women get them, especially during the last half of pregnancy.

Stretch marks aren't a sign of excessive weight gain. They're caused by a stretching of the skin along with a normal increase in the hormone cortisone, produced by the adrenal glands. The increase in cortisone can weaken elastic fibers of the skin, causing the marks. Heredity is also believed to play a big role in the development of stretch marks. Some women experience severe stretch marks even though they gain only a modest amount of weight during pregnancy.

Stretch marks usually don't disappear altogether, but after delivery they often fade gradually to light pink or white.

Prevention and self-care Contrary to popular belief, no creams or ointments will keep stretch marks from appearing. Because stretch marks develop from deep within the connective tissue underneath the skin, they can't be prevented by anything applied externally.

Stretch marks typically fade on their own over time. If you're bothered by their appearance, talk with your care provider. A number of treatments are available to help improve the texture and appearance of existing stretch marks. The best option for you may depend on how long you've had the stretch marks, your skin type, and the convenience and cost of treatment.

STUFFY NOSE

Nasal stuffiness is a common problem in pregnancy, even if you don't have a cold or allergies. Nasal congestion and nosebleeds are more frequent because of the increased flow of blood to the mucous membranes in your body. As the lining of your nose and airway swells, your airway shrinks. Your nasal tissue also becomes softer and more prone to bleeding. This nasal stuffiness is common in pregnancy, but can be annoying.

Prevention and self-care Most pregnant women can tolerate a stuffy nose and other nasal symptoms without taking medications. If there's no accompanying problem such as a cold or allergies, no treatment is generally required. These tips may help keep your stuffy nose clearer:

▶ Use a humidifier in your home to loosen nasal secretions.
▶ Use nasal saline rinses or a neti pot to help flush out dense secretions.
▶ Sleep propped up with your head elevated.

Medical care Avoid over-the-counter remedies for your stuffed-up nose. Prolonged use of these medications can cause problems, and your nasal stuffiness could last for the full length of your pregnancy. Try to deal with the stuffiness using conservative treatments. For more tips on dealing with nasal congestion related to inflammation, see page 63.

SWELLING

Swelling (edema) is common during pregnancy when your body tissues accumulate more fluid due to dilated blood vessels and increased blood volume. Warm weather also can aggravate this condition.

During the last three months of pregnancy, about half of pregnant women notice their eyelids and face becoming puffy, mostly in the morning. This is due to fluid retention and dilated blood vessels, which are expected in pregnancy. In the last few weeks of pregnancy, nearly all women have some swelling in their ankles, legs, fingers or face. By itself, swelling is annoying but is not a serious complication.

Prevention and self-care If you have problems with swelling:

▶ Use cold-water compresses on areas that are swollen.
▶ Ease off extremely salty foods, but you don't need to cut back dramatically on salt. Doing so can cause your body to conserve sodium and water, which can make swelling worse.
▶ To relieve swelling in your legs and feet, lie down and elevate your legs for an hour in the middle of the afternoon. Using a footrest also may help.
▶ Swimming or even standing in a pool may provide some relief. Water pressure will compress your ankles, and your uterus will float just a bit, easing the pressure on your veins.
▶ Wearing compression garments can help reduce swelling in the legs and ankles or prevent it from worsening.

When to seek medical help If you experience a sudden swelling of your face and hands — especially if you also have a headache that doesn't respond to acetaminophen (Tylenol, others) — contact your care provider. Occasionally, sudden swelling can be a sign of pre-eclampsia (see page 448).

SWOLLEN FEET

During pregnancy it's common for your feet to swell. Hormonal changes that relax the ligaments and joints in your pelvis in preparation for delivery also relax all the other ligaments and joints in your body, including those in your feet. While these changes are normal and necessary, they can make the arch ligament of the foot stretch under your body's extra weight. As a result, the arch may lose some of its supporting strength, and your feet grow flatter and wider. They may be as much as a full shoe size larger.

On top of these changes, your feet may swell due to fluid retention during pregnancy. If your weight gain is significant, your feet may carry a little extra fat.

The swelling from fluid in your feet should go down shortly after delivery. But it can take up to six months for the other changes in your feet to reverse themselves and your feet to return to their normal size and shape. If your arch has been stretched excessively, your feet may be permanently larger.

Prevention and self-care As your feet expand, wear shoes that will provide comfort and support. Buy a couple of pairs of shoes that fit you well now and will remain comfortable if your feet continue to change. Avoid narrow-toed or high-heeled shoes. Look for low heels, nonskid soles and plenty of space for your feet to spread out.

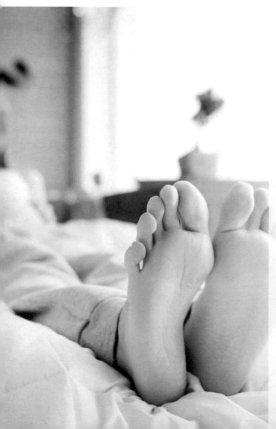

Canvas or leather shoes are good choices because they allow your feet to breathe. Good walking or running shoes are a wise choice. If your feet are aching and tired at the end of the day, try wearing supportive slippers.

Medical care Some orthotic shoe inserts are specially designed for women in pregnancy. They're meant to make your feet more comfortable and reduce back and leg pain. Ask your care provider for more information.

THIRST

You may notice you're thirstier than normal while you're pregnant. That's perfectly healthy. Increased thirst is your body's way of getting you to drink more water and other fluids. Your body needs extra fluids to maintain your increased blood volume. Drinking more fluids also helps prevent constipation and dry skin and helps your kidneys dispose of the waste products being produced by the baby.

Prevention and self-care Drink at least eight glasses a day of water or other beverages. Caffeinated beverages stimulate urine production, so they aren't the best choice. In addition to plain or sparkling water, good choices include a fruit juice fizz made with half juice and half sparkling water; vegetable juice; soup; and a fruit smoothie made with low-fat milk. If you've been vomiting or you've had trouble with feeling faint, sports drinks may be good.

When to seek medical help Although increased thirst is normal when you're expecting, thirst can also be a symptom of diabetes, which can develop during pregnancy. It can be hard to distinguish the subtle signs and symptoms of diabetes, such as fatigue, excessive thirst or excessive urination, from the typical changes of pregnancy. Talk with your care provider if you're concerned about excessive thirst.

URINARY TRACT INFECTIONS

Many of the normal changes of pregnancy can increase your risk of urinary tract infections (UTIs) — infections of the bladder, kidney or urethra. It's very important to recognize and treat UTIs during pregnancy because such infections can lead to preterm labor. What's more, UTIs during pregnancy are more likely to be severe. For example, if you have a bladder infection that goes untreated, it may result in a kidney infection.

You're also more susceptible to UTIs after giving birth. For a time after delivery, you may be unable to empty your bladder completely. The urine that's left provides a breeding ground for bacteria.

If you have a UTI, you may feel pain or burning when you urinate. You might feel a frequent, almost panicky urge to go, or you might feel like you need to go again right after you've urinated. Other signs and symptoms include blood in the urine, strong-smelling urine, mild fever and tenderness over the area of the bladder. Abdominal pain and backache also may signal an infection.

Prevention and self-care You can prevent and help clear up UTIs in several different ways:

▶ Drink plenty of liquids, especially water.
▶ Urinate often — don't hold it or wait for long periods of time before you go. Holding in your urine can result in incomplete emptying of the bladder, which can lead to a UTI. Frequent urination is also helpful in clearing up an infection.
▶ Lean forward while you urinate to help empty your bladder more fully.
▶ Always urinate after having sexual intercourse.
▶ After you urinate, wipe from front to back.

Medical care A urinary tract infection is diagnosed by testing a urine sample for bacteria. Treatment includes antibiotics to clear up the infection. If you've had several UTIs, your care provider might recommend that you continue taking antibiotic medication to lessen the chance of recurrence.

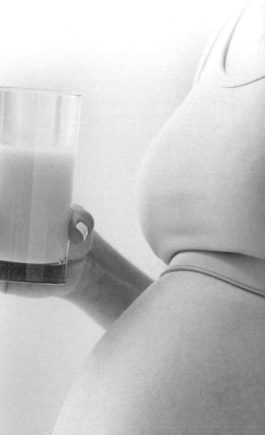

URINATING FREQUENTLY

During the first trimester of pregnancy, your growing uterus pushes on your bladder. As a result, you may find yourself running to the bathroom more often than usual. You may also leak a small amount of urine when you cough, sneeze or laugh. By the fourth month, the uterus expands up out of the pelvic cavity, easing pressure on the bladder. Then, in the last few weeks of pregnancy, you may need to urinate more frequently again when the baby's head drops into the pelvis, placing renewed pressure on your bladder. The frequent need to urinate almost always goes away after you give birth.

Prevention and self-care Try some of the following suggestions:
- Urinate as often as you need to. Holding in urine can result in incomplete emptying of the bladder, which can lead to a urinary tract infection.
- Lean forward when you urinate to help empty your bladder more fully.
- Avoid drinking anything a few hours before bedtime so that you don't have to get up as often during the night. Make sure you're still getting plenty of fluids during the rest of the day.

When to seek medical help If you're urinating frequently and are also experiencing burning, pain, fever, or a change in the odor or color of your urine, you may have a urinary tract infection. Contact your care provider.

URINE LEAKAGE

Sometimes, pregnant women and new mothers pass urine involuntarily, especially when coughing, straining or laughing. That's because during pregnancy the baby is often resting directly on your bladder — and no one is guaranteed to stay dry with a baby bouncing on her bladder. Sometimes, damage at birth to the pelvic floor muscles and nerves to the bladder will cause urine leakage for a few weeks after birth. Fortunately, this problem usually improves within three to six months of giving birth. Unfortunately, the problem tends to recur later in life.

Prevention and self-care Research shows that doing Kegel exercises may help prevent urinary incontinence during pregnancy and after childbirth. These strengthening exercises help form a stronger, thicker support for your bladder, urethra and other pelvic organs. To do Kegel exercises, squeeze the muscles around your vagina tightly, as if you were stopping the flow of urine, for a few seconds, then relax. Repeat 10 times.

If you experience incontinence, wear panty liners or other protective undergarments.

VAGINAL BLEEDING

A quarter or more of all pregnant women may experience spotting or vaginal bleeding at some point during their pregnancies, especially in the first trimester. Vaginal bleeding in pregnancy has many causes — some are serious and some aren't. The significance and possible causes of bleeding are different in each trimester.

First trimester Many women have spotting or bleeding in the first 12 weeks of pregnancy. Depending on whether it's heavy or light, how long it lasts, and if it's continuous or sporadic, bleeding can indicate many things. It may be a warning sign, but it may also be due to the normal events of pregnancy.

You may notice a small amount of spotting or bleeding very early in your pregnancy, about a week to 14 days after fertilization. Known as implantation bleeding, it happens when the fertilized egg attaches to the lining of the uterus. This type of bleeding usually doesn't last long.

Bleeding in the first trimester can also be a sign of a miscarriage. Most miscarriages take place during the first trimester. They occur less frequently later in pregnancy. However, bleeding doesn't necessarily mean you're having a miscarriage. At least half the women who bleed in the first trimester don't experience miscarriages.

Another problem that can cause bleeding and pain in early pregnancy is ectopic pregnancy, a condition in which the embryo implants itself outside the uterus, usually in a fallopian tube. An uncommon cause of bleeding in the first trimester is molar pregnancy, a rare condition in which an abnormal mass, instead of a baby, forms inside the uterus after fertilization (see page 485).

Second trimester Although miscarriage is less common in the second trimester, a risk still exists. Vaginal bleeding is the primary sign of miscarriage.

Moderate to heavy bleeding in the second trimester may also indicate a problem with the placenta. Placental problems may include placenta previa, in which the placenta lies too low in the uterus and partly or completely covers the cervix, or placental abruption, in which the placenta begins to separate from the inner wall of the uterus before birth. Both of these conditions are more frequent in the third trimester.

A cervical infection, an inflamed cervix or growths on the cervix also can cause vaginal bleeding. Cervical bleeding is usually not a risk to the baby, but if it's caused by cervical cancer, it's very important that the diagnosis be made promptly. Occasionally, bleeding from the cervix may be a sign of cervical incompetence, a condition where the cervix opens spontaneously, leading to preterm delivery. Light bleeding or spotting during intercourse can also occur if vessels on the surface of the cervix are disrupted. This is not harmful to the pregnancy.

Third trimester Vaginal bleeding in the late second or third trimester may be a sign of a problem with the placenta. In placental abruption, the placenta begins to detach from the inner wall of the uterus. Bleeding may be nonexistent, heavy or somewhere in between.

In placenta previa, the cervix is partly or completely blocked by the placenta, which is normally located near the top of the uterus. This problem is diagnosed through an ultrasound evaluation, either at a routine visit or after some vaginal bleeding. Painless vaginal bleeding is the main sign of placenta previa, typically near the end of the second trimester or the beginning of the third. The blood from placenta previa is usually bright red. The bleeding is often fairly heavy, and while it may stop on its own, it nearly always returns days or weeks later.

Light bleeding from weeks 20 to 37 may indicate preterm labor. During the last weeks of pregnancy, bleeding can be a sign of impending labor. And a few weeks before labor or at the start of it, the mucous plug that seals the opening of the uterus during pregnancy may be expelled. The discharge may include a small amount of blood.

When to seek medical help Any bleeding during pregnancy should be evaluated by your care provider. Contact your care provider if you have slight spotting or bleeding, even if it goes away within a day. Contact him or her immediately or go to a hospital emergency room if you have:

▶ Bleeding in the second or third trimester
▶ Moderate to heavy bleeding
▶ Bleeding along with pain, cramps, fever, chills or contractions

Treatment will depend on the cause. For more information on placental problems, see pages 446 and 447.

VAGINAL DISCHARGE

Many women have increased vaginal discharge throughout pregnancy. This discharge, called leukorrhea, is thin, white, and mild smelling or odorless. It's caused by the effects of hormones on the vaginal lining, which must grow dramatically during the pregnancy. Vaginal discharge may increase throughout the pregnancy, becoming quite heavy. The high acidity of the discharge is thought to play a role in suppressing growth of harmful bacteria.

You'll also have temporary vaginal discharge after giving birth. This discharge, called lochia, is caused by hormone shifts and varies in amount, appearance and duration. Initially it's bloody, and then it becomes paler or brownish after about four days and white or yellowish after about 10 days. You may occasionally pass a blood clot. This post-pregnancy discharge can last from two to eight weeks.

Vaginal discharge may also be a sign of a vaginal infection. If your vaginal discharge is greenish, yellowish, thick and cheesy, strong smelling, or accompanied by redness, itching or irritation of the vulva, you may have a vaginal infection.

Bacterial vaginosis is a common type of vaginal infection. It causes a foul-smelling gray to greenish discharge, and may be associated with preterm labor. Two other common types of vaginal infections during pregnancy are candidiasis and trichomoniasis. Neither presents a direct hazard to your baby, and both can be treated during pregnancy.

A steady or heavy watery discharge may be a sign that your membranes have ruptured — your water has broken. A vaginal discharge that's bloody or thick and mucuslike may indicate a problem with the cervix.

Prevention and self-care To deal with the normal increased discharge of pregnancy, you might want to wear panty liners or a light sanitary pad. To reduce your risk of getting an infection:

▶ Don't douche. Douching can upset the normal balance of microorganisms in the vagina and can lead to a vaginal infection called bacterial vaginosis.
▶ Wear cotton underwear.
▶ Wear comfortable, loosefitting clothing. Avoid fabrics that don't breathe, tight pants and leotards.

When to seek medical help Contact your care provider if:

▶ You have abdominal pain or fever with a discharge.
▶ The discharge becomes greenish, yellowish or foul smelling; or is thick and cheesy or curd-like; or is bloody.
▶ The discharge is accompanied by soreness, redness, burning or itching of the vulva.
▶ You have a steady or heavy discharge of watery fluid.
▶ You've just had amniocentesis, and you have an increased vaginal discharge. This could indicate an amniotic fluid leak.

If you've already given birth, call your care provider in the following situations:

- You're soaking a sanitary napkin every hour for four hours. Don't wait the four hours if you become dizzy or notice increasing blood loss. Call right away or go to the emergency room.
- The discharge has a foul, fishy odor.
- The discharge is accompanied by fever and abdominal pain.
- Your abdomen feels tender or you're passing numerous blood clots.

VARICOSE VEINS

The circulatory changes that support the growing fetus during pregnancy can also produce the unfortunate side effect of varicose veins. It's not uncommon to develop varicose veins during pregnancy. To accommodate increased blood flow during pregnancy, blood vessels often become larger. At the same time, blood flow from your legs to your pelvis may be slowed. This can cause the valves in the veins in your legs to fail, leading to dilated, bulging veins. Varicose veins tend to run in families. An inherited weakness in the valves of your veins can make you more susceptible.

Varicose veins may cause no symptoms, or they may be painful or uncomfortable, causing sore, aching legs, sometimes accompanied by a burning sensation. The size of the veins usually decreases somewhat after birth.

Prevention and self-care These measures can help prevent varicose veins, keep them from getting worse or ease their discomfort:

- Avoid standing for long periods.
- Don't sit with your legs crossed. Doing so can aggravate circulatory problems.

- Elevate your legs as often as you can. When you're sitting, rest your legs on another chair or a stool. When lying down, raise your legs and feet on a pillow.
- Exercise regularly to improve your overall circulation.
- Wear support stockings or stronger compression stockings from the time you wake up until you go to bed. These socks help to improve the circulation in your legs. Support stockings are available at medical supply stores, larger pharmacies and online retailers.
- Wear loose clothing around your thighs and waist. Socks and tight clothing on the lower legs are fine, but don't wear clothes that constrict the upper legs, such as underwear with tight openings. This can impede the return of blood from your legs and worsen varicose veins.

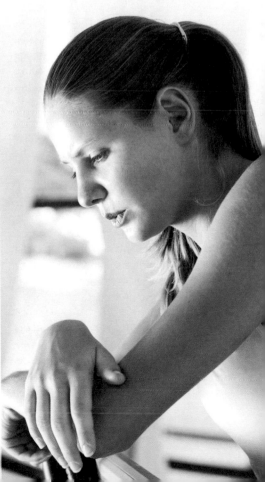

Medical care Varicose veins generally don't require treatment. In severe cases, they may need to be treated surgically, but the procedure isn't normally done until after delivery.

VOMITING

Nausea and vomiting are common during early pregnancy and can occur at any time of day. But sometimes vomiting becomes so severe that a pregnant woman can't eat or drink enough to maintain proper nutrition and stay hydrated. This condition, called hyperemesis gravidarum, is the medical term for excessive vomiting in pregnancy.

Hyperemesis gravidarum is characterized by vomiting that's frequent, persistent and severe. You may also feel faint, dizzy or lightheaded. If not treated, hyperemesis gravidarum can keep you from getting the nutrition and fluids you need, and you may become dehydrated. Rarely, the loss of fluids and salts from vomiting can be severe enough to threaten the health of the fetus.

The exact causes of hyperemesis aren't known, but it seems to occur more frequently when the level of the pregnancy hormone human chorionic gonadotropin (HCG) is very high. This is typical in a multiple pregnancy or a molar pregnancy, a rare condition in which an abnormal mass rather than a baby forms inside the uterus. Hyperemesis is more common in first pregnancies, young women and women carrying multiples.

Prevention and self-care If you're vomiting only occasionally or about once a day, follow the self-care measures listed in the section on morning sickness on page 102.

When to seek medical help Contact your care provider if:
- You have nausea and vomiting so severe you can't keep fluids down
- You're vomiting more than two or three times a day
- Vomiting persists well into the second trimester
- You have some of the signs and symptoms of early or mild dehydration, which include a flushed face, extreme thirst, dizziness, leg cramps, headache and dark yellow urine

YEAST INFECTIONS

Yeast infections (candidiasis) are caused by a type of fungus called candida, which is found in small amounts in the vagina in about 25 percent of women. Increased estrogen levels during pregnancy cause changes in the vaginal environment, which may throw off the natural balance and allow some organisms to grow faster than others.

Candida may be present without causing signs and symptoms, or it may cause an infection. Signs and symptoms of infection include a vaginal discharge that is thick, white and curd-like; itching; burning and redness around the vagina and vulva; and painful urination.

Although a yeast infection is unpleasant for you, it won't hurt your baby, and it can safely be treated during pregnancy.

Prevention and self-care To help prevent yeast infections:
- Wear underwear or pantyhose with a cotton crotch, as well as loose-fitting pants.
- Avoid wearing wet bathing suits or exercise clothes for long periods of time, and wash them after each use.

▶ Eat yogurt that contains live *Lactoba-cillus acidophilus* cultures — most yogurt does. Yogurt may help keep the right mix of bacteria flourishing in your body.

Medical care Candidiasis is treated during pregnancy with a vaginal cream or a suppository containing an antifungal cream. These medications are available without a prescription, but don't use one without consulting your care provider first. Your care provider needs to confirm the diagnosis before you start treatment. He or she may also recommend a prescription medication to clear the infection.

Once you've had a yeast infection while pregnant, it can be a recurring problem until after delivery, when it usually subsides. It may be necessary to treat yeast infections repeatedly throughout your pregnancy.

PART 6

Complications of pregnancy and childbirth

CHAPTER 27

Issues during pregnancy

If you face an unexpected problem during your pregnancy, you may be concerned, confused or frightened. This section describes some of the complications pregnant women may face and how these conditions are often treated. Many problems that develop during pregnancy can be successfully managed. Listen to your care provider's advice and ask questions until you feel that you fully understand the complication and how best to treat it.

If you're enjoying a problem-free pregnancy, feel free to skip this chapter. Try not to worry unnecessarily about things that could go wrong.

BLOOD CONCERNS

Here are some blood complications moms-to-be may experience.

Rhesus factor incompatibility Rhesus (Rh) factor incompatibility occurs when a pregnant mother has Rh negative blood and her fetus has Rh positive blood. Rh factor is a type of protein found on the surface of red blood cells. If you have this protein, you are Rh positive. If you don't, you are Rh negative. This is the "positive" or "negative" reported with your blood type. For example, if your blood type is B positive, you're Rh positive. The Rh protein is inherited from your parents.

When you're not pregnant, your Rh status has no effect on your health, unless you need a blood transfusion. If you're Rh positive, you have no cause for concern during pregnancy either. But if you're Rh negative and your baby is Rh positive — which is likely if your partner is Rh positive — a problem called Rh factor incompatibility (Rh disease) can result. During pregnancy and delivery, your baby's blood can cross into your bloodstream. Your body sees the Rh protein from your baby's blood as a foreign substance and starts making antibodies to destroy it. These antibodies can cross the placenta in subsequent pregnancies.

Because the Rh protein is on the surface of the red blood cells, destruction of the protein also results in the destruction of red blood cells, leading to anemia in your baby. Red blood cells carry oxygen to all parts of the body. If left untreated, anemia in the fetus can cause mild to severe fetal complications. In very rare cases, it can lead to death.

If you're Rh negative, your partner is Rh positive and this is your first pregnancy, Rh incompatibility is unlikely to be a problem. Antibodies may start to form, but often the baby is born before you've developed enough antibodies to harm your baby. Your risk is higher during future pregnancies, as your body can form antibodies more quickly when it encounters the Rh protein again (if your next baby is Rh positive). Fortunately, the problem is almost always preventable.

Treatment The key to "treating" Rh incompatibility is preventing it. This is possible with a medication that consists of antibodies against the Rh protein, called Rh immune globulin (RhIg). A RhIg injection will bind to any Rh positive cells that may have entered your bloodstream. Your body then does not detect the Rh protein and will not make the antibodies that cause problems. Because of the widespread use of RhIg in Rh negative mothers, fetal Rh disease is now rare.

If you are Rh negative and you test negative for Rh antibodies in early pregnancy, you will receive RhIg at about 28 weeks of pregnancy. This prevents antibodies forming late in pregnancy. At the time of delivery, cord blood will be collected from your baby. And if your baby is Rh positive, you will receive another dose of RhIg to prevent antibody formation due to any cells that might have crossed into your blood during delivery.

If you're one of the few women who does have Rh antibodies early in pregnancy, you can be tested on a regular basis throughout your pregnancy to determine the level of antibodies in your blood. In addition, testing with ultrasound may be recommended to screen for anemia in your baby. If anemia is suspected, steps can be taken to prevent harm to the baby. These steps may include blood transfusions to the fetus while still in the uterus or, possibly, early delivery. Occasionally the baby may still develop anemia after delivery.

Iron deficiency anemia Iron deficiency anemia is a condition marked by fewer than normal red blood cells in your body. It results when your body doesn't have enough iron stores to produce healthy red blood cells.

Iron deficiency anemia develops most often in the second half of pregnancy, after the 20th week. As your body makes more blood during the first 20 weeks of pregnancy, you have a lower red blood cell concentration overall. This happens because you make the fluid portion of blood (plasma) more quickly than you make red blood cells. However, about 20 percent of pregnant women don't have enough iron available in their bodies to produce the red blood cells necessary to catch up with blood volume, resulting in iron deficiency anemia.

When you're pregnant, it can be a challenge to keep your iron stores at an adequate level through diet alone. That's why many care providers prescribe iron supplements during pregnancy. If you're taking a daily prenatal vitamin with iron, you'll generally be able to steer clear of iron deficiency anemia.

Signs and symptoms If you have a mild case of iron deficiency anemia, you may not even notice any problems. However, if you have a moderate or severe case, you may be pale, weak or excessively tired, short of breath, and dizzy or lightheaded. Heart palpitations and fainting spells also may indicate iron deficiency anemia.

An unusual symptom of iron deficiency anemia is the desire to eat nonfood items such as ice chips, cornstarch and even clay (pica). If you experience pica, contact your care provider. Your baby may be struggling to get enough oxygen because there aren't enough red blood cells to transport it to your baby.

Treatment Treatment usually consists of consuming enough iron, which is prescribed in capsule or tablet form, in addition to standard prenatal vitamins. Occasionally, iron supplementation may be given intravenously if a woman is unable to tolerate taking iron by mouth. In women with severe anemia, a blood transfusion may be necessary.

Signs and symptoms Cervical incompetence occurs without pain, but it may be associated with many of the other signs and symptoms of miscarriage and preterm labor. These include spotting, bleeding or increased vaginal discharge. You may also have a feeling of pressure or heaviness in your lower abdomen.

Treatment If you experience signs and symptoms, contact your care provider. If you develop cervical incompetence and it's caught early, your care provider may be able to stitch the edges of the cervix together. This reinforces the cervix and may prolong the pregnancy. This procedure (cerclage) is most successful if it's performed before the 20th week of pregnancy.

If you've had a previous pregnancy with cervical incompetence, you'll probably have the cerclage procedure done early in subsequent pregnancies. It may happen at about 12 to 14 weeks, after the pregnancy is well established but before the cervix might begin to shorten.

CERVICAL INCOMPETENCE

Cervical incompetence is the medical term for a cervix that begins to thin and open too early in pregnancy. Instead of happening in response to uterine contractions, as in a normal pregnancy, the cervix thins and opens because its connective tissue can't withstand the pressure of the growing uterus.

Cervical incompetence is relatively rare. However, it can be associated with pregnancy loss, especially in the second trimester. You're more likely to develop cervical incompetence if you've had a previous operation on your cervix or you've had a previous pregnancy with cervical incompetence.

DEPRESSION

It's not unusual to feel sad or low once in a while. These feelings usually pass with time. But if your low mood lasts for longer than two weeks and it interferes with your ability to eat, sleep, work, concentrate, relate to others and enjoy life, you may possibly be experiencing depression. Depression is a common mood disorder that is serious but treatable. Unfortunately, it is also underdiagnosed and undertreated.

Depression can be a problem for women during pregnancy, and it's especially common after pregnancy (postpartum). It's estimated that about 1 in 10 women experiences postpartum depression after delivery. Studies suggest that number is often higher in communities with lower average incomes.

During pregnancy, factors that can contribute to depression include:

▶ Stress
▶ Insufficient social or emotional support
▶ Pregnancy and birth complications
▶ Losing a baby
▶ Having a baby with health issues or needing to be hospitalized
▶ Financial pressures
▶ Unrealistic expectations of childbirth and parenting

Certain personality traits and lifestyle choices can also make you more vulnerable. For instance, having low self-esteem or being overly self-critical, pessimistic or easily overwhelmed by stress can put you at increased risk of depression.

Signs and symptoms Two of the main symptoms of depression are loss of interest in normal daily activities and feeling sad, helpless or hopeless. Other symptoms of depression can often be mistaken for common problems of pregnancy. That can make depression during pregnancy easy to overlook. For a care provider to diagnose depression, most of the following signs and symptoms must

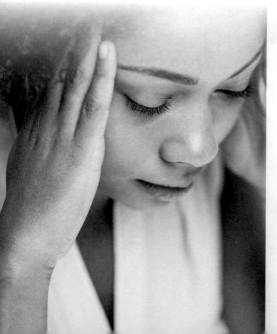

be present most of the day, nearly every day for at least two weeks:

▶ Sleep disturbances
▶ Impaired thinking or concentration
▶ Significant and unexplained weight gain or loss
▶ Agitation or slowed body movements
▶ Fatigue
▶ Low self-esteem
▶ Loss of interest in sex
▶ Thoughts of death

Many people with depression also have symptoms of anxiety such as persistent worry or a sense of impending danger.

Treatment Depression is a serious illness that requires treatment. Ignoring this diagnosis can put you and your baby at risk. Most often, depression that occurs during pregnancy is treated with counseling and behavioral therapy. Antidepressant medications may be used as well. Many of these medications appear to pose little risk to developing babies. If medication is needed, your care provider can prescribe one that's safe for you to take during pregnancy.

Having depression before or during pregnancy can increase your risk of postpartum depression (see page 476). Untreated depression can become a chronic condition that can return before or during subsequent pregnancies.

If you think you may be depressed, talk with your care provider about it. It is often helpful to reach out to people that you trust, whether a friend or loved one, a close peer or minister in your faith community if you have one, or any health professional.

Emergency help If you are having thoughts about attempting suicide or hurting yourself or others, call 911 or your local emergency number immediately. Also consider the following options:

- Call your doctor or a mental health professional.
- Go to your local emergency room for evaluation.
- Call a suicide hotline. In the United States, call the National Suicide Prevention Lifeline at 800-273-TALK (800-273-8255).
- Contact a minister, spiritual leader or someone else in your faith community.
- Reach out to a friend or loved one.

EARLY LABOR

A term pregnancy is defined as one in which birth occurs 37 to 42 weeks after the start of your last menstrual period. Preterm labor refers to regular uterine contractions that cause the cervix to open and delivery to occur before your 37th week of pregnancy.

Babies who are born this early often have low birth weights (less than $5\frac{1}{2}$ pounds). Their low weights, along with various other problems associated with preterm birth, often puts them at risk of certain health problems.

No one knows exactly what causes preterm labor. In many cases, it occurs among women who have no known risk factors. Care providers and researchers have identified factors that seem to increase risk. These include:
- Previous preterm labor or birth, particularly in the most recent pregnancy or more than one previous pregnancy
- A pregnancy with twins, triplets or other multiples
- Previous miscarriages or abortions
- Chronic conditions such as high blood pressure and diabetes
- Smoking cigarettes or using illicit drugs
- Problems with your uterus, placenta or cervix

- Being underweight or overweight before pregnancy, or gaining too little or too much weight during pregnancy
- Stressful life events such as the death of a loved one
- Vaginal bleeding during pregnancy
- Excess amniotic fluid (polyhydramnios)
- Red blood cell deficiency (anemia), particularly during early pregnancy
- Infection, especially of the genital tract
- Preeclampsia, a condition characterized by high blood pressure
- Little or no prenatal care
- An interval of less than six months since the last pregnancy

Signs and symptoms For some women, the clues that labor is starting are unmistakable. For others, the signs and symptoms are more subtle. You may have regular or frequent, painful contractions that feel like a tightening in your abdomen. If the contractions aren't painful, you may note the contractions only by feeling your abdomen with your hand. Some women go into preterm labor without feeling any uterine contractions.

Women sometimes mistake contractions for gas pain, constipation or movement of the fetus. Other signs and symptoms of labor may include:
- Lower backache that is typically constant and dull
- Increased lower abdominal, pelvic or vaginal pressure
- Menstrual-type or abdominal cramps
- Light vaginal spotting or bleeding
- A change in vaginal discharge

If you have a watery discharge, whether in a gush or a trickle, it may be amniotic fluid, a sign that the membranes surrounding the fetus have ruptured (your water has broken). If you pass the mucous plug — the mucus that builds in the cervix during pregnancy — you may

BED REST AND ACTIVITY RESTRICTION

When you're pregnant, a prescription for bed rest might seem appealing. In reality, however, restrictions on movement during pregnancy can pose challenges and even certain health risks.

Bed rest used to be prescribed frequently for pregnancy complications such as preterm labor. However, it's no longer recommended in most situations. It does not change pregnancy outcomes for complications including preterm labor, preeclampsia and placental problems. Meanwhile, bed rest during pregnancy is known to increase the risk of potentially life-threatening blood clots (deep vein thrombosis, or DVT, and pulmonary embolism). Bed rest may also lead to muscle and bone loss.

Instead of bed rest, your care provider might prescribe some level of activity restriction. You might be free to move about the house, as long as you avoid lifting children and doing heavy housework. Depending on the specific complication, many women may even be able to continue working.

Pelvic rest might be recommended if you have a condition such as placenta previa, if you're at increased risk of preterm labor or if you have abdominal surgery during pregnancy. Pelvic rest means avoiding activities that might increase pelvic pressure or pelvic muscle contractions, including sexual activity and orgasm, using tampons, heavy lifting, repetitive squatting, and brisk walking or other lower body exercises.

If your care provider does recommend activity restrictions, make sure you understand the details of the restrictions and the reasoning behind them.

---

notice this as a thick discharge tinged with blood.

If you have any concerns about what you're feeling — especially if you have vaginal bleeding along with abdominal cramps or pain — contact your care provider or your hospital immediately. Don't worry about mistaking false labor for the real thing, especially when you are less than 37 weeks pregnant. It is better to be seen and evaluated at this point in pregnancy.

Treatment Unfortunately, there is no effective treatment to stop preterm labor. There are, however, some things that can be done to help predict and prevent preterm labor from happening. If you've had an early delivery in the past, using ultra-sound to look at the length of the cervix can help determine your risk of another early delivery. A short cervix indicates a higher risk of delivering early.

To help prevent this, your care provider might suggest weekly injections of the hormone progesterone. For women with a history of preterm birth, progesterone is typically given starting around 16 weeks. Progesterone can also be placed inside the vagina daily in women with a short cervix but no history of early delivery.

If you are less than 22 to 24 weeks pregnant, have a history of preterm delivery and an ultrasound that shows your cervical length is less than 25 millimeters, your doctor may recommend a surgical procedure known as cervical cerclage.

The cervix is stitched closed with strong sutures. The sutures are typically removed when you're at or near full term, or when labor starts.

A cerclage may also be offered if the cervix is found to be open and the amniotic membranes are exposed, but this carries a higher risk of rupture of membranes and preterm labor. If the amniotic membranes are exposed, there may be a hidden or undiagnosed infection of the membranes or placenta.

Decreasing complications from preterm delivery If you're having preterm contractions before 37 weeks and there is concern that you are in labor, your care provider will likely recommend admission to the hospital. Depending on the situation, your doctor might recommend the following medications:

▶ *Tocolytics.* These medications are effective at slowing or stopping contractions, but only for a short time.
▶ *Corticosteroids.* A course of steroids may be recommended if you are less than 37 weeks pregnant and there is concern that you might deliver within the next seven days. This will help speed up your baby's lung maturity.
▶ *Magnesium sulfate.* Research has shown that magnesium sulfate given shortly before a preterm delivery may reduce the risk of cerebral palsy for babies born before 32 weeks.

Your care provider can help you weigh the risks and benefits of using any of these medications. For example, a tocolytic may not be recommended if you have certain conditions, such as bleeding or high blood pressure. In other situations, a tocolytic may be beneficial as delivery may be delayed long enough for you to be given steroids or, if necessary, be taken to a facility that can provide specialized care for your premature baby.

Sometimes, preterm labor results from other complications, such as uterine infection or premature separation of the placenta (placental abruption). Other pregnancy conditions, such as severe high blood pressure, may put both mom and baby at risk. If these complications are a greater threat to the baby than prematurity, preterm delivery may be necessary.

EXCESSIVE VOMITING

Nausea and vomiting in early pregnancy are common. But for a small subset of women, vomiting during pregnancy can become frequent, persistent and severe. This is known as hyperemesis gravidarum. The exact cause of this condition is unknown, but is widely thought to be related to the pregnancy hormones human chorionic gonadotropin (HCG), estrogen and progesterone. Hyperemesis gravidarum is more common in first pregnancies, among young women and among women carrying more than one baby.

Signs and symptoms Persistent, excessive vomiting is the main sign. In some women, vomiting can be so severe that they may experience weight loss, become lightheaded or faint, and show signs of dehydration.

If you have nausea and vomiting so severe that you can't keep food or liquids down, contact your care provider. Without treatment, hyperemesis gravidarum can keep you from getting the nutrition and fluids you need. If it lasts long enough, it can affect the development of your baby.

Before treating you for this condition, your care provider may want to rule out other possible causes of the vomiting.

These include gastrointestinal disorders, diabetes or a condition called molar pregnancy (see page 485).

Treatment Mild nausea and vomiting of pregnancy is often treated with reassurance, avoidance of foods that trigger vomiting, use of over-the-counter medications and small, frequent meals.

For hyperemesis gravidarum, the oral medications pyridoxine (vitamin B6) and doxylamine (Unisom) may be prescribed. These have been shown to effectively treat nausea in many women, and may also reduce vomiting. Severe nausea and vomiting associated with dehydration and weight loss may also require intravenous (IV) fluids and, possibly, hospitalization.

FETAL GROWTH RESTRICTION

Fetal growth restriction (FGR), also known as intrauterine growth restriction (IUGR), describes a condition in which a baby doesn't grow at the normal rate inside the uterus. Growth restriction is diagnosed using ultrasound to determine the estimated fetal weight. A baby with FGR has an estimated weight below the 10th percentile for his or her gestational age.

Each year in the United States, around 100,000 full-term babies are born with low birth weight, often associated with FGR. FGR may stem from problems with the placenta that prevent it from delivering enough oxygen and nutrients to the fetus. Other risk factors for growth restriction include:

▶ High blood pressure in the mother
▶ Cigarette smoking
▶ Severe malnutrition or poor weight gain in the mother
▶ Drug or alcohol abuse
▶ Multiple fetuses
▶ Chronic disease in the mother, such as type 1 diabetes or heart, liver or kidney disease
▶ Abnormalities of the placenta or umbilical cord

FGR may also occur because of an infection, birth defect or chromosome abnormality. Most often, the cause of the growth restriction is unknown.

Medical advances and early diagnosis have greatly reduced serious complications of growth restriction. However, these babies can still develop problems.

Signs and symptoms If you're carrying a baby with suspected growth restriction, you may have few, if any, signs and symptoms. This is why your care provider regularly checks to see if your baby is growing, including measuring your uterus at each of your prenatal visits.

If FGR is suspected, an ultrasound exam likely will be done to measure the baby's size. Blood flow measurements in the umbilical cord and fetal vessels may be measured with an ultrasound technique called Doppler analysis.

Treatment To treat growth restriction, the first step is to identify and address any contributing factors, such as smoking or poor nutrition. You and your care provider will monitor the baby's condition, and you may be asked to keep a daily record of the baby's movements. Depending on how far along you are in pregnancy, you may be scheduled for ultrasounds once or twice a week to check on the baby's well-being. Ultrasound exams are generally done every few weeks to track the baby's growth.

If tests and ultrasounds show that the baby is growing and isn't in danger, the pregnancy may continue until labor begins on its own. But if test results indicate that the fetus may be in danger or isn't growing properly, your care provider may recommend an early delivery.

Careful monitoring and early intervention may decrease the risks associated with growth restriction. A focus on good prenatal care, including getting excellent nutrition and eliminating smoking and alcohol use, will increase your chances of having a healthy baby.

If you do have a baby with growth restriction, size at birth may not be an indication of how well he or she will grow and develop. Many babies with FGR catch up to others their age by 18 to 24 months. Unless there are serious birth defects, it is most likely that babies with fetal growth restriction will have normal intellectual and physical development in the long term.

GESTATIONAL DIABETES

Diabetes is a condition in which the body can't properly regulate the level of blood sugar. When diabetes develops in a woman who didn't have it before pregnancy, it's called gestational diabetes.

Typically, your body breaks down much of the food you eat into sugar (glucose). Glucose moves from the stomach into your blood so that your cells can store and use it as energy. The hormone insulin then helps move glucose from the blood into your cells. In pregnancy, it's normal for insulin not to work as well as usual. As a result, not as much glucose can get into the cells, leaving higher levels of glucose in the blood to nourish the baby. Most women can produce extra insulin to keep their blood sugar levels in a normal range. However, if the level of glucose gets too high, this results in gestational diabetes.

Any woman can develop gestational diabetes. The risk is higher in some women, particularly those who:

- Have had gestational diabetes in a previous pregnancy or have a personal history of prediabetes
- Have a family history of diabetes
- Are older than 25
- Are obese
- Have a history of high blood pressure, high cholesterol or heart disease
- Have had polycystic ovary syndrome (PCOS) or another health condition related to problems with insulin

Latina, African-American, American Indian, Alaska Native, Asian-American, and Pacific Islander women are also at increased risk of developing gestational diabetes, just as they are at increased risk of type 2 diabetes.

Most women with well-controlled gestational diabetes have healthy pregnancies and healthy babies. However, gestational diabetes that's not carefully managed can cause problems for both mom and baby. If it goes undetected or is not carefully controlled, your baby may be at increased risk of:

- *Excessive birth weight.* The extra glucose in your blood crosses the placenta into your baby's blood and triggers baby's pancreas to make extra insulin. Your baby's cells then take in the extra glucose. This can cause your baby to grow too large (macrosomia). Very large babies are more likely to sustain birth injuries or require cesarean delivery.
- *Early (preterm) birth and breathing problems at birth.* High blood sugar in a mother may increase her risk of early labor or cause complications that could lead to early delivery. Babies who are born early may need help breathing until their lungs mature and become stronger. Babies of women

with gestational diabetes may have breathing problems even if they're not born early.

▶ *Low blood sugar.* Babies of women with gestational diabetes typically have high levels of insulin. Shortly after birth, the baby is no longer receiving extra glucose from the mother, but insulin levels remain high. This can result in low blood sugar (hypoglycemia). If untreated, severe hypoglycemia can cause seizures. Prompt feeding and sometimes an intravenous glucose solution can return the baby's blood sugar level to normal and help prevent complications. In rare instances, untreated gestational diabetes may result in a baby's death either before or shortly after birth.

▶ *Long-term health consequences.* Babies of women who have gestational diabetes have a higher risk of developing certain health problems as adults, including being overweight and developing glucose intolerance, insulin resistance or type 2 diabetes. If gestational diabetes is carefully managed, many of these health problems can be avoided. Helping your child maintain a healthy lifestyle also will help prevent long-term consequences.

Gestational diabetes may increase the mother's risk of the following:

▶ *High blood pressure.* Gestational diabetes raises your risk of developing preeclampsia, a serious pregnancy complication that causes high blood pressure and leads to issues that can, in severe cases, threaten the lives of both you and your baby.

▶ *Future diabetes.* If you have gestational diabetes, you are more likely to have gestational diabetes again during a future pregnancy. You are also more likely to develop type 2 diabetes as you get older. Making healthy lifestyle choices, such as maintaining a healthy weight, exercising and eating healthy foods can help reduce these risks.

▶ *Future heart disease and stroke.* Women with a history of gestational diabetes have a higher risk of stroke or heart attack later in life. Healthy lifestyle choices greatly reduce this risk, as well.

Signs and symptoms In general, gestational diabetes doesn't cause any noticeable symptoms, so it is now recommended that all pregnant women be screened.

Your doctor will likely evaluate your risk factors and screen for undiagnosed type 2 diabetes when you start your prenatal care early in pregnancy. Women should then be screened for gestational diabetes at 24 to 28 weeks of pregnancy, even if early screening was negative. The two-step approach is the most commonly used method to screen for and diagnose gestational diabetes:

1. Initial glucose challenge test. For the one-hour glucose challenge test, you'll be asked to drink a syrupy solution. After an hour, a sample of your blood is drawn to measure your blood sugar level. A blood sugar level below 130 to 140 milligrams per deciliter (mg/dL), or 7.2 to 7.8 millimoles per liter (mmol/L), is considered normal, although this may vary by lab. If your blood sugar level is higher than normal, you have a higher risk of gestational diabetes. Your care provider will recommend a three-hour glucose tolerance test to determine if you have gestational diabetes.

2. Three-hour glucose tolerance test. For this test, you will fast overnight and then drink another syrupy glucose solution. Blood tests are taken before the test and then hourly over a three-hour period. If at least two of the blood sugar readings are higher than normal, you'll be diagnosed with gestational diabetes (though some experts recommend making the diagnosis with just one higher reading). Gestational diabetes is diagnosed in only a small percentage of women who undergo follow-up testing.

Treatment Once you are diagnosed with gestational diabetes, your care provider will work with you to create a treatment plan, which typically includes diet and lifestyle changes to help control your glucose levels throughout pregnancy.

Controlling your blood sugar level is the key to managing gestational diabetes. A nutritionist may provide dietary counseling and tips to help you eat well and stay on track.

You'll likely be asked to monitor your blood sugar throughout each day. This is usually done before breakfast and again two hours after each meal to see how high glucose levels climb after eating. Your care provider also will likely recommend frequent checkups, especially during your last three months of pregnancy.

If you're having trouble controlling your blood sugar with diet and lifestyle changes, you may need to take insulin injections. In certain situations, oral medications may be used as an alternative to insulin, but these are not as effective, and their safety is not as well-established.

Your care provider will discuss with you the recommended best timing for delivery if you do not go into spontaneous labor by your due date. Although women with gestational diabetes have a higher risk of cesarean births, many have successful vaginal deliveries. For women with gestational diabetes and a baby suspected to be greater than 9.9 pounds (4.5 kilograms), a planned cesarean birth may be considered to help prevent birth trauma.

Gestational diabetes usually resolves after delivery. Your doctor will screen for ongoing diabetes six to 12 weeks postpartum. If your tests are normal — and most are — you'll need to have your diabetes risk assessed every one to three years thereafter.

INFECTION

Pregnancy doesn't make you immune to everyday infections and illnesses — you can still get sick, and you actually may be more susceptible because of the hormonal changes in your body. Pregnancy may also change the way an infection is managed by your care provider. The following illnesses may require special treatment and monitoring in pregnancy.

Chickenpox Chickenpox (varicella) is caused by the varicella zoster virus. A vaccine to prevent chickenpox became available in 1995 and is recommended for children starting at 1 year of age. People who had chickenpox or have been vaccinated against it are typically immune to the virus. If you're not sure whether you're immune, your care provider can perform a blood test to find out.

In childhood, chickenpox is generally a mild disease. However, in adults — and especially in pregnant women — it can be serious.

Managing chickenpox If you are not immune and you were exposed to someone with chickenpox, inform your care provider right away. An injection of a drug called varicella-zoster immune globulin (Varizig) can help prevent infection after exposure during pregnancy. Chickenpox infection early in pregnancy very rarely results in birth defects. The greatest threat to the baby is when mom develops chickenpox the week before birth. It can cause a serious, life-threatening infection in a newborn. The varicella-zoster immune globulin (VZIG) can decrease the severity of the infection if a baby is treated quickly after birth. The mother also needs protection with VZIG to diminish the severity of the disease, and will likely be given antiviral medication to decrease the severity of the infection as well.

Cytomegalovirus Cytomegalovirus (CMV) is a common viral infection. In healthy adults, almost all CMV infections go unrecognized. Between 50 and 80 percent of adults in the United States are infected with CMV by age 40. A pregnant woman with CMV can infect her baby with the virus before birth, during delivery or while breast-feeding. Women who contract CMV for the first time during pregnancy may pass a severe congenital infection on to their babies.

Managing cytomegalovirus It's important to be educated about CMV and how it's transmitted. Good hygiene, such as hand-washing, can minimize the risk of infection. An amniocentesis can test for fetal infection if CMV is diagnosed in a pregnant woman. Your care provider may recommend a series of ultrasounds to see if the fetus develops problems related to the infection. If the baby is affected, treating a mother with CMV antibody during pregnancy might be helpful.

A small percentage of infants show signs and symptoms of CMV at birth. These include severe liver problems, seizures, blindness, deafness and pneumonia. Some of these babies die. The majority of those who live have serious neurological defects.

Fifth disease (parvovirus infection) Fifth disease (erythema infectiosum) is a virus common among school-age children. The condition is caused by the human parvovirus B19. The most noticeable part of the infection in children is a bright red rash on the cheeks.

Infection often occurs without signs or symptoms, so many adults may not know if they've had parvovirus. Once you've had it, you're generally immune.

About one-half or more of all pregnant women remain susceptible to the B19 virus during pregnancy, so it's not uncommon for expectant women to contract the infection.

The great majority of these women will have healthy babies. In rare cases, however, fifth disease in the mother can cause severe, even fatal, anemia in the fetus. The anemia can cause congestive heart failure, manifested by a severe form of swelling (edema) called fetal hydrops. If a fetus develops this complication, it may be possible to give the fetus a blood transfusion through the umbilical cord.

Managing fifth disease Currently, no vaccine exists to prevent fifth disease. Antiviral therapy hasn't been shown to benefit women with the infection. If a pregnant woman has been exposed to fifth disease or is suspected of having it, blood tests can help determine immunity or confirm infection. If the tests show evidence of infection, additional ultrasounds might be done for up to 12 weeks to watch for possible signs of anemia and congestive heart failure in the fetus.

Flu (influenza) During pregnancy, you're especially susceptible to influenza if you don't receive a flu vaccination. Even if you did get a flu shot, you could become infected by an influenza strain not covered by the vaccine. However, infections in people who are vaccinated tend to be less severe. If you think you may have the flu, contact your care provider right away.

Managing influenza The Centers for Disease Control and Prevention (CDC) recommends that women who have the flu in any trimester of pregnancy receive treatment with antiviral medications. The CDC believes the benefits of antiviral therapy outweigh potential risks of the drugs. Antiviral treatment is most beneficial if it is started within two days of the onset of symptoms.

German measles German measles (rubella) is a viral infection that's sometimes confused with measles (rubeola), but each of these illnesses is caused by a different virus.

German measles is extremely rare in the United States. Most children are vaccinated against it at a young age. However, small outbreaks of rubella continue to occur in the United States. Therefore, it's possible for you to become infected during pregnancy if you aren't immune.

Managing German measles German measles is a mild infection. However, if you contract it while you're pregnant, it can be dangerous. The infection can cause miscarriage, stillbirth or birth defects. The highest risk to the fetus is during the first trimester, but exposure to rubella during the second trimester also is dangerous.

Early in their pregnancies, women are routinely tested for rubella immunity. If you're pregnant and found not to be immune, avoid contact with anyone who may have been exposed to German measles. Vaccination isn't recommended during pregnancy. However, you can be vaccinated after childbirth for rubella along with measles and mumps, through the MMR vaccine, so that you will be immune in future pregnancies.

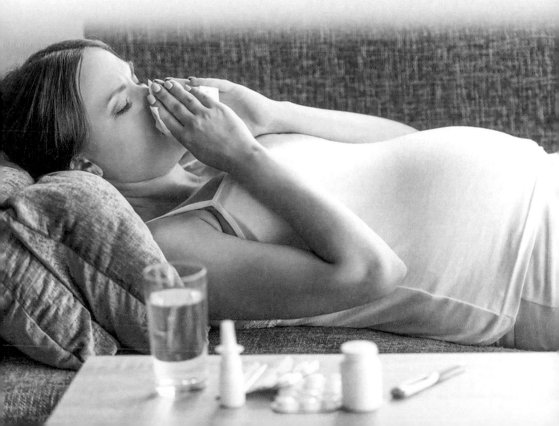

Group B streptococcus About 1 in 4 adults in the United States carries a bacterium known as group B streptococcus (GBS). For women with GBS, the organism may reside in the colon, rectum or vagina. Typically, GBS lives harmlessly in the body. However, pregnant women who harbor GBS bacteria may pass the bacteria to their babies during labor and delivery. Babies, especially preterm babies, don't handle the bacteria in the same manner as do adults. If they acquire this infection, they can become seriously ill.

Managing group B streptococcus Using antibiotics during labor to treat women who carry the bacteria prevents most fetal infections. If tests indicate you carry GBS, remind your care provider at the beginning of labor to give you antibiotics.

If GBS does infect a newborn, the resulting illness can take one of two forms: early-onset infection or late-onset infection. In early-onset infection, a baby typically becomes sick within hours after birth. Problems can include infection of the fluid in and around the brain (meningitis), inflammation and infection of the lungs (pneumonia), and a life-threatening condition called sepsis, which can cause fever, difficulty breathing and shock. Late-onset infection occurs within a week to a few months after birth and usually results in meningitis.

Listeriosis Listeriosis is an illness caused by a type of bacteria called *Listeria monocytogenes*. Most infections result from eating contaminated foods, including processed foods such as deli meats and hot dogs, unpasteurized milk and soft cheeses.

Most healthy people exposed to listeria don't become ill, but the infection can cause flu-like symptoms such as fever, fatigue, nausea, vomiting and diarrhea.

These problems are somewhat more likely during pregnancy.

Managing listeriosis If you contract listeriosis during pregnancy, the infection can be passed from you to your fetus through the placenta and lead to premature delivery, miscarriage, stillbirth or the death of the baby shortly after birth.

It's important to make every effort to prevent exposure to listeria during pregnancy. Avoid consuming unpasteurized dairy products or deli meats that haven't been well-refrigerated and reheated before consumption.

Toxoplasmosis Toxoplasmosis is a parasitic infection that is most often passed from cats to humans. Outdoor soil or sandboxes, especially those in warm climates, may contain the parasite from outdoor cats. The risk of infection from cleaning an indoor cat's litter box is low.

A pregnant woman who contracts toxoplasmosis can pass the infection on to her baby, and the baby can develop serious complications. To help avoid infection:

▶ Wear gloves when gardening or handling soil, and wash your hands thoroughly when done.
▶ Thoroughly wash the soil off all fruits and vegetables grown outdoors.
▶ If you have a cat, have someone else clean its litter box, or wear gloves if you have to handle litter.

Managing toxoplasmosis Toxoplasmosis during pregnancy may result in miscarriage, fetal growth problems or preterm labor. The majority of fetuses who acquire toxoplasmosis develop normally. However, the disease can cause problems, including blindness or impaired eyesight, an enlarged liver or spleen, jaundice, seizures, and intellectual disability.

If toxoplasmosis infection is suspected, your care provider can check for it with a blood test. Treating toxoplasmosis during pregnancy can be difficult, and it isn't clear whether the medications used to treat it are effective for baby.

Tuberculosis (TB) Tuberculosis is a potentially serious infection that mainly affects the lungs. It is usually spread by breathing in tiny infected droplets produced when someone with TB coughs or sneezes. TB infection may be latent — not causing symptoms — or active, causing symptoms including fever, night sweats, fatigue and weight loss. Latent TB is not contagious. But without treatment, some people with latent TB will develop active TB — especially those with weakened immune systems.

Although TB was once rare in developed countries, it is a modern public health concern worldwide. You might be screened or tested for TB if you've had significant exposure or if there's suspicion based on your symptoms.

Managing tuberculosis Latent TB can't be transmitted from mother to baby during pregnancy, and medications to treat latent TB can often be delayed until after pregnancy.

However, active TB in pregnancy has been associated with higher risk of maternal complications, including anemia, miscarriage, infection with another disease such as HIV and even maternal death. There is also increased risk of preterm birth, lower birth weights and fetal death. Active TB can be treated with medications considered safe in pregnancy. A doctor with expertise in infectious diseases is usually involved in the care of a pregnant woman with active TB, and the pregnant mother will be carefully monitored for response to medications.

Zika virus Zika is a viral infection that primarily occurs in tropical and subtropical areas of the world. It is spread by certain types of mosquitoes, but infection can also occur through sexual contact with an infected person. For most people the virus causes no signs and symptoms. Others report mild fever, rash, and muscle and joint pain, and sometimes headache or red eyes. Symptoms typically begin two to seven days after being bitten by an infected mosquito and clear up within a week.

Pregnant women should be especially cautious about exposure to the virus. Zika infections during pregnancy have been linked to miscarriage and fetal complications such as deformed joints and severe birth defects, including a very small head (microcephaly) and an abnormally formed brain.

Managing Zika No specific antiviral treatment for Zika exists, so it's essential to minimize your risk of exposure. To be safe, avoid visiting areas with risk of Zika virus while you're pregnant or planning for pregnancy. You can find up-to-date information on high- and low-risk areas on the website of the Centers for Disease Control and Prevention (CDC). If you must travel to an area of risk or if Zika is active where you live, talk to your care provider, and take strong precautions to prevent mosquito bites:

- *Stay in air-conditioned or well-screened housing.* The mosquitoes that carry the Zika virus are most active during the day, but they can also bite at night. Consider sleeping under a mosquito bed net, especially if you are outside.
- *Wear protective clothing.* If you are outside in mosquito-infested areas, wear a long-sleeved shirt, long pants, socks and shoes.

▶ *Use mosquito repellent.* Permethrin spray, an insecticide, can be applied to your clothing, shoes, camping gear and bed netting. For your skin, use a repellent containing up to a 50 percent concentration of DEET.

If you travel to an area with Zika risk while pregnant, you may be eligible for testing after your return. Your care provider also may perform an ultrasound to detect microcephaly or other abnormalities of the brain, or take a sample of amniotic fluid using a hollow needle inserted into the uterus (amniocentesis) to screen for Zika virus.

If your partner travels to an area of Zika virus risk, you'll need to protect yourself from becoming infected through sexual contact. Ask your care provider or check the CDC website for current recommendations of how to prevent Zika infection from a sexual partner.

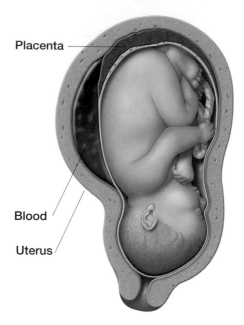

Placenta

Blood

Uterus

PLACENTAL PROBLEMS

The placenta is the organ that connects your blood supply to the baby's through the umbilical cord, providing your baby with nutrients and oxygen. In a normal pregnancy, it remains attached to the uterine wall until shortly after your baby is born. Occasionally, problems develop with the placenta that can cause serious complications if not identified early.

Placental abruption Placental abruption occurs when the placenta separates from the inner wall of the uterus before delivery. What causes this to happen is unknown, but it can be life-threatening for you and your baby. The most common condition associated with placental abruption is high blood pressure (hypertension). This is true whether the high blood pressure developed during your pregnancy or you had it before you were pregnant.

Placental abruption also appears to be more common in black women, women who are older — especially those older than age 40 — women who've had many children, women who smoke, and women who abuse alcohol or drugs during pregnancy. Very rarely, trauma or injury to the mother may cause premature placental separation (abruption).

Signs and symptoms In the early stages of placental abruption, you may not have any signs or symptoms. When they do occur, the most common sign is bleeding from the vagina. The bleeding may be light, heavy or somewhere in between. The amount of bleeding doesn't necessarily correspond to how much of the placenta has separated from the inside of the uterus. Other signs or symptoms may include:

- Back or abdominal pain
- Uterine tenderness
- Rapid or strong contractions
- A uterus that feels rigid or hard

Treatment The condition of the mother and baby, as well as the stage of the pregnancy, are taken into account. Electronic monitoring may be used to watch the baby's heart rate. If the monitoring shows no signs the baby is in immediate trouble and baby is premature, the mother may be hospitalized and her condition monitored closely.

If the baby has reached maturity and placental abruption is minimal, a vaginal delivery is possible. If an abruption progresses and signs indicate that the mother or baby is in jeopardy, immediate cesarean delivery may be necessary. A mother who experiences severe bleeding may need blood transfusions.

There's a chance that placental abruption will recur in a subsequent pregnancy. However, stopping smoking and getting treatment for substance abuse can greatly reduce that chance.

Placenta previa In some pregnancies, the placenta is located low in the uterus and covers part or all of the opening of the cervix. This is called placenta previa, and it poses a potential danger to the mother and baby because of the risk of excessive bleeding before or during delivery. Placenta previa occurs in about 1 in 200 pregnancies and may take one of two forms:
- *Low-lying placenta.* The edge of the placenta lies within 2 centimeters of the cervical opening but doesn't cover it. Vaginal delivery may be possible, although it still carries a risk of excessive bleeding.
- *Placenta previa.* The placenta covers the cervical opening, making vaginal

delivery dangerous because of the high risk of heavy bleeding.

The cause of placenta previa isn't known, but like placental abruption, it's more common in women who've had children before, older women, women who smoke and those who've had previous uterine surgery, including a cesarean delivery.

Signs and symptoms Painless vaginal bleeding is the main sign of placenta previa. You are less likely to have vaginal bleeding prior to labor if you have a low-lying placenta. Vaginal bleeding is usually bright red, and the amount may range from light to heavy. The bleeding may stop, but it nearly always recurs days or weeks later.

Placenta previa can almost always be detected by ultrasound before any bleeding has occurred. After the diagnosis is made, another ultrasound will be done later in the pregnancy to determine the

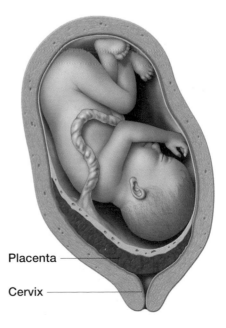

Placenta

Cervix

placental location and the best way to deliver the baby. As the uterus enlarges and the lower segment of the uterus develops, the placental edge may be found farther away from the cervix and allow for safe vaginal delivery. If the placenta remains over the cervix, pelvic exams are not done, as even a gentle cervix check can cause significant bleeding.

Treatment Treatment for placenta previa depends on several factors, including whether the fetus is mature enough to be born and whether you're experiencing vaginal bleeding. If the placenta is close to the cervix but not covering it, and there's no bleeding, you may be allowed to stay at home, avoiding any strenuous physical activity and refraining from intercourse.

If placenta previa persists until week 36 of pregnancy and bleeding episodes are recurrent, you may be kept in the hospital until the baby can be safely delivered via planned cesarean birth. Because of the chance of premature birth, steroids may be given to enhance the maturity of the baby's lungs. If bleeding starts and can't be controlled or you go into labor, an emergency cesarean delivery generally is necessary.

Women who have experienced placenta previa in a previous pregnancy have a small chance of having it again in a future pregnancy. Most often, if placenta previa occurs it can be detected early and accurately. If the placenta lies over the area in the uterus of a prior cesarean birth scar, you may be at increased risk for placenta accreta. This is a serious, possibly life-threatening condition in which the placenta grows into the muscle of the uterus. The treatment for this is usually removal of the uterus when the baby is delivered (cesarean hysterectomy).

PREECLAMPSIA AND HYPERTENSION

Preeclampsia is a disorder specific to pregnancy and is marked by:
) High blood pressure
) Protein in the urine after the 20th week of pregnancy

Preeclampsia affects 2 to 8 percent of all pregnancies and occurs most often during a woman's first pregnancy. The cause of preeclampsia still isn't known, but other risk factors include carrying two or more fetuses (multiple pregnancy), diabetes, high blood pressure (hypertension), kidney disease, rheumatic disease such as lupus, and family history. Preeclampsia is more common in very young women and women older than age 35.

Signs and symptoms Women may have preeclampsia for several weeks before signs and symptoms develop, including high blood pressure and protein in the urine. Headaches, vision problems and pain in the upper abdomen are other common symptoms of preeclampsia.

The diagnosis of preeclampsia is typically made when blood pressure is consistently elevated over a period of time. A single high blood pressure reading doesn't mean you have preeclampsia. High blood pressure has to be observed in two separate occasions at least four hours apart. In pregnant women, a blood pressure reading of 140/90 millimeters of mercury (mm Hg) or higher is considered above the normal range.

Hypertension in pregnancy has various degrees of severity. If the only sign you have is elevated blood pressure, without protein in your urine or other problems, your care provider may call your condition gestational hypertension rather than preeclampsia.

There's also a severe form of preeclampsia known as HELLP syndrome. HELLP stands for hemolysis, elevated liver enzymes and low platelets. It's distinguished from milder forms of the condition by the breakdown of red blood cells (hemolysis), abnormal liver function and a low blood platelet count. People with HELLP syndrome may also have abnormal kidney function.

Treatment The only cure for preeclampsia and other hypertensive problems in pregnancy is delivery. However, medications to treat high blood pressure in pregnancy may be used to protect the mother, helping to prevent stroke and other complications related to very high blood pressure.

Gestational hypertension or a mild case of preeclampsia is often managed at home with activity limitations and regular monitoring of your blood pressure. Although decreased activity may be recommended, bed rest is not, as this can be more dangerous to you and your baby — not moving around enough increases the likelihood of a blood clot forming in the deep veins of your legs or in the lungs. That can be life-threatening as well. Your care provider will recommend more-frequent appointments, perhaps as frequently as once or twice a week. During these appointments, your care provider will check for any changes in your blood counts, liver and kidney function, and also check on the status of your baby.

A more severe case often requires a stay in a hospital where testing of the baby's well-being can be done regularly. Left untreated, preeclampsia can result in eclampsia — a severe complication marked by seizures with possibly serious risks for both mother and baby.

If preeclampsia becomes severe, even well before the due date, labor may be in-duced or a cesarean delivery performed to protect the mother and the baby.

After delivery, blood pressure usually returns to normal within several days or weeks. Blood pressure medication may be prescribed when you're dismissed from the hospital. If blood pressure medicine is necessary, it often can be gradually decreased and then stopped a month or two after delivery. Your care provider may want to see you frequently after you go home from the hospital in order to monitor your blood pressure.

The risk that preeclampsia will happen in a subsequent pregnancy depends on how severe it was during the first pregnancy. With mild preeclampsia, the risk of recurrence is low. But if preeclampsia was severe in a first pregnancy, the risk in future pregnancies is higher.

All hypertensive disorders in pregnancy increase the risk of hypertension, stroke and heart attack later in life, as well. Women who have experienced hypertensive disorders in pregnancy should see their primary care providers each year, with close monitoring of their weight, BMI, blood pressure, cholesterol and glucose.

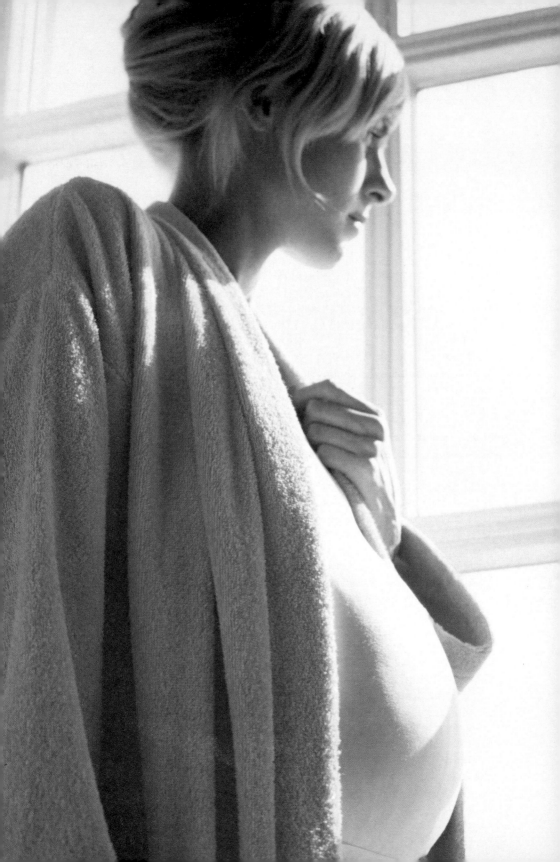

CHAPTER 28

Problems of labor and childbirth

Even if you're doing everything right as you go through labor and childbirth, complications can occur. If something does go wrong, trust that your care provider and your health care team will do the best for both you and your baby. When complications arise and things don't go as planned, it's easy to feel out of control, but be as flexible as you can and try not to panic. Your care provider can discuss concerns, possible outcomes and new courses of action with you. Ask as many questions as you need to in order to feel comfortable with the plan of care. Together, you can decide what the next steps should be.

LABOR THAT FAILS TO START

If your labor doesn't begin on its own, your care provider may recommend starting (inducing) labor. Induction stimulates contractions of the uterus to begin the process toward a vaginal birth.

Your care provider may recommend labor induction if your baby is ready to be born but contractions haven't started yet or if there's concern for your health or your baby's. Some situations in which you may be induced include:

- You've reached 41 weeks or more of pregnancy.
- Your water has broken (amniotic membranes have ruptured), but your labor hasn't started.
- There's an infection in your uterus.
- Your care provider is concerned that your baby has stopped growing or isn't active enough or that there's a decreased amount of amniotic fluid.
- You have health complications, such as high blood pressure or diabetes, that may put you or your baby at risk.

If you were hoping for labor to begin on its own but your care provider recommends induction of labor for a medical reason, try to view it in a positive light. For example, induction may allow you to be more prepared, mentally and physically, when you go to the hospital.

Inducing labor Your care provider can induce labor in several ways. Induction is most successful when the cervix is first ripened (softened and thinned). Having some degree of cervical opening (dilation) also is helpful prior to the start of induction. If needed, your care provider may use medication or mechanical techniques to help with cervical ripening. Cervical ripening and induction can be a long process, especially for first-time moms. It's not uncommon for the process to take 24 to 48 hours.

Medications Medications can be used to soften and dilate your cervix. Misoprostol (Cytotec) and dinoprostone (Cervidil, Prepidil) are commonly used for this purpose. These drugs often work to begin labor as well, and they may reduce the need for other labor-inducing agents, such as oxytocin (Pitocin). If you need to have your cervix ripened, you may go to the hospital the night before your labor induction to give the medication time to work.

Mechanical techniques Mechanical techniques can also be used to help ripen the cervix. One commonly used technique is placing a small catheter with a balloon through the cervix. The balloon is then inflated with water or saline. It applies pressure on the cervix and is gradually expelled through the cervix, softening and opening it 2 to 4 centimeters (cm).

Breaking your water When your water breaks, the amniotic sac that envelops your baby develops an opening or a tear, and the fluid begins to flow out. Normally, this signals that delivery will happen fairly soon. Often, uterine contractions increase after the water breaks.

Once the cervix is ripened, one way to induce or accelerate labor is to artificially break your water. To do this, your care provider inserts a long, thin plastic hook through the cervix and creates a small tear in the membranes of the amniotic sac. This procedure will feel just like a vaginal exam, and you'll probably sense the warm fluid flowing out. It isn't harmful or painful to you or your baby.

Oxytocin A common method for inducing labor is with a drug called oxytocin (Pitocin), which is a synthetic version of the hormone oxytocin. Your body normally produces low levels of oxytocin throughout pregnancy. The levels rise in active labor.

Oxytocin is generally administered intravenously after your cervix is dilated somewhat and thinned (effaced). An intravenous (IV) catheter is inserted into a vein in your arm or on the back of your hand. A pump is connected to your IV that delivers small, regulated doses of the drug into your bloodstream. These doses may be adjusted throughout your induction to change the strength and frequency of your contractions until they're occurring regularly. The contractions may be more regular and stronger than those with a naturally occurring labor.

Oxytocin is one of the most commonly used drugs in pregnancy and childbirth. It can initiate labor that may not have started otherwise, and it can also speed things up if contractions or dilation stalls in the middle of labor. Uterine contractions and your baby's heart rate are monitored closely to reduce the risk of complications.

If labor induction is successful, you'll begin to experience signs of active, progressive labor, such as longer lasting contractions that are stronger and more frequent, dilation of your cervix, and rupture of your amniotic sac — if it hasn't broken or been broken already. But keep in mind that induction can take many hours, especially for a first-time mom.

Induction of labor should be done only for good medical reasons. If your health or your baby's is in question, your care provider may decide to take further intervention, such as a cesarean delivery.

LABOR THAT FAILS TO PROGRESS

If your labor isn't progressing as it should, a condition called dystocia, it's usually due to a problem with one or more components of the birth process. Progress in labor is measured by how well your cervix opens (dilates) and the descent of your baby through the pelvis. This requires the following:

▶ Regular and strong contractions
▶ A baby that can fit through the mother's pelvis and is in the correct position for descent
▶ A pelvis that's roomy enough to allow for the passage of the baby

If your contractions aren't forceful enough to open the cervix, you may be given medication to make your uterus contract. Contractions can sometimes start regularly but then stop during your labor. If this happens and the progress of your labor halts for a few hours, your care provider may suggest breaking your water, if it hasn't already broken, or stimulating your labor with oxytocin (Pitocin).

Problems that can occur during labor include:

Prolonged early labor The latent phase of labor lasts from the onset of contractions until your cervix is dilating at a faster rate, usually after 5 to 6 cm. This phase can last for the better part of a day or more, particularly for first-time moms. Your contractions may still be mild during this time, so try to relax.

Sometimes, progress is slow because you're not in true labor. The contractions you feel are those of false labor (Braxton Hicks contractions), and they're not effective at opening your cervix.

Treatment Whatever the cause, if your cervix is still fairly closed when you arrive at the hospital or birthing center and your contractions aren't very strong, your care provider may suggest some options to promote labor. You may be told to walk or to return home and rest. Often, the most effective treatment for a prolonged early phase is rest. A medication may be given to help you rest.

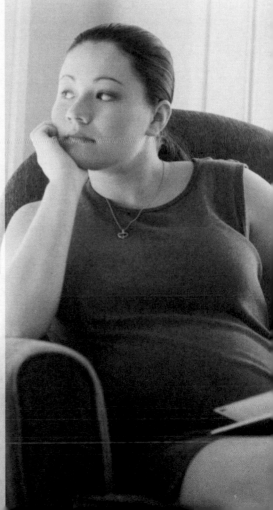

ASSISTED BIRTH

If labor is prolonged or complications develop, you may require some medical assistance. Instruments — such as forceps or a vacuum extractor — can be used to help with delivery if your cervix is fully dilated and the baby has descended but is having difficulty making the last step to delivery. An assisted delivery may also be necessary if your baby's head is facing the wrong direction and is wedged in your pelvis. If your baby's heart rate is too low and the baby must be delivered quickly or you're too exhausted to push any longer, your care provider may intervene medically with a forceps- or vacuum-assisted birth. A forceps- or vacuum-assisted delivery can be the quickest and safest means of delivering a baby.

Forceps-assisted birth Forceps are shaped like a pair of spoons that, when hooked together, resemble a pair of salad tongs. Your care provider gently slides one spoon at a time into your vagina and around the side of the baby's head. The two pieces lock together, and the curved tongs cradle the baby's head. While your uterus contracts and you push, the care provider gently guides the baby through the birth canal, which usually happens on the very next push or two.

Forceps are used today only when the baby's head has descended well into the mother's pelvis or is near the pelvic outlet. If the head hasn't descended enough and the baby needs to be delivered quickly, a cesarean birth may be necessary.

Vacuum-assisted birth A vacuum extractor may be used instead of forceps if the baby has descended into the pelvis. A rubber or plastic cup is placed against the baby's head, a pump creates suction, and the care provider gently guides the instrument to ease the baby down the birth canal while the mother pushes. The vacuum extractor cup doesn't take as much room as forceps and is associated with fewer injuries to the mother. But a vacuum-assisted birth is slightly riskier for the baby.

What to expect An assisted delivery doesn't take very long, but it may take 30 to 45 minutes to get you ready for the procedure. You may need an epidural or spinal anesthetic and a catheter placed in your bladder to empty the urine. Your care provider may make a cut to enlarge the opening of the vagina (episiotomy) to help ease the delivery of the baby.

Instruments to help deliver babies are important tools and are generally safe. Still, you should be aware that forceps may leave bruises or red marks on the sides of your baby's head. A vacuum extractor may leave a bruise or bump on the top of the head or cause bleeding in the baby's scalp. The bruises take about a week to go away. A bump or red marks disappear within a few days. Serious damage with either technique is rare.

The choice of which approach to use — forceps or a vacuum extractor, if either — is best left to your care provider. Experience with the instrument is the greatest defense against complications.

If you are told to return home in early labor, remember that the goal is a natural progression of labor with fewer medical interventions.

Prolonged active labor Your labor may go smoothly during the early phase, only to slow down during the active phase of labor. Labor is considered prolonged if the cervix doesn't dilate approximately 1 to 2 cm an hour in active labor. Progress may continue but take too long or it may stop or dwindle. An abrupt halt in progress following good contractions can suggest an incompatibility between the size of your pelvis and the size of your baby's head.

Treatment If you're making progress in active labor, your care provider may allow your labor to continue naturally. He or she may suggest that you walk or change positions to assist in labor.

In the event that you've been in active labor and haven't made progress for several hours, your care provider may start oxytocin, rupture the amniotic sac or do both in an attempt to move things along. These steps are often enough to restart contractions and allow you to deliver without complications.

Prolonged pushing At times, efforts to push the baby through the birth canal are slow or aren't effective, which can result in exhaustion on the mother's part. If this is your first baby, pushing for more than three hours is generally considered to be prolonged. If you've already had a child, pushing more than two hours is considered prolonged.

Treatment Your care provider will evaluate how far down the birth canal the baby has descended and if the problem can be corrected by readjusting the baby's

head position. If you're able to continue and your baby isn't showing signs of distress, you may be allowed to push for a longer time. Sometimes, if the baby has descended far enough, his or her head can be eased out with the gentle use of forceps or a vacuum extractor (see "Assisted birth" on page 454). You may be asked to try a semisitting, squatting or kneeling position, which can help push the baby out. If your baby is too high in the birth canal and other measures won't help, cesarean delivery may be needed.

BABY IN AN ABNORMAL POSITION

Your labor and delivery may become complicated if your baby is in an abnormal position within your uterus — making a vaginal delivery difficult or, sometimes, impossible.

Right around the 32nd to 34th weeks of pregnancy, most babies settle into a head-down position for descent into the birth canal. As your due date nears, your care provider may determine the position of your baby simply by feeling your abdomen for clues as to the baby's placement. He or she may also perform a vaginal exam or an ultrasound. Sometimes an ultrasound exam is also done during labor to determine the baby's position.

If your baby isn't positioned for an easy exit through your pelvis during labor, problems can develop.

Facing up (occiput posterior) A baby's head is widest from the front to the back. Ideally, its head should turn to one side once it enters the top of the pelvis. The chin is then forced down to the chest so that the more narrow back of the head leads the way. After descending to the

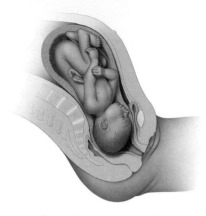

Occiput posterior position

midpelvis, the baby needs to turn either facedown or faceup to align with the lower pelvis. Most babies turn facedown, but when a baby is facing up, labor may progress more slowly. Care providers call this the occiput posterior position. Intense back labor and prolonged labor may accompany this position.

Treatment Sometimes, changing your position can help rotate the baby. Your care provider might have you get on your hands and knees, or place a pillow or ball between your knees. Repositioning may allow your baby to rotate to the facedown position.

If this doesn't work, your care provider might try to rotate the baby manually. By reaching through your vagina and using his or her hand as a guide, he or she can encourage the baby's head to turn facedown. If this technique isn't successful, your health care team can monitor your labor to determine whether your baby is likely to fit through your pelvis faceup or whether a cesarean birth would be safer. Most babies can be born faceup, but it may take a bit longer.

Abnormal angle When a baby's head enters the pelvis, ideally the chin should be pressed down onto the chest. If the chin isn't down, a larger diameter of the head has to fit through the pelvis. However, a baby can enter the birth canal with the top of the head, the forehead or even the face presenting first — none of which is a preferred position.

If your baby's head moves through your pelvis at an abnormal angle, it can affect the location and intensity of your discomfort and the length of your labor.

Treatment A cesarean birth (C-section) may be necessary if your baby isn't progressing down the birth canal or shows signs he or she isn't tolerating labor.

Head too big When a baby's head can't fit through the pelvis, the problem is called cephalopelvic disproportion. It may be that the baby's head is too big or the mother's pelvis is too small. Also, the baby's head may not be properly aligned, with the smallest width leading the way through the birth canal. No matter what's causing the problem, labor can't progress or the cervix may not dilate normally. The result is prolonged labor.

Treatment Size alone isn't the only factor to determine if your baby will fit through your pelvis. The forces of labor can temporarily mold a baby's head, even when poorly positioned, to fit through the pelvis, and loosened ligaments that occur with pregnancy allow the bones of the pelvis to open wider. Because of these variables, the best way for your care provider to determine whether your baby's head matches the roominess of your pelvis is to monitor your labor as it progresses. If necessary, a C-section may be performed.

Breech A baby is in the breech position (presentation) when the buttocks or one or both feet enter the pelvis first (see the illustration below). Breech presentation poses potential problems for the baby during birth, which can, in turn, create complications for you. A prolapsed umbilical cord is a serious complication that's more common in breech births. In addition, it's impossible to be certain whether the baby's head will fit through the pelvis. The head is the largest and least compressible part of the baby. Even if the baby's body has already delivered, the head could become trapped.

Treatment If your care provider knows prior to labor and delivery that your baby is breech, he or she may try to turn the baby into the proper position. This technique is called an external cephalic version. The procedure is usually done at approximately 37 weeks in a monitored area, such as a labor and delivery unit.

For an external cephalic version, a medication may be administered to temporarily relax your uterus. Then your care provider will apply pressure to your abdomen, guiding the baby into a somersault to reach a head-down position. This is done with ultrasound guidance, and your baby's heart rate will be monitored after the procedure.

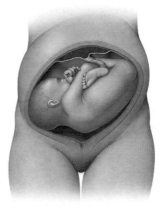

Transverse lie

If external cephalic version isn't an option or doesn't work, a C-section is the safest way to deliver a breech fetus. An exception may be a breech second baby in a set of twins, if the first baby is head down.

Lying sideways A baby lying crosswise in the uterus is in a position called transverse lie (see the illustration above).

Treatment Just as in breech presentation, your doctor may try to turn the baby. This step is often successful. Babies who remain in this position need to be delivered by C-section.

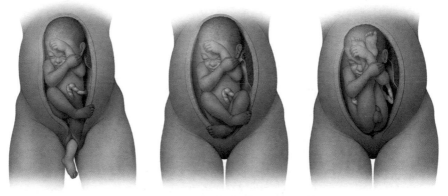

Three examples of breech presentation

INTOLERANCE OF LABOR

A baby is considered to be intolerant of labor if there are persistent signs that he or she may not have an adequate oxygen supply. These signs are usually detected by studying the fetal heart rate on an electronic monitor. Decreased oxygen to the baby usually occurs when blood flow from the placenta to the baby is reduced, meaning that he or she isn't receiving enough oxygen from the mother.

Potential causes for this problem include compression of the umbilical cord, decreased blood flow to the uterus from the mother and a placenta that's not functioning correctly.

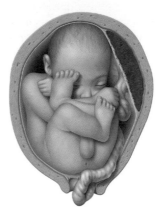

Umbilical cord prolapse

Umbilical cord prolapse If the umbilical cord slips out through the opening of the cervix (see the illustration at upper right), blood flow to the baby may be slowed or stopped. Umbilical cord prolapse is most likely to occur with a small or premature baby, with a baby who is breech, with a very high amount of amniotic fluid, or when the amniotic sac breaks before the baby is down far enough in the pelvis.

Treatment If the cord slips out after you're fully dilated and ready to push, a vaginal delivery may still be possible. Otherwise, a C-section is usually the safest option.

Umbilical cord compression If the umbilical cord becomes squeezed between any part of the baby and the mother's pelvis, or if there's a decreased amount of amniotic fluid, the umbilical cord can become pinched (compressed). Blood flow to the baby is slowed or, very rarely, stopped, for a very short period during a contraction. The condition usually develops when the baby is well down the birth canal. If cord compression is prolonged or severe, the baby may show signs of decreased oxygen supply.

Treatment To minimize the problem, you may be asked to change positions during labor in order to move the position of the baby or the umbilical cord. You may be given oxygen to increase the amount of oxygen the baby gets. Your care provider may also try to infuse fluid into your uterus to reduce the cord compression, a therapy called amnioinfusion. It may be necessary for your care provider to deliver the baby with forceps or a vacuum extractor. If the baby is too high in the birth canal or you aren't completely dilated, a C-section may be necessary.

Decreased fetal heart rate With uterine contractions, the flow of blood through the uterus decreases as the contraction strength peaks. Babies can generally tolerate these temporary changes in blood flow, thanks to natural oxygen reserves. But if the reserves become depleted, changes in the fetal heart rate may signal that the baby can no longer compensate for the interruption in oxygen supply. That's why your baby's heartbeat is monitored regularly during labor. If your baby's heartbeat is persistently too rapid or too slow, it may mean that he or she isn't receiving enough oxygen.

By using an electronic fetal monitor, your care provider can detect heartbeat irregularities that may indicate concern. Methods of fetal monitoring include:

External monitoring In external monitoring, two wide belts are placed around your abdomen. One is put high on your uterus to measure and record the length and frequency of your contractions. The other is secured across your lower abdomen to record the baby's heart rate. The two belts are connected to a monitor that displays and prints both readings at the same time so that their interactions can be observed.

Internal monitoring Internal monitoring can be done only after your water has broken. Once your amniotic sac has ruptured, your care provider can actually reach inside your vagina and through the dilated cervix to touch the baby. To more accurately monitor the baby's heart rate, a tiny wire is attached to the baby's scalp. To measure the strength of contractions, the doctor inserts a narrow, pressure-sensitive tube (catheter) between the wall of your uterus and the baby. The tube records the pressure of each contraction. As with external monitoring, these devices are connected to a monitor that displays and records the readings, as well as amplifies the sound of your baby's heartbeat.

Fetal stimulation test Ordinarily, when a baby's scalp is touched or tickled by a care provider's touch, the baby will move around, and his or her heart rate will go up. Sound may also be used to stimulate the fetus. A baby who is stimulated but doesn't experience an increase in heart rate may not be getting enough oxygen.

Treatment *There are ways to help a baby get more oxygen.* Your care provider may give you medication during labor to slow or stop your contractions, which increases blood flow to the fetus. If your blood pressure is low, you may be given a medication to increase it. You may also be given extra oxygen to breathe.

Most of the time, labor should be allowed to continue, even when there are signs the baby is responding to temporary stress.

In extreme situations, low oxygen levels can be life-threatening. Your care provider is trained to identify the signs of severe distress and take immediate action, which generally involves emergency cesarean delivery.

If you're concerned by what you see on a fetal monitor, ask a member of your health care team.

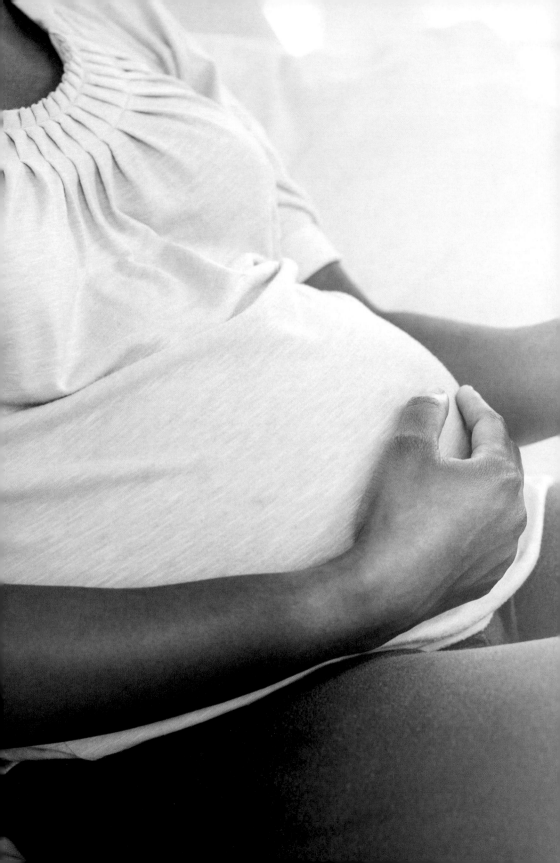

CHAPTER 29

Managing mom's health concerns

In addition to caring for baby, pregnancy involves making sure you stay healthy — both during pregnancy and afterward. Your care can be more complicated if you enter pregnancy with existing medical issues. These issues could also increase the risk of certain problems after your baby is born.

PRE-EXISTING HEALTH ISSUES

Women who have a health condition before becoming pregnant may receive different care during their pregnancies, depending on the condition. That's because a pre-existing health condition can affect the outcome of a pregnancy. The good news is, with a doctor's help and guidance, most problems can be managed in a way that's safe for both you and your baby.

Asthma Asthma occurs when the main air passages of the lungs (bronchial tubes)

become inflamed and constricted. Production of extra mucus can further narrow the airways. This can lead to signs and symptoms ranging from minor wheezing to severe difficulty breathing. Although asthma attacks can be life-threatening, asthma is a highly treatable condition. With the right care and medication, problems can be prevented during pregnancy.

Managing asthma If your asthma is well-controlled during pregnancy, there's little chance you and your baby will have an increased risk of health complications. In general, women with mild asthma have few difficulties during pregnancy, while women with severe asthma need to be followed more closely. Talk with your care provider about what steps to take. The medical profession has extensive experience with treating asthma during pregnancy. Most asthma medications can be safely used by pregnant women.

Left uncontrolled, asthma can cause problems for both you and your baby. If you experience low oxygen levels, oxygen to the fetus may decrease, possibly resulting in slowed fetal growth and even fetal brain damage. If you experience an attack, extra oxygen and inhaled medications (nebulizer treatments) are commonly used to increase oxygen levels and help open up lung airways.

To control your signs and symptoms, it's important to continue taking medications as directed. Don't stop any medication for asthma unless directed to do so by your care provider. For some pregnant women, asthma worsens in the second and third trimesters. Rarely, it can worsen during labor.

Cancer Cancer in pregnancy is rare, and there's no evidence that the risk of cancer increases during pregnancy. However, cancer can — and does — occur in women of childbearing age, including during pregnancy.

If you're being treated for cancer or you have a history of it, you may be advised to delay becoming pregnant. Women diagnosed with breast cancer, for example, usually are encouraged to take steps to prevent pregnancy until after treatment is complete. Those who have had breast cancer in the past also may be advised to wait and see if it recurs before trying to conceive. In some women, cancer treatment can affect fertility.

If you receive a diagnosis of breast cancer while you're pregnant, the prognosis generally is the same as that of women with breast cancer who aren't pregnant. However, it's important that treatment begins right away. Treatment during pregnancy can improve your odds of survival and give you the opportunity to raise your child.

Managing cancer Your treatment will be based on several factors. These include the type of cancer, how advanced the

cancer is, what the best treatment would be and how far along you are in pregnancy. Various treatment options may be considered.

Chemotherapy, a common cancer treatment, is most dangerous during the first trimester of pregnancy. At that time, it has a risk of causing birth defects or miscarriage. In the second and third trimesters, chemotherapy may lower your baby's birth weight. The risk of causing other problems varies according to the medications used.

Radiation therapy might or might not affect your baby. It depends on the type of exposure, the location of the radiation site — the distance from the baby — the timing of the treatment and the age of the fetus. Radiation applied to your chest or abdominal area is more likely to affect the fetus than radiation applied to your head or a lower leg. The most vulnerable period for a fetus is between week eight and week 15 of pregnancy. Depending on your circumstances, it may be best to postpone treatment or delay it until the baby can be safely delivered.

Surgical procedures are often possible while you're pregnant. If surgery is needed for cancer and it doesn't involve the uterus, it's probably best to do the surgery during the pregnancy rather than wait until your baby is born. However, if surgery causes inflammation or infection in the abdomen, the risk of early delivery increases.

It's not clear whether pregnancy directly affects the progression of cancer. However, it often can complicate treatment or reduce treatment options. If you'll be undergoing cancer treatment after delivery, talk with your health care team about measures to preserve your ability to have additional children, if that's important to you. Techniques are available that help allow for future pregnancies.

Depression Depression is a serious mental health condition. It can interfere with the ability to eat, sleep, work, interact with others, care for yourself and others, and enjoy life. It may be a one-time problem, triggered by a stressful event such as the death of a loved one, or it may be a chronic condition. The illness often runs in families, and genetics likely play a role. Experts think this genetic vulnerability, along with environmental factors such as stress, may trigger an imbalance in brain chemicals and result in depression.

Pregnancy can affect depression. For a woman with depression, body changes during pregnancy can trigger a wide range of emotions that can make coping more difficult. Changes in fluid volume during pregnancy and labor also can alter the effectiveness of antidepressant medications. In addition, women with histories of major depression can have repeated episodes of it during and after pregnancy. This is especially true if they stop using antidepressant medications during pregnancy. The good news is, with proper medical care, most women with depression have healthy pregnancies.

Managing depression Treatment of depression is very important during pregnancy. If you don't take proper care of depression during pregnancy, you may put your health — and your baby's health — at risk. While emotions in pregnancy can make it more difficult for you to cope with depression, untreated depression may affect your baby's well-being. Some studies associate signs and symptoms of maternal depression with preterm birth, lower birth weight and intrauterine growth restriction.

Make sure to tell your care provider about any medication you take for depression. Depending on what you're taking, your doctor may suggest switching to a different drug. That's because some antidepressants are thought to be safer during pregnancy than others. Overall, the risk of birth defects and other problems for babies of women who take antidepressants during pregnancy is very low.

During the last trimester of pregnancy, some doctors suggest tapering antidepressant doses until after birth to minimize newborn withdrawal symptoms, though it's unclear whether this method can substantially reduce harmful effects. Such an approach needs to be closely monitored. It may be unsafe for new mothers as they enter the postpartum period, when the risk of mood and anxiety problems is typically increased.

The decision to continue or change your antidepressant medication is up to you and your care provider. Follow your care provider's advice on how to best manage depression during pregnancy.

Diabetes Diabetes affects the regulation of blood sugar (glucose), the body's main source of energy. Foods you eat are broken down to glucose, which is stored in the liver and released into the bloodstream. Insulin, a hormone secreted by the pancreas, helps glucose enter your cells, especially muscle cells. In people with diabetes, this system doesn't function properly.

There are two main types of diabetes, type 1 and type 2:

- *Type 1.* With this type, the insulin-producing cells in the pancreas are destroyed. The individual needs injections of insulin every day to survive. Type 1 diabetes is often diagnosed in childhood.
- *Type 2.* With type 2, there's limited insulin activity, mostly because the body has developed a resistance to insulin. When cells become resistant, they don't take in sufficient insulin

from the bloodstream. As a result, sugar stays in the bloodstream and accumulates there. Type 2 diabetes is usually diagnosed in adulthood.

During pregnancy, some women develop a temporary condition known as gestational diabetes (page 439). It resembles type 2 diabetes, but usually goes away after pregnancy. Women who develop gestational diabetes are at increased risk of diabetes later in life.

Managing diabetes There is no cure for diabetes. However, blood sugar can be controlled with proper medication and lifestyle management, which includes eating a well-balanced diet, maintaining a healthy weight and getting plenty of exercise. If you have diabetes and you keep your blood sugar levels under control before conception and during pregnancy, you're likely to have a healthy pregnancy and give birth to a healthy baby. If your diabetes isn't under control, you're at higher risk of having a baby with a birth defect of the brain or spinal cord, heart, or kidneys. The risk of miscarriage and stillbirth also increases significantly.

Poor control of your diabetes also puts you at increased risk of having a baby that weighs 10 pounds or more. That's because when blood sugar becomes too high, the baby receives higher-than-normal levels of glucose and produces extra insulin to use the sugar and to store it as fat. The fat tends to accumulate and produce an infant that's larger than normal — a medical condition known as macrosomia. Monitoring your baby's growth during pregnancy can give advanced warning if the baby appears to be adversely affected by diabetes.

Insulin requirements tend to increase for pregnant women with diabetes because hormones from the placenta impair the normal response to insulin. Some women may need two to three times their usual dose of insulin to control their blood sugar. Most women taking insulin before pregnancy will require multiple daily doses of insulin or an insulin pump. Frequent adjustments of dosage will likely be needed throughout the pregnancy. Eating properly also is an important part of diabetes care during pregnancy.

It's important to work closely with your doctor to protect your health and the health of your baby.

Epilepsy Epilepsy is a seizure disorder that results from abnormal electrical activity in the brain. These abnormal signals may cause temporary changes in sensation, behavior, movement or consciousness. In some cases, seizures may have a known cause, such as a disease or an accident that affects the brain. In others, seizures may occur for no apparent reason.

Anti-epileptic drugs can eliminate or reduce the amount and intensity of seizures in the majority of people with epilepsy. The great majority of women with epilepsy who become pregnant will have healthy pregnancies.

Managing epilepsy It's important to continue treatment for seizures during pregnancy, as seizures could be harmful to your baby. Before you conceive, talk with your doctor about your treatment. Some anti-seizure medications have been associated with birth defects. If you are taking one of these medications, your doctor may recommend a different drug that's safer for you and your baby.

Most women continue taking the same medications they used before becoming pregnant, because changing medications increases the risk of new seizures. Some anti-epileptic drugs affect the way the body uses folic acid, an important source of protection against birth defects. Therefore, your doctor may ask you to take a higher dosage of folic acid with your medications.

Because your blood volume increases during pregnancy and your kidneys can remove medications faster, you may need to monitor blood levels more frequently and increase your medication dosage as your pregnancy progresses. Be sure to follow your doctor's orders.

Heart disease Heart disease can include a range of conditions, including coronary artery disease, congenital heart problems and valve disease. Although some conditions are more serious than others, all can affect how blood is moved around the body.

For the most part, women with heart disease who are pregnant can be monitored and managed so that they and their babies will do well. There are exceptions, however. So it's always best to consult your doctor about the specifics of your condition before becoming pregnant and to work with a specialist during your pregnancy to manage your condition.

Managing heart disease Pregnancy can put additional stress on the heart and circulatory system, as early as during the first trimester. You'll be closely monitored during pregnancy for possible worsening of your underlying condition. This may mean more-frequent tests and exams. In addition, some of the common changes accompanying pregnancy may be of special concern for you. Anemia, for example, poses a greater risk to people with some types of heart conditions. Fluid retention, typically first noticed as sudden swelling in the lower extremities or weight gain, needs to be monitored and managed carefully. Though typical during pregnancy, it could also indicate worsening of the underlying heart problem.

During labor, you may require special evaluation, including cardiac monitoring. Pain relief medications are used, in part, to decrease stress on the mother's heart. Epidural or spinal anesthesia is commonly used. In addition, forceps or vacuum extractors are more likely to be used during a vaginal birth to minimize prolonged pushing, which also puts stress on the mother's heart. Women with certain heart conditions might even need to have C-sections to avoid labor, but vaginal delivery is preferred for most women.

Hepatitis B Hepatitis B is a serious liver infection caused by the hepatitis B virus (HBV). The virus is transmitted by way of the blood and body fluids of someone who's infected — similar to the way the human immunodeficiency virus (HIV) that causes AIDS is transmitted. But HBV is much more infectious than HIV.

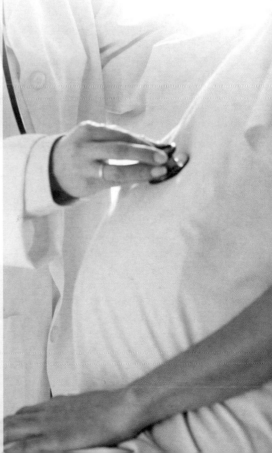

Women with hepatitis B can pass the infection to their babies during childbirth. Newborn babies can also become infected with the virus from contact with household members who are HBV positive. In the United States, pregnant women who receive prenatal care are routinely screened for HBV.

Most people infected with HBV as adults recover fully. Infants and children are much more likely to develop a chronic infection.

Managing hepatitis B The greatest risk of hepatitis infection during pregnancy is that of infecting the baby with HBV. The risk of pregnancy complications and infection of your newborn appear to be related to the activity of your HBV disease. If your disease activity is high, you may be given medication to reduce the risk of complications to you and your baby. Your newborn can be given antibodies against the virus after birth.

Vaccination against HBV is a common part of infant immunizations. In some states, HBV vaccination is mandatory. The hepatitis B vaccination is administered as a series of shots, which may be given to newborns as well as to premature infants. For optimal protection, an individual needs to receive all of the shots in the series.

High blood pressure Blood pressure is the force with which flowing blood pushes against the walls of the arteries. When the pressure becomes too high, the condition is called high blood pressure (hypertension).

High blood pressure that develops before pregnancy can occur for various reasons. Genetic factors, diet and lifestyle are thought to play a role in the condition, but other chronic conditions also can account for its development.

Most women with high blood pressure can have healthy pregnancies. However, the condition does require careful management throughout the pregnancy. High blood pressure can worsen significantly, leading to problems for both the mother and the baby.

Managing high blood pressure If you have high blood pressure, it's best to see your doctor before trying to become pregnant so that he or she can see if your condition is under control and review your medications. Some medications used to lower blood pressure are safe to take during pregnancy, but others, such as angiotensin-converting enzyme (ACE) inhibitors, can harm your baby. For that reason, your doctor may want to change the type or dosage of medications you take while pregnant. Treatment is important during pregnancy.

Blood pressure usually changes as the body adapts to pregnancy. High blood pressure that existed before pregnancy can worsen during pregnancy, especially in the last trimester. In some women, pregnancy can reveal previously unrecognized hypertension.

To monitor baby's health and development, frequent visits and repeated ultrasounds will usually be done to assess fetal growth and monitor the baby's well-being. Most often, women with high blood pressure will need to deliver by their due dates to avoid complications.

Immune thrombocytopenic purpura Also known as idiopathic thrombocytopenic purpura (ITP), this disease results in an abnormally low number of platelets in the blood. Platelets are a type of blood cell essential to clotting, which stops bleeding from cuts or bruises. If the level of platelets becomes too low, bleeding can occur even after a minor injury or even through normal wear and tear. With ITP, the body destroys platelets due to a malfunction of the immune system.

Pregnancy itself doesn't affect the course or severity of ITP. But the antibodies that can destroy platelets occasionally cross the placenta and can decrease the platelet count in your baby. Unfortunately, the baby's platelet count can't be predicted by your platelet count or even by the length of time you've had a low platelet level. The baby's platelet count may be low even if yours is fine.

Managing ITP Because the risk of bleeding in the baby is very low, cesarean birth isn't routine for this condition, unless you've had a pervious birth in which your child experienced complications related to low platelet counts. Efforts should be made to provide the baby with appropriate treatment at delivery with a team approach. If your platelet count is very low, medications may be given to try and raise your platelet count before your baby is born.

Inflammatory bowel disease Inflammatory bowel disease (IBD) is a chronic inflammation of the digestive tract. Ulcerative colitis and Crohn's disease are the two most common forms of IBD. Both can cause repeated episodes of fever, diarrhea, rectal bleeding and abdominal pain. The exact cause of IBD is unknown. Heredity, environment and the immune system may play a role.

Although there's no cure for ulcerative colitis or Crohn's disease, medications and other treatments are available. IBD conditions can arise during pregnancy. But the diagnosis is more likely to be made before pregnancy.

Women whose IBD has affected their weight or nutritional condition may have difficulty getting pregnant or having a healthy pregnancy. Women with Crohn's disease may be at increased risk of giving birth prematurely. However, if you have your disease under control before and during your pregnancy, you're much more likely to have a healthy pregnancy and full-term delivery.

Managing IBD If you have IBD, pregnancy shouldn't significantly affect your treatment. Most of the medications commonly used to treat IBD don't harm the fetus. Improving your condition is likely to benefit both you and baby, outweighing potential concern for a drug's effect on the fetus.

However, some immunosuppressive medications used to treat people with IBD might cause harm to the fetus. If you take one of these medications, discuss it with your doctor. Also discuss the use of anti-diarrheal medications, especially during the first trimester of pregnancy.

If you have Crohn's disease and it was inactive before pregnancy, it's likely to stay inactive while you're pregnant. When it's active, it's likely to remain active or even worsen during pregnancy. With ulcerative colitis, about one-third of the women who become pregnant while the disease is in remission will experience a flare-up. If the colitis is active when you become pregnant, it's likely to remain active or possibly worsen.

If diagnostic testing becomes necessary to deal with IBD during pregnancy, it's likely that the procedures can be done safely. Extra precautions may be taken to minimize risk to the fetus.

Lupus Lupus can cause chronic inflammation of many organ systems. It can affect your skin, joints, kidneys, blood cells, heart and lungs. The disease commonly results in a rash and arthritis of varying severity. Several types of lupus exist. The most common type is systemic lupus erythematosus (SLE).

Lupus sometimes shows up for the first time during pregnancy or shortly after giving birth. Women who already have lupus may note an increase in symptoms during pregnancy — even if the condition hasn't been active. If lupus is active at the start of pregnancy, there's a much higher risk of it worsening during pregnancy.

Managing lupus If you have active lupus during your pregnancy, you're at risk of problems, including the development of high blood pressure and preeclampsia. You may need to adjust the use of certain medications that could harm your baby. Work closely with your doctor before and during your pregnancy to take proper care of your health and to protect the health of your baby. Your pregnancy care team should be led by a specialist.

Phenylketonuria This is an inherited disease that affects how the body processes phenylalanine, one of the amino acid building blocks of proteins. Phenylalanine is found in milk, cheeses, eggs, meat, fish and other high-protein foods. If the level of phenylalanine in the bloodstream becomes too high, it can cause brain injury. A special diet low in phenylalanine can prevent or minimize brain damage in those with phenylketonuria (PKU).

Managing PKU If you have PKU and it's been kept under control both before and during pregnancy, you can have a healthy baby. If your blood levels of phenylalanine aren't well-regulated, you could give birth to an infant with mild to severe intellectual disability. Affected infants may also be born with a small head and congenital heart disease.

If you have a family history of the disease or were treated for PKU as a child, tell your doctor. Ideally, you'll want to have your blood levels of phenylalanine measured before trying to conceive. If necessary, you can begin a special diet to help keep levels low and prevent birth defects.

During pregnancy, the dietary restrictions needed to keep down the levels of phenylalanine can be hard to manage. Your diet may be reviewed and adjusted if phenylalanine levels are too high.

Rheumatoid arthritis Rheumatoid arthritis causes chronic inflammation of the joints, most often the wrists, hands, feet and ankles. Problems can vary from occasional flares of pain to serious joint damage. The disease is most common in women between the ages of 30 and 60.

Managing rheumatoid arthritis This condition can be managed with proper medical treatment and self-care. Rheumatoid arthritis is unlikely to affect your pregnancy, but the medications you use to treat the condition may need to be adjusted. For example, aspirin and other anti-inflammatory medications generally aren't recommended during pregnancy.

During your pregnancy you may experience some improvement in your rheumatoid arthritis. This can result from a change in your immune system while you're carrying a child. However, almost all women who experience improvement during pregnancy will experience a relapse after delivery.

Sexually transmitted infections If sexually transmitted infections (STIs) aren't diagnosed and treated, they can affect the health of a pregnant woman and her baby. Unfortunately, many STIs have mild signs and symptoms that may go unnoticed, and a woman may be unaware that she's infected.

Chlamydia It is the most common bacterial STI in the United States. The majority of women who contract it have no signs or symptoms. If you have untreated chlamydia, you may face an increased risk of miscarriage and premature rupturing of the membranes surrounding your baby in the uterus. It's also possible for you to spread chlamydia from your vaginal canal to your child during delivery. This can cause pneumonia or an eye infection in the child, which may lead to blindness.

Gonorrhea This highly contagious STI also has few recognizable signs and symptoms. Sometimes, there's a slight increase in vaginal discharge. Gonorrhea, like chlamydia, can increase your risk of miscarriage and premature rupture of the membranes if the disease is left untreated. In addition, you can infect your infant during vaginal delivery. A baby who becomes infected can develop a severe eye infection. Because gonorrhea and chlamydia can go undetected in women and because these infections pose a serious risk to a newborn's eyes, all newborns are given medication at birth to prevent development of eye infection.

Genital warts There are many kinds of genital warts, some invisible and some hard to miss. Genital warts can appear one month to several years after sexual contact with an infected person. They appear in the moist areas of the genitals and may look like small, flesh-colored bumps.

If you have genital warts, they can enlarge during pregnancy, causing increased itching and sometimes spotting. If the warts are severe, they may cause difficulty urinating, profuse bleeding or even obstruct the birth canal. Your doctor may remove these warts using one of several procedures, including medication or surgery. Most often, though, the warts don't cause significant problems and it's not necessary to have them removed. Very rarely, an infant born to an infected mother may develop warts in the throat and voice box, which may require surgery to prevent obstruction of the airway.

The presence of warts isn't a reason for a cesarean delivery, unless the warts are extremely large and could interfere with vaginal delivery of the infant.

Herpes Herpes is a contagious disease caused by the herpes simplex virus. The virus comes in two forms: herpes simplex virus type 1 (HSV-1) and type 2 (HSV-2). Type 1 causes cold sores around the mouth or nose, but it may also involve the genital area. Type 2 causes painful genital, and sometimes oral, blisters that rupture and become sores. Both types are passed on through direct contact with an infected person.

The initial (primary) infection may be obvious, with serious signs and symptoms lasting a week or more. After the initial outbreak, the virus remains dormant in infected areas, periodically reactivating. These episodes last about 10 days. They may start with tingling, itching or pain before sores become visible.

Antiviral drugs can help reduce the number of reactivations or shorten the duration. Sometimes, antiviral drugs are used to help avoid recurrences in late pregnancy. If you have genital herpes, your baby potentially can become infected with the virus during delivery through the birth canal. The most serious risk to a newborn exists when the mother has her first (primary) herpes infection just before labor. A recurring episode of herpes at childbirth poses much less risk to the baby.

Preventing newborn herpes infection can be difficult. In the majority of newborn infections, the mother has no signs or symptoms suggesting herpes during labor or birth. Still, prevention is important because herpes infection can be life-threatening for a newborn. In addition, newborns who contract herpes can develop serious infections that damage the eyes, internal organs or brain, despite treatment with antiviral drugs.

If you've had genital herpes, your baby is unlikely to have a serious infection acquired at birth. Women who've had the disease develop antibodies that they pass to their babies, and the antibodies provide some temporary protection. Nevertheless, there's a small risk. If sores are present, cesarean birth might lessen this very small risk of newborn infection. For this reason, cesarean delivery is the standard of care in the United States for women with active herpes lesions at the time of delivery.

HIV and AIDS Acquired immunodeficiency syndrome (AIDS) is a chronic, life-threatening condition caused by the human immunodeficiency virus (HIV). HIV is most commonly spread by sexual contact with an infected partner. It can also spread through infected blood and shared needles or syringes contaminated with the virus. Untreated women with HIV can pass the infection to their babies during pregnancy and delivery or through their breast milk.

Testing for HIV is now a routine part of prenatal care. If you feel you may have become infected during your pregnancy, consider having your HIV status tested again. Although a positive diagnosis can be devastating, treatments are available that can greatly improve a mother's health and reduce the risk of passing on the infection to her baby. Drug treatments begun before or during pregnancy can benefit both mom and baby.

If you know you have HIV or AIDS, tell your doctor. A doctor who knows about your condition can monitor your health and help you to avoid procedures that could increase your baby's exposure to your blood. The medical treatment you receive can greatly influence the risk of transmission of the infection to your baby. Your doctor can also make sure that your baby is promptly tested and treated for infection after birth. Early testing can make it possible for infants diagnosed with HIV to be treated with HIV-fighting drugs, which have been shown to slow the progression of the disease and improve survival rates.

Syphilis Syphilis is a bacterial infection that commonly begins as a small sore (ulcer), usually in the genital region, where the infection first enters the body. Signs and symptoms then vary, as syphilis develops in stages. Typically, syphilis in pregnancy is acquired through sexual contact with exposure to an infected open sore.

If you have syphilis while pregnant, the infection can pass through the placenta. Syphilis in pregnancy is associated with miscarriage, preterm delivery, stillbirth, problems with fetal growth and symptoms in the baby after delivery. The number of syphilis cases reported in both adults and newborns in the United States has increased in recent years. Screening early in pregnancy is recommended for all women, and some clinics will test more frequently, depending on the number of cases in the area and recommendations of local health departments.

Syphilis is diagnosed with a blood test or a series of blood tests, and it is typically treated with penicillin. If possible, patients with syphilis during pregnancy should see a doctor with expertise in infectious disease and a doctor who manages high-risk pregnancy. After delivery, the baby will also be followed closely for signs of syphilis.

Sickle cell disease Sickle cell disease is an inherited blood disease that often results in anemia, pain, frequent infections and damage to vital organs. It's caused by a defective form of the protein in red blood cells that carries oxygen from the lungs to other parts of the body (hemoglobin). In people with the disease, red blood cells change from healthy, round cells to crescent-shaped cells. These unusual cells can block blood flow through smaller blood vessels, causing pain.

Sickle cell disease typically is diagnosed in infancy with a screening test. In the United States, it most commonly affects black Americans and Latinos. Women with sickle cell disease have a greater risk of developing serious pregnancy-related complications, such as pregnancy-induced high blood pressure. In addition, they have an increased risk of preterm labor and of delivering a baby with a low birth weight. During pregnancy, infections such as pneumonia and urinary tract infection can occur more frequently and lead to painful sickle cell crises.

Managing sickle cell disease Women with sickle cell disease may need to have a team of medical specialists involved in their prenatal care. They often are closely monitored for complications of the disease, such as seizures, congestive heart failure and severe anemia. Anemia is likely to be most severe during the final two months of pregnancy, and may require blood transfusions. If a mother-to-be has a sickle cell crisis or another com-

plication, the baby's health will likely be closely monitored.

Thyroid disease The thyroid is a butterfly-shaped gland located at the base of the neck, just below the Adam's apple. The hormones it produces regulate your metabolism, which is related to everything from your heart rate to how quickly you burn calories. Problems can occur from too much or too little hormone production.

Hyperthyroidism When your thyroid gland produces too much of the hormone thyroxine, it can cause overactive thyroid disease known as hyperthyroidism. This can prompt your body's metabolism to speed up, and it may lead to sudden weight loss, a rapid or irregular heartbeat, and nervousness or irritability.

Most pregnancies proceed normally in women with hyperthyroidism, but the disease can be difficult to control. In addition, some medications commonly used to treat hyperthyroidism may need to be avoided or readjusted during pregnancy or while breast-feeding. For example, radioactive iodine medications shouldn't be used during pregnancy.

If you have hyperthyroidism or a history of the condition, review your medications with your doctor. He or she can monitor your condition throughout your pregnancy. Management of hyperthyroidism is important for the health of both you and your baby. If you develop a fever or feel ill, contact your care provider immediately. Follow his or her instructions carefully and report signs and symptoms that return or worsen.

During pregnancy, hyperthyroidism sometimes worsens during the first trimester, often associated with the significant hormonal changes taking place. It can improve during the second half of the pregnancy. In some women, hyperthyroidism develops or worsens after birth (postpartum thyroiditis). It can cause excessive fatigue, nervousness and increased sensitivity to heat. Sometimes it's mistaken for other problems, such as postpartum depression. Report such symptoms to your care provider.

Hypothyroidism Hypothyroidism is the opposite of hyperthyroidism; it occurs when the thyroid doesn't produce enough hormones. When the thyroid is underactive, you may feel tired and sluggish. Left untreated, signs and symptoms can include increased sensitivity to cold, constipation, pale and dry skin, a puffy face, weight gain, a hoarse voice, and depression. The signs and symptoms of hypothyroidism can easily be mistaken for pregnancy fatigue.

Women with hypothyroidism may have difficulty becoming pregnant. If they do become pregnant and their hypothyroidism is left untreated or undertreated, they have an increased risk of miscarriage, preeclampsia, problems with the placenta and slowed growth for their babies. Proper thyroid hormone replacement is required for normal fetal growth and development.

If you have hypothyroidism, your dosage of replacement hormone will probably increase as your pregnancy progresses. Your care provider will likely check your thyroid levels throughout pregnancy.

Uterine fibroids Uterine fibroids are noncancerous tumors of the uterus that are common in women in their childbearing years. They can appear on the inside or outside lining of the uterus, or within its muscular wall. They usually develop from a single smooth muscle cell that continues to grow. Some can be as small as a pea. Others can grow as large as a grapefruit, or even bigger. Most cause no symptoms and are discovered only during a routine pelvic exam or during a prenatal ultrasound.

When symptoms do occur, they may include abnormally heavy or prolonged menstrual bleeding, abdominal or lower back pain, pain during sexual intercourse, difficult or more frequent urination, and pelvic pressure. Medication or surgery may be recommended prior to conception to shrink or remove fibroids that cause discomfort or could result in complications, including infertility.

Rarely, uterine fibroids can interfere with the ability of a fertilized egg to implant on the uterine lining, making it difficult to become pregnant. Fibroids can also increase the risk of miscarriage during the first and second trimesters of pregnancy or increase the likelihood of preterm labor. Sometimes they can obstruct the birth canal, complicating labor and delivery.

Managing uterine fibroids Fibroids can enlarge during pregnancy, possibly because of increased levels of estrogen in the body. Occasionally, larger fibroids may outgrow or become cut off from their blood supply and degenerate, resulting in pelvic or abdominal pain. If you experience pelvic or abdominal pain or abnormal bleeding, contact your doctor immediately. If the fibroids are painful, your care provider may recommend medication for pain management. During pregnancy, surgery for fibroids is generally avoided because it can lead to preterm delivery and extensive blood loss.

The vast majority of pregnancies involving uterine fibroids have few or no problems. Depending on the size and location of the fibroids, the fetus may be positioned abnormally at the time of delivery, possibly requiring the need for cesarean delivery. Fibroid removal generally is avoided during cesarean delivery because of bleeding risk (hemorrhage).

POSTPARTUM CONCERNS

After your child is born, you enter the postpartum period. It's a transition time for you, both physically and emotionally. This section explains problems that can develop during the postpartum weeks.

Blood clots A blood clot inside an internal vein, called deep vein thrombosis (DVT), is one of the most serious potential complications after birth. Most often the clot develops in a leg. If it's left untreated, a portion of the clot can break off and travel to your heart and lungs. There, it can obstruct blood flow, causing chest pain, shortness of breath and, rarely, even death.

The hormonal changes of pregnancy increase your risk of developing DVT during or after pregnancy. That said, the condition is rare. However, your risk of developing DVT is about four times greater after a cesarean birth than after a vaginal birth. You're at increased risk of developing DVT if you smoke, have a body mass index (BMI) of 25 or greater, are over age 35, or can't walk after surgery as much as recommended. Studies indicate that many people with DVT have a genetic predisposition for DVT formation.

Clotting often occurs in the legs but can also occur in the pelvic veins. Signs and symptoms of DVT include tenderness, pain or swelling in your leg, particularly around your calf. DVT typically appears within the first few days after delivery and is often detected in the hospital. It can, however, occur up to several weeks after you've been discharged. Although less common, blood clots may also develop during pregnancy.

Treatment If you have a blood clot, you'll likely be given blood-thinning medication (anticoagulant) to help prevent more clots from forming. Initially, this may require that you be admitted to a hospital to be monitored. Depending on whether DVT occurs before or after delivery, you may have to give yourself anticoagulant injections or take anticoagulant medications orally.

Excessive bleeding Serious bleeding (hemorrhaging) after birth is not normal. It occurs in a small percentage of all births, and generally takes place during childbirth or within 24 hours of giving birth. Less commonly, bleeding can occur up to six weeks after childbirth.

A number of problems can cause serious bleeding after birth. Blood loss is most often caused by one of the following:

▶ ***Uterine atony.*** After you've given birth, your uterus must contract to control bleeding from where the placenta was attached. The reason your nurse periodically massages your abdomen after delivery is to encourage your uterus to contract. With uterine atony, the uterine muscle doesn't contract well. The condition is slightly more likely to occur when the uterus has been stretched by a large baby or twins, if you've already had several babies, or if labor has been lengthy. To reduce the chance of atony, you may be given oxytocin (Pitocin) — a synthetic form of the hormone oxytocin — after the baby is delivered. Other medications may also be given if atony occurs.

- *Retained placenta.* If your placenta doesn't expel on its own within 30 minutes after your baby is born, you can experience excessive bleeding. Even when the placenta does expel on its own, your doctor carefully examines it to make sure it's intact. If tissue is missing, there's a risk of bleeding.
- *Tearing (laceration).* If your vagina or cervix tears during birth, excessive bleeding can result. Tearing might be caused by a large baby, a forceps- or vacuum-assisted birth, a baby that came through the birth canal too rapidly, or an episiotomy that tears.

Other, less common, causes of postpartum bleeding include:
- *Abnormal placental attachment.* Very rarely, the placenta attaches to the uterine wall more deeply than it should. When this happens, the placenta doesn't readily detach after birth. An abnormal placental attachment can cause severe bleeding.
- *Uterine inversion.* The uterus turns inside out after the baby is born and the placenta is removed. This is somewhat more likely when there's abnormal attachment of the placenta.
- *Uterine rupture.* Rarely, the uterus can tear during pregnancy or labor. If this happens, the mother loses blood, and the baby's oxygen supply is decreased. Uterine rupture is most common in women attempting trial of labor after cesarean (TOLAC), also called vaginal birth after cesarean (VBAC). Uterine rupture is extremely rare in patients with no history of uterine surgery.

Your risk of bleeding may be higher if you've had bleeding problems with past births. Your risk is also increased if you have a complication such as placenta previa, in which the placenta is located low in the uterus and may partly or completely cover the opening of the cervix.

In addition to blood loss, signs and symptoms of heavy postpartum bleeding include pale skin, chills, dizziness or fainting, clammy hands, nausea and vomiting, and a racing heart. Excessive blood loss requires immediate action.

Treatment Your medical team can take several steps to respond to excessive bleeding, including massaging your uterus. They may also give you intravenous (IV) fluids and oxytocin. Oxytocin stimulates uterine contractions. Other treatments may include additional medications to stimulate contractions, surgical intervention and blood transfusions. Rarely, medications and other treatments are not able to control the bleeding. In this situation, hysterectomy may be considered. Treatment depends on the cause and severity of the problem.

Infection Infections can occasionally occur after delivery. The most common are:

Endometritis Endometritis is an inflammation and infection of the lining of the uterus (endometrium). The bacteria that cause the infection initially grow in the lining of the uterus but may extend beyond the lining of the uterus. The infection sometimes can spread to the ovarian and pelvic blood vessels.

Endometritis is one of the most common infections that occurs after childbirth. It can develop after a vaginal or cesarean birth, but it's far more common after a cesarean delivery. A long labor or a long length of time between when your water breaks and delivery occurs can contribute to endometritis. Other factors that increase risk include smoking, diabetes and obesity.

Signs and symptoms can vary depending on the severity of the infection. They may include fever, an enlarged and tender uterus, abnormal or foul-smelling vaginal discharge, general abdominal discomfort, chills, and a headache.

To diagnose the condition, your care provider may press on your lower abdomen and uterus to check for tenderness. If an infection is suspected, a pelvic exam, blood tests and urine tests may be done. Most often, the infection is diagnosed during labor or within the first 24 hours after delivery. It's much less common to develop endometritis after being discharged from the hospital.

Treatment. Women with endometritis are commonly hospitalized and given intravenous (IV) antibiotics. Fluids are given either orally or intravenously. For mild endometritis, treatment may occur on an outpatient basis.

Antibiotics clear up most endometritis infections. However, if the infection goes untreated, it can lead to other serious problems, including infertility and chronic pelvic pain. Contact your care provider if you develop signs or symptoms of endometritis.

Mastitis Mastitis is an infection of the breast that occurs when bacteria accumulate in the breast tissue. It may result if you have a blocked milk duct, if you don't empty the breast of milk, or if bacteria enter cracked skin on the nipple. Sometimes, bacteria can enter the breast without any signs of nipple problems. If you do have problems with cracked nipples or inadequate emptying of the breasts, it could be a sign that the baby isn't well-positioned or latched appropriately when breast-feeding.

Mastitis can affect one or both breasts. When a breast becomes infected, you'll develop a fever and feel sick, like you have the flu. The breast may feel sore, hard and hot. It may swell and redden. Typically, the diagnosis is based on personal history and a physical examination with no further testing required. An ultrasound may be performed if your doctor suspects a breast abscess.

Treatment. Antibiotics are generally prescribed for mastitis. Because mastitis can be painful, you may be tempted to stop breast-feeding. It's best to keep breast-feeding or breast pumping, which will help empty your breast and relieve pressure. The infection won't spread to the milk your baby consumes, and the antibiotics you take won't harm your baby, although you may notice a change in the color of your baby's bowel movements.

Applying warm compresses to the infected breast several times a day can help. Acetaminophen (Tylenol, others) or ibuprofen (Advil, Motrin IB, others) may be used to relieve fever and pain. Dry your breasts between feedings and compresses so that they can heal properly.

Post-cesarean wound infection Most cesarean incisions heal with no problem at all, but sometimes an incision can become infected. Wound infection rates after cesarean births vary. Your chances of developing a wound infection after a cesarean birth are higher if you abuse alcohol or drugs or smoke. Your risk is also higher if you have diabetes or are obese, as fat tissue tends to heal poorly.

If the skin on the sides of your incision becomes painful, red and swollen, it may be infected, especially if the wound is draining in any way. Wound infection can also cause a fever. If you suspect your incision has become infected, contact your care provider.

Treatment. Your care provider may need to open and drain the incision to release trapped bacteria. You may also be treated with antibiotics.

Urinary tract infection (UTI) An infection of your bladder, kidneys or urethra — the tube that transports urine from the bladder — develops when bacteria travel up the urethra. This can occur after you give birth, especially if you had a catheter inserted before or after delivery. You're at increased risk of developing a UTI if you have diabetes or if you keep a catheter in longer than necessary after surgery.

With a urinary tract infection, you may have a frequent, almost panicky urge to urinate, pain while urinating, a fever and tenderness over the area of the bladder. If you experience any of these signs and symptoms, contact your care provider.

Treatment. Treating a UTI generally involves taking antibiotics, drinking plenty of fluids, emptying your bladder regularly and taking medication to relieve the fever.

Postpartum depression The birth of a baby can bring on many powerful emotions, including excitement, joy and even fear. But there's another emotion many new moms experience: depression.

Within days of delivery, many new mothers experience a mild depression that's often called the baby blues. The baby blues may last for a few hours or up to two weeks after delivery. However, some new mothers experience a more severe form of the baby blues called postpartum depression, which can occur

---

SELF-CARE FOR POSTPARTUM DEPRESSION

If you're diagnosed with postpartum depression, or you think you may have the condition, it's very important that you seek professional care. To aid in your recovery, try these tips:

▶ Get a healthy amount of rest. Make a habit of resting while your baby sleeps.
▶ Eat a range of nutritious foods. Emphasize whole grains, vegetables and fruits.
▶ Get some physical activity every day.
▶ Stay connected with family and friends.
▶ Ask for occasional help with child care and household responsibilities from friends and family.
▶ Take some time for yourself. Get dressed, leave the house, and visit a friend or run an errand.
▶ Talk with other women who have children. Ask your care provider about groups for new moms in your community.
▶ Spend time alone with your partner.

from weeks to months after giving birth. Left untreated, postpartum depression can last for a year or longer.

There's no clear cause of postpartum depression. A combination of body, mind and social interactions likely plays a role. The levels of the hormones estrogen and progesterone drop dramatically immediately after childbirth. In addition, changes occur in the body's blood volume, blood pressure, immune system and metabolism. All of these changes can impact how a woman feels, both physically and emotionally.

Other factors that can contribute to postpartum depression and increase the risk in new mothers include:

▶ A personal or family history of depression
▶ An unsatisfying birth experience
▶ A problematic or high-risk pregnancy
▶ Postpartum pain or complications from delivery
▶ A baby with a high level of needs
▶ Exhaustion from caring for a new baby or multiple children
▶ Anxiety or unrealistic expectations about parenthood
▶ Stress from changes at home or work
▶ Feeling a loss of identity
▶ Lack of social support
▶ Relationship difficulties

Signs and symptoms Signs and symptoms of the baby blues include episodes of anxiety, sadness, irritability, crying, headaches, exhaustion and feelings of unworthiness. Often, these signs and symptoms pass within a few days or weeks. Sometimes, though, the baby blues turn into postpartum depression.

With postpartum depression, the signs and symptoms of depression are more intense and can last longer. They include:

▶ Constant fatigue
▶ Changes in appetite

▶ Lack of joy in life
▶ A sense of emotional numbness or feeling trapped
▶ Withdrawal from family and friends
▶ Lack of concern for yourself or baby
▶ Severe insomnia
▶ Excessive concern for your baby
▶ Loss of sexual interest or sexual responsiveness
▶ A strong sense of failure or inadequacy
▶ Severe mood swings
▶ High expectations and an overly demanding attitude
▶ Difficulty making sense of things

If you're feeling depressed after your baby's birth, you may be reluctant or embarrassed to admit it. But it's important to inform your care provider if you experience signs or symptoms of postpartum depression.

Treatment Your care provider most likely will want to review your signs and symptoms in person. Because a great number of women feel tired and overwhelmed after having a baby, your care provider may use a depression-screening scale to distinguish a short-term case of the blues from a more severe form of depression.

Postpartum depression is a recognized and treatable medical problem. Treatment varies according to individual needs. It may include:

▶ Support groups
▶ Individual counseling or psychotherapy
▶ Antidepressants or other medications

If you experience depression after childbirth, you have an increased risk of depression after a subsequent pregnancy. In fact, postpartum depression is more common in second-time mothers. With early intervention and proper treatment, however, there is less of a chance for serious problems and a greater chance of a rapid recovery.

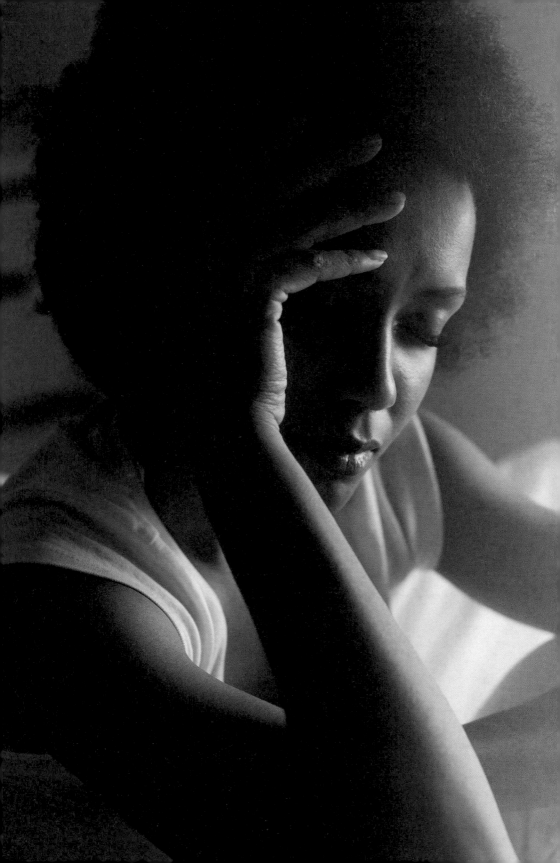

CHAPTER 30

Pregnancy loss

Unfortunately, sometimes a pregnancy ends without the dreamed-of outcome. There is no new baby to hold in your arms.

If this is your situation, it's likely a time of grief, confusion and fear. While understanding why miscarriage and other forms of pregnancy loss occur won't stop the emotional pain, it may help you understand why your care provider recommends certain types of care.

In addition to miscarriage, pregnancy loss can take many forms, including ectopic pregnancy, molar pregnancy, preterm birth and stillbirth. Each has different causes and treatments.

MISCARRIAGE

Miscarriage is the spontaneous loss of a pregnancy before 20 weeks. About 10 to 20 percent of known pregnancies end in miscarriage. However, the actual number is probably much higher because many miscarriages occur so early in pregnancy that a woman doesn't even know that she's pregnant. Most miscarriages occur because the fetus isn't developing normally.

Miscarriage is a relatively common experience — but that doesn't make it any easier. Pregnancy that ends without a baby to hold in your arms is heartbreaking.

Signs and symptoms Signs and symptoms of miscarriage include:
- Vaginal spotting or bleeding
- Pain or cramping in your abdomen or lower back
- Fluid or tissue passing from your vagina

Keep in mind that spotting or bleeding in early pregnancy is fairly common. In most cases, women who experience light bleeding in the first trimester go on to have successful pregnancies. Sometimes even heavier bleeding doesn't result in miscarriage.

Some women who miscarry develop an infection in their uterus. If you experience this infection, called a septic miscarriage, you may also experience a fever, chills, body aches and vaginal discharge that has a foul odor.

Call your doctor if you experience:

▸ Bleeding, even light spotting
▸ A gush of fluid from your vagina without pain or bleeding
▸ Passing of tissue from the vagina

You may bring tissue that's passed into your doctor's office in a clean container. It's unlikely that testing could identify a cause for the miscarriage, but confirming the passage of placental tissue helps your doctor determine that your symptoms aren't related to a tubal (ectopic) pregnancy.

Causes Most miscarriages occur because the fetus isn't developing normally. Problems with the baby's chromosomes account for about 50 percent of all miscarriages. And these problems typically result from errors that occur by chance as the embryo divides and grows — not problems inherited from the parents. Some examples of abnormalities include:

▸ *Empty gestational sac.* Empty gestational sac is common. It's the cause of about half of all miscarriages in the first 12 weeks. It occurs when development of the embryo stops very early or does not occur at all.
▸ *Intrauterine fetal demise.* In this situation the embryo is present but has died before any symptoms of pregnancy loss have occurred. This situation may also be due to genetic abnormalities within the embryo.
▸ *Molar pregnancy.* A molar pregnancy, also called gestational trophoblastic disease, is less common. It's an abnormality of the placenta caused by a problem at the time of fertilization. In a molar pregnancy, the early placenta develops into a fast-growing mass of cysts in the uterus, which may or may not contain an embryo. If it does contain an embryo, the embryo will not reach maturity. For more on molar pregnancy, see page 485.

In a few cases, a health condition in the mother may play a role. Uncontrolled diabetes, thyroid disease, infections, and hormonal, uterine or cervical problems can sometimes lead to a miscarriage. Other factors that increase a woman's risk of miscarriage include:

▸ *Age.* Women older than age 35 have a higher risk of miscarriage than younger women do. At age 35, you have about a 20 percent risk. At age 40, the risk is about 40 percent. And at age 45, it's about 80 percent. Paternal age also may play a role. Some studies indicate that the chance of miscarriage is higher after a woman's partner is age 40 or 45, with the chance increasing as men age.
▸ *Two or more previous miscarriages.* The risk of miscarriage is higher in women with a history of two or more previous miscarriages. After one miscarriage, your risk of miscarriage is only slightly higher than that of a woman who's never had a miscarriage.
▸ *Smoking, alcohol and illicit drugs.* Women who smoke or drink alcohol during pregnancy have a greater risk

---

WHAT DOESN'T CAUSE MISCARRIAGE

Routine activities such as these don't provoke a miscarriage:

▸ Exercise
▸ Lifting or straining
▸ Having sex
▸ Working, provided you're not exposed to harmful chemicals

TYPES OF MISCARRIAGES

There are specific names for the different types of miscarriage. Your care provider may use one of these terms in discussing your symptoms with you:

▶ *Threatened miscarriage.* If you're bleeding but your cervix hasn't begun to dilate, you're experiencing a threatened miscarriage. Such pregnancies often proceed without any further problems.

▶ *Inevitable miscarriage.* If you're bleeding, your uterus is contracting and your cervix is dilated, a miscarriage is inevitable.

▶ *Incomplete miscarriage.* If you pass some of the fetal or placental material but some remains in your uterus, it's considered an incomplete miscarriage.

▶ *Missed miscarriage.* The placental and embryonic tissues remain in the uterus, but the embryo has died or was never formed.

▶ *Complete miscarriage.* If you've passed all of the pregnancy tissues, it's considered a complete miscarriage. This is common for miscarriages occurring before 12 weeks.

▶ *Septic miscarriage.* If you develop an infection in your uterus, it's known as a septic miscarriage. This may require immediate care.

---

of miscarriage than do nonsmokers and women who avoid alcohol during pregnancy. Illicit drug use also increases the risk of miscarriage.

Seeing a doctor If you're experiencing symptoms or you feel that you may have experienced a miscarriage, contact your care provider. He or she will instruct you on who you need to see and when. In some circumstances, you may be instructed to go to a hospital emergency room.

Your doctor is likely to ask you a number of questions, including the date of your last menstrual period, when you began experiencing symptoms, and whether you've had a miscarriage before. He or she may also perform one or more of the following tests:

▶ *Pelvic exam.* Your doctor will check to see if your cervix has begun to dilate.

▶ *Ultrasound.* This helps your doctor check for a fetal heartbeat and deter-

mine if the embryo is developing normally.

▶ *Blood tests.* If you've miscarried, measurements of the pregnancy hormone, HCG, can help determine if you've completely passed all placental tissue. Your doctor may also recommend additional testing, such as a complete blood count (CBC) to check for anemia and a blood type test with an antibody screen to identify possible Rh factor incompatibility (see page 431).

▶ *Tissue tests.* If you have passed tissue, it can be sent to the laboratory to confirm that a miscarriage has occurred — and that your symptoms aren't related to another cause of pregnancy bleeding. In certain situations, your care provider may also recommend genetic testing of the tissue.

Treatment If you haven't miscarried but are at risk, your doctor may recommend careful observation until the bleeding or pain subsides. It's also a good idea to avoid traveling — especially to areas where it would be difficult to receive prompt medical care.

With the use of ultrasound, a doctor can usually determine whether the embryo has died or was never formed. In this situation, there are several options to consider. Before the use of ultrasound in early pregnancy, most women didn't know they were destined to have a miscarriage until it was already in process.

Expectant management If you choose to let the miscarriage progress naturally, it usually happens within a couple of weeks after determining that the embryo has died, although it may take up to three to four weeks. This option is known as expectant management. At the time of the

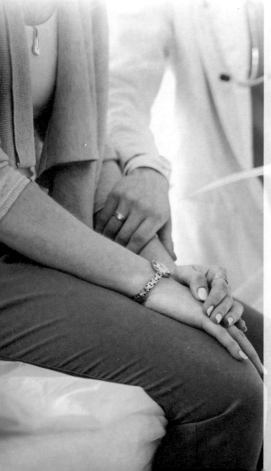

miscarriage, you may experience heavy bleeding and cramping, like a period, which could last for several hours. You may also pass some tissue. Your care provider can recommend what you should do with this tissue. Usually the heavy bleeding subsides within a few hours and light bleeding continues for several days to weeks. This can be an emotionally difficult time. If the miscarriage doesn't happen spontaneously, medical or surgical treatment may be necessary.

Medical treatment If after a diagnosis of pregnancy loss you prefer to speed the process, medication may be used to help your body expel the pregnancy tissue and placenta. You can take the medication by mouth, but your care provider may recommend applying the medication vaginally to increase its effectiveness and minimize side effects, such as nausea, stomach pain and diarrhea. The miscarriage will likely happen at home. The specific timing may vary, and you need more than one dose of the medication. For most women, treatment works within 24 hours.

Surgical treatment Another option is a minor surgical procedure called dilation and curettage (D&C). During this procedure, the doctor dilates your cervix and removes the tissue from your uterus using a long metal instrument called a curette. Curettes may use suction or have a scoop or loop on the end to gently scrape the uterine walls. Complications are rare, but they may include damage to the connective tissue of your cervix or the uterine wall. Sometimes further surgical treatment is necessary to stop the bleeding.

Recovery Physical recovery from miscarriage generally takes a few hours to a couple of days. Expect your period to return within four to six weeks. Call your care provider if you experience heavy bleeding, a fever, chills or severe pain. These signs and symptoms could indicate an infection. Avoid having sex or putting anything in your vagina — such as a tampon or douche — for two weeks after a miscarriage.

If you experience multiple miscarriages, generally more than two to three in a row, consider testing to identify any underlying causes — such as uterine abnormalities, coagulation problems or chromosomal abnormalities. In some cases, a care provider may suggest testing after two consecutive miscarriages. If the cause of your miscarriages can't be identified, don't lose hope. Even without treatment, most women with recurrent miscarriages go on to have successful pregnancies.

RECURRENT PREGNANCY LOSS

Recurrent pregnancy loss is the consecutive loss of two or more pregnancies in the first trimester or very early in the second trimester. As many as 1 couple in 20 experiences two pregnancy losses in a row. Up to 1 in 100 has three or more consecutive losses. Losses after the first weeks of the second trimester are much less common.

In the rare circumstance where more than two miscarriages have occurred, a specific cause may be identified, and in some situations, treatment may be available. Possible causes include:

▶ *Chromosomal alterations.* One parent may have a chromosomal alteration, most commonly a translocation, resulting in an increased risk of recurrent miscarriage. This problem could be addressed with in vitro fertilization and preimplantation genetic testing, or with the use of an egg or sperm donor.

▶ *Problems with the uterus or cervix.* If the woman has an unusually shaped uterus or weakened cervix, it may lead to miscarriage. Surgery may be able to correct some problems with the uterus and cervix.

▶ *Blood-clotting problems.* Women with anticardiolipin antibodies, antiphospholipid antibodies or certain hereditary conditions are more likely to form blood clots, which can result in poor placental function and miscarriage. Testing can determine whether a woman carries any of these conditions, which are associated with an increased risk of miscarriage. A variety of approaches may be used to reduce the risk of miscarriage.

Other factors have been suggested as causes of recurrent miscarriages. They include progesterone deficiency in early pregnancy, problems with implantation of the placenta and certain infections. However, there's no firm evidence that treating these problems affects the outcome of subsequent pregnancies. Most often, the cause of recurrent miscarriage is not identified.

Don't give up hope. Even if you've had repeated miscarriages, you still have a good chance of a successful future pregnancy. This is true even if the causes of the past losses cannot be found. Future pregnancies may need early attention, so talk to your care provider about special care you may need as your baby develops.

Emotional healing may take much longer than physical healing. Miscarriage can be a heart-wrenching loss that others around you may not fully understand. Your emotions may range from anger to despair. Give yourself time to grieve the loss of your pregnancy, and seek help from those who love you. Talk to your care provider if you're feeling profound sadness or depression.

Most women who've had a miscarriage go on to have successful pregnancies. Recent studies suggest that couples who try again soon after a miscarriage may have similar or even better chances of a successful pregnancy compared with those who wait longer. Talk with your care provider about when the best time would be for you to attempt pregnancy after a miscarriage.

ECTOPIC PREGNANCY

An ectopic pregnancy is one in which the fertilized egg implants itself somewhere other than inside the uterus. The vast majority of ectopic pregnancies occur in a fallopian tube. Pregnancies outside of the uterus cannot proceed normally, however. And if the growing pregnancy causes a fallopian tube to bleed or burst, the loss of blood can be life-threatening to the mother.

Certain factors are known to increase the risk of ectopic pregnancy. These include:

▶ An infection or inflammation of the tube that's caused it to become partly or entirely blocked
▶ Previous surgery in the pelvic area or on the fallopian tubes
▶ Endometriosis, in which the tissue that normally lines the uterus is found outside the uterus
▶ An abnormally shaped fallopian tube

The risk of ectopic pregnancy is also higher in women who've had any of the following:

▶ A previous ectopic pregnancy
▶ Surgery on a fallopian tube
▶ Infertility problems
▶ Pregnancy after a tubal ligation

Signs and symptoms Pain is generally the first sign of an ectopic pregnancy, but abnormal bleeding usually is present, too. You may feel sharp, stabbing pain in your pelvis, abdomen, or even your shoulder and neck. It may come and go, or get better and worse. Other warning signs of ectopic pregnancy include gastrointestinal symptoms, dizziness and lightheadedness. If you experience any of these signs or symptoms, contact your care provider right away. There may be other possible causes for the signs and symptoms, but your care provider may first want to rule out an ectopic pregnancy.

Treatment If your care provider suspects an ectopic pregnancy, he or she will likely perform a pelvic exam to locate the tenderness or a mass. Unless your condition is obvious or you're in an emergency situation, lab tests and ultrasound are typically used to confirm the diagnosis.

The embryo must be removed to prevent rupture of the tube and other complications. Small ectopic pregnancies may be treated with the medication methotrexate, which is highly toxic to placental tissue and causes the pregnancy to stop developing. After methotrexate therapy, your doctor will recommend follow-up to make sure that the pregnancy is resolving. In many cases, surgery is required to remove the embryo. A small incision is made in the lower abdomen and a long, thin instrument inserted into the pelvic area to remove the mass.

On rare occasions, a care provider may recommend no treatment except observation to see if an ectopic pregnancy will end on its own, through spontaneous absorption, before any damage is done to the fallopian tube.

Future pregnancies If you've had one ectopic pregnancy, you're more likely to have another. Still, successful pregnancy after an ectopic pregnancy is often possible. Even if one tube was injured or removed, an egg may be fertilized in the other fallopian tube before entering the uterus. If both tubes were injured or removed, in vitro fertilization (IVF) may be an option. This involves retrieving mature eggs from the ovaries, fertilizing them with sperm in a laboratory and implanting the fertilized eggs in the uterus.

If you've had an ectopic pregnancy, talk to your care provider before becoming pregnant again so that together you can decide on the best strategy.

MOLAR PREGNANCY

Molar pregnancy occurs when the tiny, finger-like projections that attach the placenta to the uterine lining (chorionic villi) don't develop properly. A complete molar pregnancy most often results in an abnormal placenta without any formation of a baby. In a partial molar pregnancy, an abnormal placenta may form along with an incomplete fetus that's not able to survive pregnancy. Molar pregnancies are relatively rare and are most often associated with genetic abnormalities in the embryo that don't usually recur.

Signs and symptoms The main sign of molar pregnancy is bleeding by the 12th week of pregnancy. The uterus may also be larger than expected. Severe nausea and other problems of pregnancy are common. Molar pregnancies are diagnosed with an ultrasound examination.

Treatment A molar pregnancy is treated using the dilation and curettage procedure, which is done in the operating room. After an anesthetic is given, the cervix is dilated and the contents of the uterus are gently removed by suction.

After the procedure, your care provider will monitor your levels of the pregnancy hormone HCG for an extended time. This is because occasionally, abnormal cells will remain after the placenta is removed, causing HCG to remain high or increase. If the abnormal cells become cancerous (malignant), treatment with chemotherapy is recommended. This type of tumor usually responds well to treatment.

Future pregnancies Women who've had a molar pregnancy are advised not to become pregnant again for 6 to 12 months, and to use a reliable form of contraception during this time. After a woman experiences a molar pregnancy, the risk of a second molar pregnancy is 1 to 1.5 percent. While that's higher than the risk for a woman without a previous molar pregnancy, chances are still very good that future pregnancies will be normal.

STILLBIRTH

In rare situations, a baby dies during the course of late pregnancy or in the process of labor and childbirth. When this happens at 20 weeks or more into pregnancy, it's known as a stillbirth, or fetal death.

The term *stillbirth* refers to an end result, not a cause of death. It may be caused by specific problems with the mother's or baby's health, or it may be unexplained. However, a fetal death usually isn't caused by anything the mother did or didn't do.

There are certain factors that appear to increase the risk of stillbirth. These include:

▶ Obesity
▶ Being a teenager
▶ Being 35 or older
▶ Abusing drugs
▶ Identifying as black
▶ Smoking during pregnancy
▶ Carrying multiples
▶ Having diabetes before pregnancy

Stillbirth is a devastating loss for expectant parents. Fortunately, it's much less common than early pregnancy loss. In the United States, stillbirth affects about 1 percent of all pregnancies, around 24,000 babies each year.

Signs and symptoms Often, the first hint that something is wrong may be noticing that your baby is moving less than before, or not at all. Keeping track of baby's normal movement and sleep patterns can help you notice a potential problem sooner. If you think there's been a sudden decrease in movement, let your care provider know. He or she will likely want to check your baby's heartbeat. In the unfortunate event of finding no signs of life, a stillbirth will be diagnosed.

Causes Stillbirth may be the result of genetic problems or other congenital defects in the baby, problems with the placenta or umbilical cord, health issues in the mother, or other unknown factors.

When a baby dies between 20 and 28 weeks of pregnancy, it's called an early stillbirth. The cause is often related to genetic problems, infections or maternal health complications. Placenta or cord problems that lead to fetal growth re-

striction may also cause complications during this period.

Fetal death between 28 and 36 weeks of pregnancy is known as late stillbirth. Loss of a baby at this point is more likely due to maternal health issues or to pregnancy problems, such as placental abruption or placenta previa, cord prolapse, or other complications of labor and delivery.

Stillbirths at term (37 weeks or later) are rare. However, when they occur, they are often due to unexplained causes.

Treatment Treatment following a stillbirth will depend on how far along your pregnancy is, your history of C-sections or uterine surgery, and your preference for delivery. Most often, your care provider will recommend induction of labor with vaginal delivery. Your provider may also discuss other possible methods of delivery, including dilation of the cervix and surgical removal through the birth canal (dilation and evacuation). Or, if you're near term and have no signs of infection, you may be able to wait for labor to start naturally. In certain cases, a C-section may be performed if there's concern for the mother's safety during a vaginal birth.

If you'd like to, you'll usually have a chance to hold your baby after delivery. While this is a time of intense grief, it may be helpful to have those moments of closeness.

Future pregnancies Your care provider may recommend certain procedures to evaluate the cause of stillbirth. Amniocentesis, analysis of other tissue, a placenta exam or an autopsy of the baby may all provide helpful information about the cause of death. You may not think you want to know these details right away. Even so, consider having an evaluation done so that you can discuss

COPING WITH PREGNANCY LOSS

When a baby dies in pregnancy, particularly late in pregnancy, the loss is immense and the grief may be hard to overcome. The baby that you've carried for many months, dreamed about and planned for is suddenly gone.

You may feel as if your world has come crashing down. Maybe you can't even think of life continuing as normal. But there are some things you can do to make the future more bearable and to ease your pain. It may help you to:

Say goodbye to the baby Grieving is a vital step in accepting and recovering from your loss. But you may not be able to grieve for a baby you've never seen, held or named. It may be easier for you to deal with the death if it's more real to you. You may feel better if you arrange a funeral or burial for the child.

Save a memento of the baby Experts say it helps to have a photo or memento from someone who has died so that you have a tangible reminder of him or her to cherish now and in the future. Ask well-intentioned family and friends not to clear out the baby's nursery, if you want and need more time to process the loss.

Grieve Cry as often and for as long as you need to. Talk about your feelings and allow yourself to experience them fully. It's best not to avoid the mourning process, and there's no need to hide it from others.

Seek support Lean on your partner, family and friends for support. Although nothing can banish the hurt you're feeling, you may gain strength from others who love you and support you. You may also benefit from professional counseling after the loss of a child or from joining a support group of parents who have experienced a loss.

You and your partner will likely wonder why you had to experience this loss. You will never have a satisfactory answer, but it may help you to learn about the possible causes of the baby's death. You may want to discuss the findings from an autopsy with your care provider, after the initial shock has passed. Knowing a cause of death or details of what happened may help you better accept the loss. In addition, it may help you and your care provider to prevent future losses.

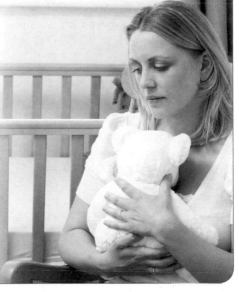

the outcome with your care provider when you're ready. An evaluation can help identify any underlying issues that may affect future pregnancies. Many times, a stillbirth will remain unexplained even after an evaluation.

In future pregnancies, make sure your care provider knows your complete obstetrical history. If the cause of a previous stillbirth is known, your provider will take precautions to check for similar issues and manage any complications throughout your pregnancy. When a previous stillbirth remains unexplained, testing may be available later in pregnancy to assess the risk of repeat problems. For most women, the risk of another stillbirth is very low, and they'll go on to have a healthy pregnancy and healthy baby.

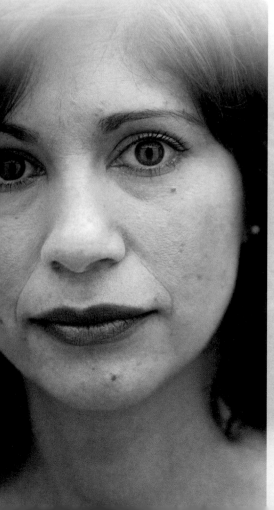

TRYING AGAIN

A pregnancy loss can be an extremely difficult experience. Even if the pregnancy was only a few weeks along, you may feel as if all your hope for a baby — or another baby — has disappeared.

There's no set of rules about what you will or will not feel after a pregnancy loss. You may even feel numb for a while. Allow yourself to have your feelings and try to work through them.

Grieving a pregnancy loss takes time. Some couples think that they must try to conceive again right away in order to fix the problem or replace the hurt. And for many people, a subsequent pregnancy won't carry the same feelings of excitement and bliss. A pregnancy after a loss can be stressful because of anxiety and fear that something may go wrong.

Although a pregnancy loss can be extremely difficult, it doesn't mean that you won't be able to have another baby. In most cases, your chances of having a normal, healthy pregnancy are still excellent, even if you've had more than one or two losses. Your decision on whether and when to try again rests on the type of pregnancy you had, as well as your physical and emotional recovery. There's no perfect time to try to conceive again. In some cases, you may wish to consult a specialist before attempting to conceive again.

Emotional recovery If you find yourself grieving deeply after a pregnancy loss, allow yourself the time to do so. Emotional recovery can, and usually does, take much longer than physical recovery.

Some people may wonder why you mourn for a child you've never known. But in many ways you may have already bonded with the baby growing inside

You and your partner may deal with a pregnancy loss in different ways. It may not always be easy to recognize that the other person is hurting. You may wish to talk things out, and your partner may prefer to stay silent. In addition, one may feel the need to move on before the other is ready.

Now more than ever you need to rely on each other for support. Try to listen and respond to each other while accepting the other person's feelings. You may consider seeing a counselor or therapist for help in expressing your emotions and expectations in more neutral territory.

you. You and your partner may have shared many moments imagining the days when you would hold your baby in your arms. The missed opportunity of watching your child grow and develop can be difficult to accept. Even if no embryo was ever present, you will still grieve when your dreams and expectations were to have a baby. Grieving is the process of letting go of the emotional attachment you've developed.

Stages of grief No one goes through the grieving process the same way, but certain emotional stages are common to people who've had an important loss.

▶ *Shock and denial.* Immediately after a traumatic event, people often feel numb and devoid of emotion. This is normal and doesn't mean you're uncaring. As reality sets in, these feelings often change.

▶ *Guilt and anger.* After a pregnancy loss, you may be tempted to blame yourself for what happened. But a pregnancy loss is rarely preventable. It's highly unlikely that anything you did or didn't do contributed to the pregnancy loss. You may also feel angry — with yourself, family, friends or simply with the circumstances. This is

normal. It may help to just let yourself be angry for a while.

▶ *Depression and despair.* Depression isn't always easy to recognize. You may find that you feel profoundly tired or that you lose interest in things you used to enjoy. Your appetite or sleeping patterns may change. Or you may find yourself crying over things that might otherwise seem very minor.

▶ *Acceptance.* Eventually, you'll come to terms with your loss. This doesn't mean you'll be free from hurt, but you will find that it becomes easier to function.

These stages have no timetable. Some may take longer than others. Even after you've come to accept your loss, feelings of sorrow and pain may recur on an anniversary or another important date. During these times, the loss may feel fresh in your mind.

If you find that your feelings are so overwhelming that you can't function or that they make you hostile or violent or interfere with your relationships with loved ones, talk with your care provider or seek the help of a mental health professional. He or she can help you deal with some of the issues you're facing.

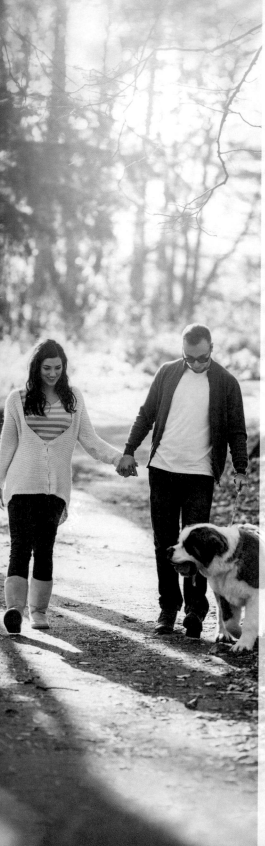

Physical recovery How long it takes to recover physically from a pregnancy loss often depends on the type of loss.

Miscarriage Physically speaking, it often takes only a few days for a woman to recover from a miscarriage. It usually takes four to six weeks after a miscarriage before your period comes back. Keep in mind that it's possible to conceive in those weeks between the miscarriage and your first menstrual cycle. If you're not yet ready to try again, during this time you may wish to use a form of birth control that's instantly reversible, such as a condom or diaphragm.

If you and your partner feel ready to become pregnant again, there are several issues to consider. Before conceiving, talk to your care provider about your plans. He or she can help you come up with a strategy that will optimize your chances of a healthy pregnancy and delivery. If you had a single miscarriage, your chances of a subsequent healthy pregnancy are virtually the same as someone who has never had a miscarriage. If you've had recurrent miscarriages, your care provider may suggest that you wait longer or have additional testing or monitoring.

Ectopic pregnancy Typically, the chances for a successful pregnancy after an ectopic pregnancy are good. Based on the cause of your ectopic pregnancy, how the ectopic pregnancy was treated and the condition of your fallopian tubes, your care provider may be able to provide additional information and recommendations for a successful future pregnancy. He or she will also likely recommend having an early ultrasound in any future pregnancy, to determine the baby's location.

Molar pregnancy After a molar pregnancy there's a slight risk of further abnormal tissue growth, which in rare cases may be cancerous (malignant). This tissue growth is usually marked by high levels of the pregnancy hormone human chorionic gonadotropin (HCG). For this reason, it's important that you not become pregnant for up to a full year after a molar pregnancy. If you conceive during this time, the rising levels of HCG in early pregnancy may be confused with recurrent disease. Your care provider may recommend that you have an ultrasound early in your next pregnancy to make sure that the pregnancy is normal.

Stillbirth Your physical recovery after experiencing a stillbirth will depend in part on the method of delivery of your baby. Give your body time to heal, as it would need to after any birth. You may have some bleeding for a few weeks, and your breasts may fill with milk in the days after delivery. While this can be a painful reminder — in multiple ways — it will resolve in several days if you avoid expressing milk.

For the best chance of a healthy future pregnancy, talk with your care provider about how long to wait before getting pregnant again. Recovering emotionally may take much longer than your physical recovery, so don't rush things. Trust that in time, you'll be ready.

Additional resources

AMERICAN ACADEMY OF PEDIATRICS
www.aap.org
The latest news and research, helpful tips, and more from the AAP.

AMERICAN COLLEGE OF OBSTETRICIANS AND GYNECOLOGISTS
www.acog.org/patients
Fact sheets, videos and many FAQs from this group of experts.

CENTERS FOR DISEASE CONTROL AND PREVENTION — PREGNANCY
www.cdc.gov/pregnancy
Health information for before, during and after pregnancy.

DONA INTERNATIONAL
www.dona.org
Information about doulas from an international professional organization of doulas.

FIRST CANDLE
http://firstcandle.org
Information about SIDS and safe infant sleep practices.

HEALTHYCHILDREN.ORG FROM THE AMERICAN ACADEMY OF PEDIATRICS
www.healthychildren.org
Information on nutrition, safety and other areas of well-being for pregnancy up through a child's young-adult years.

INTERNATIONAL CHILDBIRTH EDUCATION ASSOCIATION
www.icea.org
Search function for finding a childbirth educator or doula; other resources.

LACTMED DRUGS AND LACTATION DATABASE
https:// toxnet.nlm.nih.gov/newtoxnet/ lactmed.htm
Database of information on the safety and risks of various drugs and substances while breast-feeding.

LA LECHE LEAGUE INTERNATIONAL
www.llli.org
Supportive information and resources for breast-feeding. You may also find support by searching separately for a La Leche League group in your area.

LAMAZE INTERNATIONAL
www.lamaze.org
Information on pregnancy, labor and
Lamaze classes near you or online.

MARCH OF DIMES
www.marchofdimes.org
Information on many problems of
pregnancy and resources for pregnancy,
baby and pregnancy loss.

MAYO CLINIC
www.MayoClinic.org
Mayo Clinic's online health information
portal, which includes articles on many
pregnancy-related topics.

MULTIPLES OF AMERICA
www.multiplesofamerica.org
Education and resources for parents of
twins or other multiples.

**NATIONAL HIGHWAY TRAFFIC SAFETY
ADMINISTRATION — CAR SEATS**
888-327-4236
*https://www.nhtsa.gov/equipment/car-seats-
and-booster-seats*

An interactive guide to find the right car
seat; tips for installation.

**NATIONAL SOCIETY OF GENETIC
COUNSELORS**
www.nsgc.org
Searchable directory to find a genetic
counselor in your area.

OFFICE ON WOMEN'S HEALTH
800-994-9662
www.womenshealth.gov/breastfeeding
A wealth of information for breast-
feeding and maternal health.

OUR MOMENT OF TRUTH
http://ourmomentoftruth.com
Information about midwifery and
pregnancy from the American College of
Nurse-Midwives; searchable directory to
find a midwife in your area.

**SHARE PREGNANCY & INFANT LOSS
SUPPORT**
http://nationalshare.org
Information and online or local support
after pregnancy loss.

Glossary

A

active labor. Phase of labor, often accompanied by strong contractions, when the cervix dilates more quickly from 6 centimeters (cm) to 10 cm.

afterbirth. The placenta and membranes delivered from the uterus after childbirth.

afterbirth pains (afterpains). Uterine contractions that help deliver the placenta and control bleeding.

alpha-fetoprotein (AFP). A specific protein produced by the fetus that has implications for the baby's well-being.

amniocentesis. Procedure in which a small amount of amniotic fluid is removed from the mother. Used to test for various genetic characteristics, evidence of infection or lung maturity of the unborn baby.

amniotic sac. Sac filled with watery fluid (amniotic fluid) in which the fetus develops inside the uterus. Also called bag of water.

analgesic. Medication that relieves pain without causing loss of feeling or consciousness.

anemia. Condition in which the blood has too few red blood cells. It can cause fatigue and lowered resistance to infection.

anencephaly. Neural tube defect that results in the abnormal development of the baby's brain and skull.

anesthetic. Medication that relieves pain by blocking all sensation in a localized or regional area or throughout the body.

antibodies. Protein substances that the body makes to help protect itself against foreign cells and infections.

Apgar score. Rating (score) given to a newborn at one and five minutes after birth to assess color, heart rate, muscle tone, respiration and reflexes.

apnea. Cessation of breathing.

areola. Circular, pigmented area around the nipple of the breast.

assisted birth. Vaginal delivery assisted by medical intervention, such as a forceps-assisted birth or vacuum-assisted birth.

assisted reproductive technologies. Fertility treatments, such as in vitro fertilization, that combine sperm and eggs outside the body to aid conception and achieve a pregnancy.

B

baby blues. Period of low mood that's common in new mothers. It typically resolves within two weeks of delivery.

biophysical profile. Assessment of fetal health based on heart rate testing and ultrasound findings.

birth plan. Written record of your preferences for labor, delivery and postpartum care.

blastocyst. Rapidly dividing fertilized egg that enters the uterus and has cells committed to placental and fetal development.

bloody show. Blood-tinged mucous discharge from the vagina either before or during labor.

bradycardia. Sustained period during which the heart rate is slower than normal.

Braxton Hicks contractions. Irregular uterine contractions that don't result in changes in the cervix. Also called false labor.

breech position. Delivery position in which baby's bottom or feet are toward the cervix.

C

cephalopelvic disproportion. Circumstance in which baby's head is too large to pass through the mother's pelvis.

cervical incompetence. Condition in which the cervix begins to open without contractions before the pregnancy has come to term; a cause of miscarriage and preterm delivery in the second and third trimesters.

cervix. Necklike lower part of the uterus, which dilates and thins during labor.

cesarean birth. Birth in which an incision is made through the abdominal wall and uterus to deliver the baby. Also called cesarean section (C-section).

chorionic villus sampling (CVS). Procedure that removes a small sample of chorionic villi from the placenta where it joins the uterus. Used to test for chromosomal or other abnormalities.

circumcision. Procedure on male infants that removes the foreskin from the penis.

colostrum. Yellowish fluid produced by the breasts until the breast milk comes in after birth.

congenital disorder. Condition that a person is born with.

contraction stress test. One of several tests to evaluate the condition of the fetus and placenta. It measures the fetal heart rate in response to contractions of the uterus.

contractions (labor pains). Tightening of the uterine muscles.

D

deep vein thrombosis (DVT). Blood clot inside a vein deep in the body, often in the legs. DVT is a potential complication of pregnancy and childbirth.

dilation. The opening of the cervix, measured in centimeters (cm); 10 cm is fully dilated.

Doppler. Device with which a doctor can hear a fetal heartbeat by about the 12th week of pregnancy.

dystocia. Difficult labor for any reason.

E

early (latent) labor. Earliest phase of childbirth, during which uterine contractions gradually change the cervix. This phase generally lasts until the cervix reaches 6 cm dilation.

ectopic pregnancy. Pregnancy that implants outside the uterus, typically in the fallopian tube.

effacement. Progressive thinning of the cervix during labor as it dilates. 100 percent indicates total effacement.

embryo. Fertilized ovum from shortly after the time of fertilization until eight weeks after conception (10 weeks of pregnancy).

endometrium. Lining of the uterus, in which the fertilized egg embeds itself.

epidural. Anesthetic method used to decrease or eliminate discomfort during labor; sometimes called an epidural block.

episiotomy. Surgical incision in the perineum to enlarge the vaginal opening, performed to facilitate delivery as the baby is crowning.

external cephalic version. Procedure in which a doctor attempts to turn a baby from breech or transverse presentation to head down.

F

fallopian tubes. Structures that transport eggs as they are released from the ovaries. Sperm travel down the tubes, where fertilization can take place. Fertilized eggs are transported through the tubes to the uterus.

fetal growth restriction (FGR). Condition in which the estimated fetal weight is below the 10th percentile for the baby's gestational age.

fetus. An unborn baby after the first 10 weeks of pregnancy.

follicle-stimulating hormone. Hormone that fosters the development of eggs in the ovaries.

fontanels. Soft spots on a baby's head where the skull hasn't fused together. The different spots close between about two months and two years after birth.

forceps. Obstetrical instrument that fits around the baby's head to guide the baby through the birth canal in an operative vaginal delivery.

fundal height. Distance from the top of the uterus to the pubic bone; used to assess fetal growth in the uterus.

G

genetic disorder. Condition that may be inherited from one or both parents and that may be passed on to offspring.

gestational age. Age of the baby measured from the first day of the last menstrual period.

gestational diabetes. Form of diabetes that develops during pregnancy and usually resolves after delivery.

glucose challenge test. Test that screens for gestational diabetes by measuring your blood sugar (glucose) level after drinking a glucose solution.

group B streptococcus (GBS). Bacterium that's part of the genital tract in many women that can cause severe infection in a newborn if passed to the baby during birth.

H

human chorionic gonadotropin (HCG). Hormone produced by the placenta. Pregnancy tests measure or test for HCG in urine or blood.

hydramnios. Excess of amniotic fluid. Also called polyhydramnios.

hypoglycemia. Condition in which the sugar (glucose) concentration in the bloodstream is lower than normal.

I

induction of labor. Artificially starting labor; usually done by administering medication or rupturing the amniotic sac.

intrauterine growth restriction (IUGR). *See* fetal growth restriction.

in vitro fertilization (IVF). Process by which eggs and sperm are combined in an artificial environment outside the body, then transferred into the uterus to grow.

J

jaundice. Yellow tinge to the skin and whites of the eyes caused by too much bilirubin in the bloodstream.

K

Kegel exercises. Exercises done to strengthen pelvic floor muscles.

L

labia. Sets of skin folds that surround the opening to the vagina and urethra.

lanugo. Fine, downy hair growing on the skin of a fetus; replaced by other hairs during the third trimester.

lightening. Repositioning of baby lower in the pelvis. It may occur several weeks before or just prior to the onset of labor.

linea nigra. A line from the abdomen to the pubic area that typically darkens during pregnancy.

lochia. Discharge of blood, mucus and tissue from the uterus that's normal during the weeks after childbirth.

luteinizing hormone. Pituitary hormone that causes an ovarian follicle to swell, rupture and release an egg.

M

macrosomia. Higher than normal birth weight, often defined as more than 9 pounds, 15 ounces (4,500 grams).

mastitis. Infection of the breast that occurs when bacteria enter the breast tissue. It may be associated with a blocked milk duct.

meconium. Product of a baby's first bowel movements, which may occur before or after birth. Characteristically green in color.

meconium aspiration. In the uterus or just after birth, a baby inhales amniotic fluid mixed with meconium from a bowel movement before birth. May cause inflammation and airway blockage.

miscarriage. Spontaneous pregnancy loss before 20 weeks of gestation.

molding. Temporarily elongated shaping of the baby's skull while passing through the birth canal.

mucous plug. Collection of mucus that blocks the cervical canal during pregnancy to help prevent bacteria from entering the uterus.

N

neonatologist. Physician with advanced training in the diagnosis, treatment and care of newborn health problems.

neural tube. Structure in an embryo that develops into the brain, spinal cord, spinal nerves and backbone.

nonstress test. Test that helps a doctor examine the health of a fetus by measuring the heart rate in response to the baby's own movements.

O

occiput posterior position. Position in which baby faces the mother's abdomen during delivery.

ovulation. Release of an egg from an ovary. Fertilization can occur within about 24 hours of ovulation.

P

pelvic floor muscles, female. Muscles at the base of the pelvis that support the bladder, urethra, rectum, uterus and vagina.

perinatologist. Obstetrician who specializes in diagnosis and treatment of pregnancy problems; also called a maternal-fetal medicine specialist.

perineum. In women, this is the area between vaginal and anal openings.

pica. Uncommon craving to eat nonfood items such as laundry starch, dirt, baking powder or frost from the freezer. Pica is a sign of an iron deficiency.

placenta. Circular, flat organ that's responsible for oxygen and nutrient exchange and the elimination of wastes between mother and fetus.

placenta accreta. Abnormal placental attachment in which the placenta grows too deeply into the uterine wall.

placental abruption. Term for the separation of the placenta from the inner wall of the uterus before delivery of the baby.

placenta previa. Abnormal location of the placenta in which it partially or completely covers the cervix.

postpartum depression. Type of depression that can afflict a mother in the first 12 months after giving birth.

preeclampsia. Disease occurring during pregnancy marked by hypertension and protein in the urine.

premature labor, or preterm labor. Contractions that start opening the cervix before week 37.

progesterone. Hormone that increases throughout pregnancy; it promotes the growth of blood vessels in the uterine wall and inhibits the uterus from contracting.

prostaglandin. Chemical produced by the uterine lining and fetal membranes at or near the onset of labor.

Q

quickening. Earliest fetal movements that can be felt, usually between weeks 18 and 20 for first-time mothers but often earlier in women with a prior pregnancy.

R

regional anesthesia. Pain relief to a region of the body provided by a pain-blocking agent injected near a nerve.

relaxin. Hormone produced by the placenta to soften connective tissue and widen the pelvis for childbirth.

respiratory distress syndrome (RDS). Difficulty in breathing, caused by lack of surfactant in premature babies.

retained placenta. Failure of the placenta to deliver within 30 minutes after birth.

rhesus (Rh) factor. Red blood cell protein similar to the proteins that determine blood types A, B and O. Rh blood types are positive or negative.

Rh immunoglobulin (RhIg). Drug used in Rh negative women to prevent the immune system from recognizing Rh positive blood.

S

sciatica. Temporary condition caused by extra pressure on one or both sciatic nerves, causing pain, tingling or numbness in the low back, buttocks, thighs and lower legs.

spina bifida. Neural tube defect that results in failure of the vertebrae to close completely around the spinal cord. It may cause mobility issues and other complications.

spinal block. Anesthetic technique in which medication is injected into the fluid surrounding the spinal nerves.

station. Measurement of the descent of a fetus in the birth canal.

stillbirth. Pregnancy loss after 20 weeks of gestation.

surfactant. Substance covering the inner lining of the air sacs in the lungs that allows the lungs to expand normally during breathing.

T

teratogens. Substances or factors that can cause defects in a developing fetus, such as alcohol, certain medications and high blood sugar levels in uncontrolled diabetes.

transient tachypnea. Mild, temporary respiratory condition of newborns characterized by rapid breathing.

transition. Portion of active labor in which contractions are most intense, typically when the cervix is between 7 centimeters and full dilation.

transverse lie. Position in which a baby lies crossways in the uterus before birth; requires a cesarean birth.

twin-twin transfusion. Passage of blood from one identical twin to the other through connections of blood vessels within the placenta, which may cause significant complications.

U

umbilical cord. The tubular structure that connects the placenta to the fetus, delivering oxygen and nutrients and removing waste products.

umbilical cord compression. A complication in which the umbilical cord becomes compressed or pinched, which may cause blood flow to and from the baby to slow or even stop.

umbilical cord prolapse. A complication in which the umbilical cord slips out through the opening of the cervix, often followed by compression of the cord by the baby's presenting part.

uterine atony. Lack of muscle tone in the uterus after birth that prevents typical afterbirth contractions. Atony may result in significant postpartum bleeding (hemorrhaging).

uterus (womb). The female organ inside of which the unborn baby develops.

V

vacuum extractor. A tool with a rubber or plastic cup that can be held gently to the baby's head, providing suction to aid in delivery during an assisted vaginal birth.

vernix caseosa (vernix). A slippery, white substance covering a fetus until the last weeks of pregnancy. Vernix helps protect and moisturize the baby's skin.

Z

zygote. The result of the union of an egg (ovum) and sperm; a fertilized egg before it begins to divide and grow.

Index

medication use, 369
overview, 365
previous incision and, 366–367
reason for previous C-section and, 367–368
risks of, 366
tips for planning, 368–369
vaginal bleeding
bright red, 169
first trimester, 424–425
as implantation bleeding, 25
second trimester, 425
as sign or symptom, 82, 168, 425
third trimester, 194, 425
when to seek help, 425–426
vaginal discharge
in C-section recovery, 234
increase in pregnancy, 128, 140, 156
postpartum, 279
prevention and self-care, 412, 426
as sign or symptom, 82, 129, 140, 426
when to seek medical help, 426–427
vaginal dryness, 374
vaginal infections, 129, 140
vaginal seeding, 232
varicose veins, 166, 182, 427–428
vascular spiders, 182
vasectomy, 382
vegetarian diet tips, 37–40
veins, enlarged, 397–398
vision, blurry, 389–390
vitamin D, 20, 43, 329
vitamins and supplements, 19, 20, 105, 328
vomiting
excessive, 437–438
prevention and care, 428
treatment, 438
troubleshooting, 82
See also morning sickness

W

walking, 46
warmed-up effect, 104
water, breaking of, 203
water parks, 67
weeks
1 to 4, 84–95
5 to 8, 96–111
9 to 12, 112–121

13 to 16, 122–133
17 to 20, 134–141
21 to 24, 142–151
25 to 28, 152–161
29 to 32, 162–177
33 to 36, 178–187
37 to 40, 188–197
weight gain
distribution, 45
eating disorders and, 45
healthy, 43
overweight and, 43–45
recommended, 44
underweight and, 45
See also body changes
weight goal, 44
weight loss, postpartum, 280–281
work and family balance, 132–133
working, 56–57
workouts, 46–47
worries and concerns, 106

X

X-linked disorders, 301–303
X-rays, 65
X sex chromosomes, 88

Y

yeast infections, 428–429
Y sex chromosomes, 88

Z

Zika virus, 445–446
zygote, 87, 98

IMAGE CREDITS

The individuals pictured are models, and the photos are used for illustrative purposes only. There is no correlation between the individuals portrayed and the subjects being discussed.

All photographs and illustrations are copyright of MFMER, except for the following: